THE ETHICS OF
PALLIATIVE CARE

European perspectives

Edited by

HENK TEN HAVE
DAVID CLARK

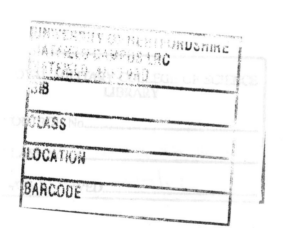

OPEN UNIVERSITY PRESS
Buckingham · Philadelphia

Open University Press
Celtic Court
22 Ballmoor
Buckingham
MK18 1XW

email: enquiries@openup.co.uk
world wide web: www.openup.co.uk

and
325 Chestnut Street
Philadelphia, PA 19106, USA

First Published 2002

A catalogue record of this book is available from the British Library

ISBN 0 335 21140 2 (pb)   0 335 21141 0 (hb)

Library of Congress Cataloging-in-Publication Data
The ethics of palliative care: European perspectives / edited by Henk ten Have
and David Clark.
       p.   cm. – (Facing death)
     Includes bibliographical references and index.
     ISBN 0-335-21141-0 – ISBN 0-335-21140-2 (pbk.)
     1. Palliative treatment – Moral and ethical aspects – Europe.   2. Terminal
care – Moral and ethical aspects – Europe.   3. Euthanasia – Moral and ethical
aspects – Europe.   I. Have, H. ten.   II. Clark, David, 1953.   III. Series.

R726.8 E885 2002
179.7 – dc21   2001056002

Typeset by Graphicraft Limited, Hong Kong
Printed in Great Britain by Biddles Limited, Guildford and Kings Lynn

Contents

Notes on the contributors

Bert Broeckaert is Professor of Comparative Religion in the Faculty of Theology of the Catholic University of Leuven, Belgium, where he also works in the Centre for Biomedical Ethics and Law. He is an ethical adviser to the Flemish Palliative Care Federation and a member of the Belgian Bioethics Advisory Commission. He has published on multiculturalism, discrimination, comparative religious ethics, euthanasia, and organizational and ethical issues in palliative care.

David Clark is Professor of Medical Sociology within the Palliative Medicine Academic Unit of the University of Sheffield, UK. He has written widely on the sociology of religion, family life and end-of-life care. He has been involved in research and teaching in palliative care since 1989. His current interests include the history of hospice, palliative care and related fields, policy development and international issues in the growth of palliative care, and palliative care ethics. He is the editor of the Facing Death series for Open University Press.

Ben Crul is an anaesthesiologist, Professor of Pain Management and Head of the Pain Unit at the University Medical Centre Nijmegen, the Netherlands. He was involved in the founding of a regional palliative care service within a nationwide network. He has published on various issues in pain management with an emphasis on cancer pain.

Wim Dekkers studied medicine and philosophy at the Catholic University at Nijmegen. Until 1992 he worked part-time as a general practitioner. At the moment he works at the Department of Ethics, Philosophy and History of Medicine of the University Medical Centre Nijmegen, the Netherlands. He is also a senior researcher at the Centre for Ethics of the same university.

He is interested in philosophical and ethical aspects of palliative medicine, especially in conceptual and ethical questions relating to the care of the chronically and terminally ill.

Bert Gordijn has been Clinical Ethicist at the University Medical Centre Nijmegen, the Netherlands, since 1996. He is secretary of the Hospital Ethics Committee and a member of the Institutional Review Board. He is involved in teaching and research in medical ethics. His interests include clinical ethics, ethics of palliative care and euthanasia.

Diego Gracia is Professor of History of Medicine and Bioethics and Director of the Department of Public Health and History of Science at the Complutense University of Madrid, Spain. He works especially in the history of medical ethics and clinical ethics. His main works are *Fundamentos de bioética* (Madrid: Eudema, 1989), *Primum non nocere* (Madrid: Real Academia de Medicine, 1990), *Procedimientos de decisión en ética clinica* (Madrid: Eudema, 1991) and *Ética y vida: Estudios de bioética* (4 vols, Bogotá: El Buho, 1998). He is Director of the Masters in Bioethics organized at the School of Medicine of the Complutense University, and Director of the Latin-American Health Organization (since 1996). He is a member of the Royal National Academy of Medicine of Spain.

Henk ten Have is Professor of Medical Ethics and Chair of the Department of Ethics, Philosophy and History of Medicine in the University Medical Centre Nijmegen, the Netherlands. He has been the coordinator of the EU-funded *Pallium* project on palliative care ethics. He has published on many issues in bioethics and philosophy of medicine, with particular emphasis on end-of-life care and palliative care. His recent publications are *Palliative Care in Europe: Concepts and Policies* (Amsterdam: IOS Press, 2001) and *Bioethics in a European Perspective* (Dordrecht: Kluwer, 2001).

Franz-Josef Illhardt worked, following his 'Habilitation' in medical ethics, at the Centre of Geriatrics and Gerontology of Freiburg University Hospital, Germany. Since 1996 he has been the Executive Director of the Ethics Committee of Freiburg University and its hospital. His major publications discuss some bioethical issues of geriatrics and gerontology, pain relief, transcultural medicine, the body in medical perspective and medical research.

Rien (Marinus Johannes Petrus Antonius) Janssens took his MA in theology in 1996. In the same year, he started to work on his thesis as junior researcher at the Department of Ethics, Philosophy and History of Medicine of the University Medical Centre Nijmegen, the Netherlands. From March 1998 until March 2001, he was the project manager of the European *Pallium* project on palliative care ethics. In June 2001 he took his PhD degree at the Catholic University of Nijmegen on his thesis *Palliative Care: Concepts and Ethics*.

Göran Lantz is Professor of Healthcare Ethics at Uppsala University, Sweden and Director of the Ersta Institute for Health Care Ethics in Stockholm. Educated as a theologian, his main field of research concerns the interface between ethics and jurisprudence.

Juan Manuel Núñez Olarte is Associate Professor of Medicine and a practising physician at the Palliative Care Unit, Hospital General Gregoria Maranon of the University Complutense of Madrid. He has written widely on symptom management in palliative medicine, history of medicine and cultural issues in end-of-life care. He has been involved in research and teaching in palliative care since 1990. He has also been actively involved in work within palliative care associations (EAPC, SECPAL and AMADECUPAL). His current research interests include opioid-induced myoclonus, ethical issues in terminal sedation and cultural issues in the delivery of palliative care.

Salvatore Privitera graduated in theology and philosophy. He is Professor of Moral Theology at the University of Palermo, Italy; founder and Director of the Istituto Siciliano di Bioetica; and Editor-in-Chief of the journal *Bioetica e Cultura*. His main interest is in the methodological aspects of ethical reflection.

Lars Sandman is a doctoral student in practical philosophy at the Department of Philosophy, University of Gothenburg, Sweden. His thesis *A Good Death* critically discussed different ideas about what makes for a good death and he is involved in research about autonomy and good death within palliative home care as well as research about turning points between curative and palliative care.

Paul Schotsmans is Professor of Medical Ethics in the Faculty of Medicine of the Catholic University of Leuven, Belgium. He has written widely on personalism and medical ethics. He is a member of the Belgian National Advisory Committee on Bioethics and currently the President of the European Association of Centres of Medical Ethics. He is also a member of the Board of the International Association of Bioethics.

Pat Webb is Lecturer in Palliative Care in the Faculty of Health and Social Care Sciences of Kingston University, London, UK and previously worked at Trinity Hospice, London. Trained as a nurse, she is editor of *The European Journal of Cancer Care*.

Simon Woods is Lecturer in Bioethics and Fellow of the Institute of Medicine, Law and Bioethics, School of Law, University of Manchester, UK. He is qualified as a nurse and holds bachelor's and doctoral degrees in philosophy. As a nurse he worked at a major cancer centre and as a Macmillan Lecturer at the University of Liverpool. He is currently involved in an innovative project funded by the NHS to provide ethics and law education for health professionals in practice. His publications cover bioethics, palliative care ethics, end-of-life issues and nursing ethics.

Zbigniew Zylicz was born in Poland and moved to the Netherlands after his medical studies. He trained in internal medicine and oncology. Since 1993 he has been Medical Director of Hospice Rozenheuvel, one of the pioneer units of this kind in the Netherlands. He has authored and co-authored about one hundred publications in the field of palliative medicine, pain treatment and ethics.

Series editor's preface

This new addition to the Facing Death series represents a major contribution to ethics and palliative care. It is the product of a three-year collaboration between scholars and clinicians working in seven European countries under the leadership of Professor Henk ten Have as part of the well known *Pallium* project. This work not only brings together perspectives from northern and southern Europe, but also combines the skills of philosophers, ethicists, doctors, nurses, theologians, historians and social scientists. The outcome of the project is quite the most detailed and challenging examination yet produced of the ethical dimensions of palliative care in the European context, making this book a work of major importance.

The Ethics of Palliative Care differs from other writings on this subject in several crucial respects. It is built on two interrelated views of its subject matter. One of these sees ethics in the service of palliative care, as an applied discipline which can be set to work in delivering 'answers' to crucial dilemmas that occur in clinical work and in the organization of services. The other sees palliative care as a field of activity which in its own right requires ethical reflection and analysis. We thereby have the distinction between ethics *in* and *of* palliative care, and the creative tension which this generates is present throughout the book.

Also important is the priority which the contributors give to an understanding of the historical development of palliative care and the varied organizational settings in which it is delivered. We are therefore offered a detailed account of key intellectual influences on palliative care, especially those deriving from innovations in twentieth century clinical medicine, theology and philosophy. We also see how these took hold and were shaped in different European contexts – where values apparently held in common were transformed and modified in local settings. As a result, service innovations and growth in provision have not proceeded evenly in the seven countries described here. Contributors from the Netherlands, the United Kingdom, Sweden, Spain, Germany, Belgium and Italy each add detail to the overall picture of palliative care development and provision, and at times striking differences are revealed. Institutional heterogeneity prompts questions in turn about the underlying concepts of palliative care which are adopted by practitioners and are manifested in the different countries. Close scrutiny here reveals some major conceptual difficulties which require clarification, not least if palliative care is to gain greater endorsement by governments and policy-makers.

Building on this detailed analysis of institutional development and the underpinning concepts, several chapters of the book then go on to discuss important cross-cutting themes relating to the moral values of palliative care. There is much here to take the reader beyond the four principles of bio-medical ethics (beneficence, non-maleficence, justice and autonomy). We see an analysis of Weber's distinction between 'conviction' and 'responsibility' ethics as they link to palliative care. There is an examination of a 'relational model' based on the ideas of Emmanuel Levinas. A wide-ranging discussion of 'the good death' draws on philosophical and sociological ideas. By such means we are offered a broadly-based assessment of key moral influences on contemporary palliative care in Europe.

From here we go on to some fascinating chapters which examine pressing issues of the moment: sedation of the terminally ill patient; responding to requests for euthanasia; the ethics of research in palliative care; the complexities of respecting autonomy at the end of life; and concerns about futile treatment. There is a depth of analysis here which, when combined with case presentations and sophisticated clinical insight, brings forth some challenging arguments.

The Ethics of Palliative Care is rich in empirical detail. It contains the results of a major European review of service developments and policy influences. It draws on a large survey of beliefs and attitudes among practitioners across Europe. It incorporates detailed case studies. Readers of the Facing Death series will recognize the mixture of critical reflection and evidence-based argument. This book also relates closely to several others in the series which have examined issues of policy and practice in palliative care (Clark, Hockley and Ahmedzai 1997; Clark and Seymour 1999; Cobb 2001) as well as volumes concerned with palliative care research (Field, Corner, Clark and Davis 2001) and with the perspectives of patients and families (Costain Schou and Hewison 1998; Riches and Dawson 2000; Seymour 2001).

Overall, *The Ethics of Palliative Care* is the eleventh book in the series. It is the first volume we have dedicated entirely to ethical issues, though it will not be the last, as other related works are now being written and planned. *The Ethics of Palliative Care* deserves to be widely read and should find an extensive readership within the palliative care community, where there is growing interest in such matters and where its rich multi-disciplinary perspective and European audience will, I am sure, make it extremely welcome.

David Clark

References

Clark, D., Hockley, J. and Ahmedzai, S. (eds) (1997) *New Themes in Palliative Care*. Buckingham: Open University Press.

Clark, D. and Seymour, J.E. (1999) *Reflections on Palliative Care: Sociological and Policy Perspectives*. Buckingham: Open University Press.

Cobb, M. (2001) *The Dying Soul: Spiritual Care at the End of Life*. Buckingham: Open University Press.

Costain Schou, K. and Hewison, J. (1998) *Experiencing Cancer: Quality of Life in Treatment*. Buckingham: Open University Press.

Field, D., Clark, D., Corner, J. and Davis, C. (2001) *Researching Palliative Care*. Buckingham: Open University Press.

Riches, G. and Dawson, P. (2000) *An Intimate Loneliness: Supporting Bereaved Parents and Siblings*. Buckingham: Open University Press.

Seymour, J.E. (2001) *Critical Moments: Death and Dying in Intensive Care*. Buckingham: Open University Press.

Acknowledgements

This book is one of the outcomes of the *Pallium* project. In March 1998, an international consortium of scholars in ethics and palliative care received funding from the European Commission to explore and analyse the conceptual and ethical issues of palliative care in seven participating European countries. For the next three years these scholars worked together intensively in order to meet the planned objectives of the project. First of all, we wish to thank the European Commission for funding our research as part of the BIOMED programme. The project could not have been a success without the engagement and enthusiasm of all our participating colleagues. We especially wish to thank the project manager, Dr Rien Janssens, for his support and encouragement to all the participants in their collaborative research activities. Finalizing the manuscript and completing the drafts of several contributions has been made possible through a fellowship awarded to one of the editors. Henk ten Have is grateful for the opportunity provided by the Center for Health Policy and Ethics at Creighton University, Omaha, USA. The visiting fellowship during the spring of 2001 not only allowed the time and energy to work on these manuscripts, but also offered an academic atmosphere of scholarship and friendship which made it a pleasure to read and write. Special thanks go to Ruth Purtilo, Director of the Center, as well as the Faculty and Staff of the Center, Jos Welie, Richard O'Brien, Judith Kissell, Oscar Punla, Winnifred Pinch, Amy Haddad, Helen Shew, Rita Nutty and Jaimy Waters. At the University of Sheffield, David Clark has benefited from the continuing support of friends and colleagues in the Sheffield Palliative Care Studies Group, particularly Jane Seymour and Mark Cobb, who have assisted his understanding of ethical issues. Immense practical support was also provided by Margaret Jane, who dealt with the detailed preparation of the final manuscript and to whom both editors express their thanks.

Henk ten Have and David Clark

Introduction: the work of the *Pallium* project

HENK TEN HAVE AND DAVID CLARK

Around the world, palliative care services are expanding rapidly. The practice of palliative care is recognized increasingly as a legitimate area of specialization in modern healthcare and experts in the field have worked hard to establish an evidence base for their activities. Several major centres of palliative care research and education now exist and palliative care services are operating in some 80 different countries. What began in the 1950s and 1960s as 'terminal' care and which soon adopted the term 'hospice' care has now evolved into an internationally recognized field of work concerned with dying people and others facing life-threatening illness, as well as their companions and family members. Palliative care encompasses a range of activities: advanced pain and symptom management; attention to psychological, social and spiritual concerns; and the deployment of multidisciplinary teams. While its origins might be traced back to some of the oldest aspects of medicine, it also constitutes a particularly modern development, which in a very short period has made enormous advances.

Although palliative care attends to a human experience which is universal, the manner of its organization is heterogeneous. In many of the countries which have developed palliative care, some of the underlying issues facing the healthcare system are held in common. One of these is the significance of an ageing population which will face death at the end of a long life and with expectations of good care throughout. At the same time the character of medical problems is changing, with an increasing burden of chronic illnesses, where the possibilities of cure are limited. The prolonged lifespan is associated in turn with longer average stays in medical institutions and an increasing need for formalized care and assistance. Likewise, in the west, the manner of death has changed from a sudden, acute episode to a longer process of dying, perhaps accompanied by mental and physical deterioration and a wider sense of suffering. New and different medical services are being developed in order to respond to these changes appropriately. However, even in western European countries, wide differences occur in the structure and organization of the healthcare system. Palliative care services must therefore adapt to the characteristics of the system, depending on the focus on specialist hospital-based medicine or home care services and general practice. It is also relevant that palliation has always had a place within medical care, albeit one which has been given diminishing attention until recently. Although the current emphasis on palliative care is more articulated and identified as a separate activity, the development of palliative care services often starts from existing structures. As a result palliative care has developed from various settings, such as oncology, geriatrics, anaesthesiology or nursing home medicine and also from the independent, not-for-profit healthcare sector. This heterogeneity has led to different concepts and modes of organizing palliative care in different countries.

The variety of palliative care also stems from some ambiguity in the palliative care movement itself. Initially, hospices were established because of dissatisfaction with the medical care provided in the mainstream hospital setting with insufficient attention to the needs of dying persons, indeed a sense of neglect. Separate institutions were therefore considered necessary in order to focus on this particular category of patients and their families. Palliative care from this perspective was seen as a complementary, more or less alternative arrangement that could make the healthcare system more encompassing and attentive to the needs of modern patients. However, at the same time, hospice and palliative care philosophy also emphasized that care and compassion cannot be the monopoly of any one individual setting, but need to be a basic component of all healthcare. Rather than creating an entirely separate system of services, it became necessary to introduce the ideas of palliative care into other healthcare services, and to transform medicine into a human activity of caring. The impact of these different tendencies within the palliative care movement has also led to divergent responses within various healthcare systems.

At the beginning of the twenty-first century we can see palliative care taking heterogeneous institutional forms in different countries, with these in turn related to the specifics of the healthcare system. Those involved in palliative care, however, argue that the concept of palliative care is unique and homogeneous. Palliative care, they suggest, differs from curative and preventive medicine because it not only has specific goals, but also specific underlying moral values. Clarifying these underlying goals and values is therefore important for the future development of palliative care: should it be integrated into medicine giving a new dimension to current practices, or should it be a new discipline or medical specialty complementing the existing range of professional activities? The answers to such questions are also a necessary basis for formulating norms and standards for good palliative care practice in the future.

Comparative research

This set of interrelationships between concepts and moral values in palliative care has been the stimulus for an international research project, entitled *Palliative Care Ethics* (*Pallium*). The project, awarded by the European Commission in the context of its BIOMED programme, united 26 researchers from seven European countries: Belgium, Germany, Italy, the Netherlands, Spain, Sweden and the United Kingdom. In each country, teams of ethicists, theologians, historians, social scientists and philosophers cooperated with healthcare practitioners in palliative care to develop the work of the project. A core group, including the project coordinator and manager, met on a regular basis over three years to assess the progress and organization of the work and all researchers came together for annual plenary meetings. The chapters in this book have all resulted directly from the project and its various meetings.

Objectives

The *Pallium* project had the following objectives:

- to examine and compare the organization of palliative care in each country
- to clarify the concepts of palliative care in each participating country
- to explain the relationships between palliative care concepts and organizational heterogeneity
- to analyse the ethical debates in palliative care and the moral implications for further development.

These objectives have a specific methodological order and assume that the moral dimensions of a healthcare practice are not pregiven, but need to be identified through analysing the particular characteristics of the practice in question. Especially when a practice (such as palliative care) is still developing and is not yet generally established, it is important to study its organizational and institutional characteristics, as well as the various concepts and definitions used to typify and to demarcate it from existing healthcare practices. This approach is particularly important when the development and implementation of a practice is different in various countries. The approach therefore provided a continuous theme to the practical and methodological ordering of our project.

Methods

In order to accomplish the objectives of the project, we adopted an eclectic combination of empirical studies and theoretical analysis:

- *Literature review*   In the various countries the available literature concerning the range of organizational systems for the delivery of palliative care was analysed, not only in scientific journals but also in policy documents, and the 'grey literature' of various national and professional organizations and associations. In each country the researchers used a similar format to analyse and describe the organization and functions of palliative care services in order to allow as much comparability as possible. In particular, preliminary analysis focused on identifying similarities and differences in the organization of palliative care in the participating countries.

- *Questionnaire survey* In order to explore the responses of palliative care practitioners to a number of conceptual and moral issues, we developed a questionnaire which was mailed in a French and English version to over 2000 participants of the Congress of the European Association for Palliative Care, held in Geneva, September 1999.

- *Conceptual analysis* The professional literature of palliative care was analysed in order to identify and clarify concepts underlying the various organizations of services in specific healthcare systems. Clarification of the concepts in each participating country meant making explicit what often is implicit in the self-understanding of palliative care practices. The researchers studied the available literature on the concept(s) of palliative care in their countries, analysing the definitions, terminology and notions used, as well as the determinants of palliative care. The concept(s) of palliative care, identified in the literature, was seen to determine how palliative care is demarcated from other activities and endeavours in healthcare.

- *Ethical analysis* The underlying assumption of the project from the outset was that what is considered as palliative care is frequently related to specific moral values (for example, dying as a normal human process; life as an intrinsic good; acceptance of unavoidable death; a focus on quality of life; the significance of interpersonal relations; integrated care of the 'total' person). We therefore made an explicit examination of the moral values implied in the various concepts of palliative care. These values were then further examined in light of the available bioethics literature, although this literature is generally not specific to the context of palliative care. The analysis of moral values implied in the concepts of palliative care allowed us to study in more detail some of the major moral problems in palliative care practice which were identified in the literature as well as in the questionnaire survey.

The organization of palliative care

During the first year of the project, the participants described, analysed and compared organizational structures of palliative care in their respective countries. The comparative character of the project was helpful at this time in obtaining a clearer picture. First, a framework of items was developed to describe the situation in the various settings. Since palliative care was already in a mature stage of development in some countries it was possible to use and adapt the experiences of evaluating palliative care services in countries like the United Kingdom and Sweden. In order to generate a comparable view of the situation in all the participating countries, similar country reports were written. The focus of these reports was on

- general background issues, such as the population structure and the health-care system
- the development of palliative care services over time (distinguishing between inpatient facilities, home care, hospital and nursing home care)
- palliative care education
- specialization and academic development
- relevant policy documents.

These reports drew on a wide range of documentary sources, including not only national and regional statistics relating to population, healthcare and service provision, but also publications concerning palliative care services in each country such as official publications and also informal reports and documents issued by palliative care organizations and non-government bodies.

Although a comparative framework was used, meeting the first objective proved a difficult task. Information was available to a varying degree in all seven countries and data were often presented in forms which made comparison difficult. While some countries had extensive documentation on the growth of palliative care services, in other countries such information was more difficult to obtain, and had to be reordered for comparative purposes. Similarly, the structure of the healthcare system was often quite different. What we produced however was a set of detailed descriptions of the status of palliative care services in the seven countries and, at least for some countries, this description was the first of its kind. The various country reports have been published in one volume (ten Have and Janssens 2001) and this volume (Chapter 2) contains a comparative overview of palliative care organization in the seven countries which made up the *Pallium* project.

Concepts of palliative care

In the second year of the project, our emphasis turned to the conceptual aspects of palliative care. The hospice movement in the United Kingdom has been a paradigm for many palliative care services in other European countries, and in the early days, it seemed that the movement had a clearly outlined concept and philosophy. From the beginning, it was argued that palliative care should be seen first and foremost as a concept of care that is different from standard (medical) practice. The difference derives from specific moral values (concerning life and death, pain and suffering, views of the individual person and the social context); but at the same time, the concept is homogeneous since the same moral values are shared, regardless of the specific palliative care setting. Yet, as our comparison of different countries showed, the concept of palliative care is shaped into different institutional forms. This raised the question of whether the range of organizational systems is an expression of one identical concept, or whether different concepts of palliative care are at work. Comparative research at this stage of the project therefore concentrated on analysing the conceptual self-understanding and the underlying moral values of palliative care, since these values were considered the distinctive core of palliative care. The analysis showed that palliative care is in a crucial phase of development in many countries. Although it has been recognized as a medical specialty in the United Kingdom, most other countries are struggling with the issue of how to relate palliative care to the healthcare system. Palliative care is increasingly organized within the setting of the formal healthcare system, but it is still open as to whether this implies specialization (developing a specific discipline with university departments and chairs, inpatient units, with all the paraphernalia of a medical specialty) or integration (incorporating palliative care in established clinical departments, and cooperating with existing medical disciplines). In view of this dilemma, the concept of palliative care has become ambiguous. Palliative care philosophy emphasizes care and communication rather than intervention and treatment. Mainstream medicine is still largely dominated by the values of technology and active intervention. In such antagonistic contexts, separation and development as a distinct new discipline is apparently more feasible than permeating all medical disciplines with a new ethos. At the same time, the increasing interrelations with mainstream medicine have also changed the initial concept of palliative care. First, the identification of palliative care with the terminal phase of illness is rejected now by most participants in the debate, who hold instead that palliative care starts from the time of diagnosis. Second, the identification of palliative care with cancer care is more and more a question of debate; and it is increasingly acknowledged that patients suffering from Alzheimer's disease, heart failure, AIDS, multiple sclerosis and other chronic diseases have been neglected by palliative care practitioners for too long. Third, the moral notions initially motivating palliative care practitioners have been strongly associated with the western Christian tradition ('love', 'sympathy', 'sanctity of life'); these notions are now 'translated' into universal, bioethical notions ('quality of life', 'human dignity', 'total care'). Fourth, the ethical norms that should prevail in palliative care practice are more and more subject to debate. In the Netherlands, the majority of physicians providing palliative care accept euthanasia as a means of last resort and in many other countries, there is no consensus that euthanasia should be excluded from palliative care. Debates on the validity of the doctrine of double effect, withholding and withdrawing life-prolonging treatment, terminal sedation, and research in palliative care have intensified and again there is little consensus of views. The integration process of palliative care into mainstream healthcare systems has created ambiguity, there is a lack of clarity about the scope of palliative care and its demarcation from other medical practices has become problematic. The values underpinning the concept of palliative care are therefore under debate as too are the ethical norms for good palliative care practice.

The methodological approach adopted in this phase of the project was similar to phase one: a common framework, focusing on analysing the definitions in use and the relevant concepts; analysis of demarcation from other healthcare activities, assessment of the nature of the primary activity (medical, nursing or other); and consideration of whether it should be integrated into all care activities or specialized as a separate expertise and discipline. Using this framework, the researchers produced reports describing the conceptual discussions and problems in their respective countries. Finally, a comparative review of all country reports was made (see Chapter 3 in this volume) in which the conceptual debates are clarified through an analysis of the goals of palliative care. It seems that there is some consensus about these goals, but considerable discussion concerning the character, significance, priority and implementation of each.

Ethics of palliative care

In the final phase of the project, we turned to an analysis of moral dilemmas relating to medical decision-making at the end of life. The assumption here was that moral dilemmas in palliative care practice could be examined and analysed only after conceptual issues of palliative care had been assessed. Thus, it was only in the third year of the project that issues regarding the withholding and withdrawal of medical treatment, terminal sedation and euthanasia were scrutinized. The approach of the ethics of palliative care in the project has been twofold. First, the focus was on the clarification of the underlying value structure of palliative care. Second, analyses were made of moral dilemmas specific to the practice of palliative care.

Research into the ethics of palliative care is facilitated by the fact that the concept of palliative care is apparently itself morally motivated. The roots of palliative care lie in the hospice movement which in the 1960s arose from a public moral discomfort with mainstream medicine of that time. Nowadays, medicine itself as well as palliative care have changed significantly. Medicine is more attentive to the needs of the dying person and palliative care no longer opposes mainstream medicine as stringently as it once did. The literature on palliative care, and specifically the literature on care for the dying, indicates that divergent approaches exist in the moral debate. One line of argument is that mainstream medicine is still dominated by an interventionist and activist attitude in the care of the dying, using biomedical, invasive technologies in the terminal phase. Furthermore, pain and symptom management are in many countries still insufficiently developed in many areas of medicine. Likewise, communication skills and the development of an authentic sympathetic attitude are still not major subjects in many medical education programmes. In other words, the concept of care is marginal to modern medicine, which remains identified predominantly with the possibility of cure. Another line of argument, however, holds that palliative care has already become routine practice. Furthermore, recent research in pain and symptom management has improved the quality of life of terminal cancer patients substantially. It is also argued that present-day medical doctors have developed a more authentic caring attitude than some decades ago. Studying the literature on palliative care ethics it is hard to avoid the conclusion that the ethical debate between palliative care and mainstream medicine has not been subject to thorough investigation. On the one hand, palliative care criticizes the moral principles of mainstream medicine. On the other hand, mainstream medicine is regarded as the basis for further development. Moreover, mainstream medicine claims to have already introduced palliative care into daily practice and has a considerable interest in its further development. It is plausible to argue that these discrepancies are based on mutual misunderstandings, arising from the ambiguity of the concept of palliative care and from a lack of insight into the organization of palliative care in respective countries. It therefore becomes necessary to examine the underlying value structure of palliative care, focusing on the following questions. What is the moral motivation of palliative care in the various countries? What is the relation of this moral motivation to its current institutional forms? What are the moral differences between palliative care and mainstream medicine? How can the moral motivation of palliative care itself be ethically evaluated in relation to mainstream medicine? Assuming that implementation of the concept of palliative care leads to a specific medical practice, is there a moral surplus of palliative care in relation to mainstream medicine? What are the moral criteria to evaluate this moral surplus? One of the activities in the final phase of the project was therefore to analyse and clarify the ethical perspectives which are incorporated in palliative care. Three ethical theories were used explicitly: conviction ethics, consequentialist ethics, and responsibility ethics. Although palliative care nowadays is more characterized by the notion of 'responsibility', conviction ethics was more pervasive in the earlier days with its emphasis on duties, principles and intentions (see Chapter 5). It is now argued, for example, that the central concept in palliative care is 'practical wisdom' (what Aristotle called *phrónesis*) (Randall and Downie 1996). It is also stated that palliative care is characterized not so much by the notion of individual autonomy but rather by interpersonal relationships (see Chapter 7).

Finally, we turn to specific moral dilemmas in palliative care practice. In the context of care for incurably and often terminally ill persons, particular moral problems emerge more frequently than in some other healthcare settings. In the project, four specific problems were analysed: sedation, euthanasia, research and futility. Terminal sedation is frequently used, for example, in palliative care in Spain, yet it can be associated with hastening of the patient's death. Thorough moral analysis shows that it is primarily a means of relief for refractory pain (see Chapter 9). Yet, making a suffering patient unconscious in the face of death is not easily accepted in other countries, such as the Netherlands, where a debate on terminal sedation is almost absent. On the other hand, the Netherlands has legalized euthanasia and physician-assisted suicide under specific conditions, while the practice of palliative care has only recently started to unfold. This raises an issue concerning the compatibility of palliative care and euthanasia (discussed in Chapter 10). Research in palliative care is also a matter of increasing debate. Palliative care will improve only if clinical research continues to be executed. At the same time, research with severely ill and dying patients is considered ethically problematic. The current guidelines and standards for clinical research need to be adapted to the necessities of better palliative care, but moral reflection has hardly begun (see Chapter 11). A final and not frequently addressed issue is the question of where are the limits to palliative care. It is often taken for granted that care itself is unlimited. Palliative care in particular starts at a time when medical interventions have become futile; cure is no longer a feasible goal, and other goals should prevail. However, improving quality of life or relieving suffering cannot be restricted in principle. The notion of 'futility' therefore has a limited use in the context of palliative care. On the other hand, it is imperative, also in this context, to make specific arrangements and policies for withholding and withdrawing treatment (see Chapter 12).

The benefits of comparative research

Comparative research, as we have experienced in the *Pallium* project, confronts the participants in a very direct way with the organizational and conceptual context of palliative care. Comparison of organizations, concepts, current strategies and the implied moral values helps to elucidate the sociological, normative and applied clinical determinants of ideas and developments of palliative care in specific countries. It also leads to a critical assessment of (moral and other) arguments justifying current practices and approaches. We can thereby create a broader view of the care of the dying in modern societies. Problems can be more easily identified and blank spots, deficiencies, or undesirable developments in a country's palliative care practice can be revealed when identified and evaluated by analysis and comparison with experiences from other countries. After three years of intensive international cooperation and research within the *Pallium* project, several conclusions can be formulated.

Palliative care has intrinsic importance

Palliative care has value in itself. It is important that future healthcare is well adapted to the changing needs of patients. Good care will at least be as important as high-technology, cure-orientated medical intervention. Also the search for a good death is likely to permeate future societies as people seek to avoid suffering and a loss of dignity. Further attention to palliative care modalities can be one of the answers to requests for euthanasia, although it does not imply that palliative care needs to be developed first and foremost in order to provide an antidote for euthanasia. The major goal of palliative care is to provide good care and to improve the quality of life of the patients and their families, not to avoid euthanasia. This may be a secondary goal, ethically imperative, but the first internal goal of palliative care practice is to care for those who are about to lose human existence.

Conceptual clarification remains necessary

The project has been important in addressing essential questions relating to the concept of palliative care. In particular, our questionnaire survey identified issues that palliative care workers experience in their daily practice. From this it has been impossible to argue for one single concept of palliative care. Further ethical, philosophical, theological and historical research will be necessary in order to understand notions that are used in these debates and in order to introduce new notions which reflect the demarcation of palliative care from other medical practices and the overall scope of palliative care and its terminology. This work will also need to recognize the different social and cultural backgrounds within the countries of western Europe.

Specific training for palliative care is imperative

If palliative care is to develop further, specific training is necessary. In many countries palliative care is taught as a part of oncology, anaesthesiology, nursing home medicine or general practice. However, care for the dying requires specific expertise. In the light of the scarcity of specific training programmes for palliative care in Europe, further development of educational initiatives focusing on adequate pain and symptom control, communication skills, spiritual guidance, care for caregivers, complementary therapies, and also on the ethics of medical decision-making at the end of life is imperative.

Palliative care ethics needs further specification

The ethics of medical decision-making at the end of life is extremely complex. New issues are emerging, for instance in relation to terminal sedation and the role of the principle of double effect as well as research with terminally ill patients. In many European countries, the issue of euthanasia is now discussed extensively. In Belgium and the Netherlands a process of legalization is taking place, though this is viewed critically in most European countries. Further debate on alternative palliative modalities, as well as on the morality of euthanasia, is therefore imperative. Although palliative care practitioners frequently discuss moral problems in their professional journals, the input and contribution to this of professional bioethicists are rather limited (Hermsen and ten Have 2001). The ethics of palliative care is not at the moment an object of research for many ethicists. Many important theoretical questions however are awaiting thorough scholarly analysis.

Ethical consultation needs to be available

Caregivers in palliative care are often confronted with moral dilemmas. Up to now, there has been little opportunity for clinical-ethical consultation. Such consultation is not theoretical in orientation but primarily practical and supportive of good clinical practice. In order to make caregivers more aware of the complexity of moral dilemmas in end-of-life care as well to provide models and mechanisms for analysing and managing these dilemmas, ethical expertise should be more widely available. Ethicists who are trained in moral deliberation need to be on call if moral dilemmas occur. Their expertise is not so much a technical expertise in the sense that ethicists know the right answers and can provide solutions, but they can point to morally relevant issues within the decisions that are taken and the perspectives that are significant and should be considered in order to make the best decision in the particular circumstances of a specific case. Thus, an ethical 'observatory' that can always be contacted, would be useful for caregivers in palliative care.

Further development of good clinical practice standards is important

Clarifying the concepts of palliative care in various countries, and identifying and analysing the moral values underlying these concepts, is a necessary step towards formulating norms and standards for good palliative care practice internationally. The process of reaching agreement on standards can start only with the analysis of differences in existing practices and the clarification, if possible, of the rationales which underpin diversity.

Palliative care requires further recognition at the policy level

A great deal of work needs to be done in many countries to bring palliative care higher up the policy agenda. There is evidence of widespread variation in levels of palliative care provision across the countries of Europe. These discrepancies raise serious questions about equity and justice within the European Union and will no doubt draw increasing attention in the next few years.

In the chapters that follow we present in detail the results of this important European collaboration on the ethics of palliative care. Through empirical analysis, literature review, case exploration and ethical argumentation we draw attention to some of the well known, as well as less frequently considered problems in the field. We hope that readers will find justification for our approach and trust that our book adds something further to the ethical culture of palliative care organization and practice.

References

Hermsen, M. and ten Have, H.A.M.J. (2001) Moral problems in palliative care journals, *Palliative Medicine*, 15(5): 425–31.

Randall, F. and Downie, R.S. (1996) *Palliative Care Ethics: A Good Companion.* Oxford: Oxford University Press.

Ten Have, H.A.M.J. and Janssens, M. (eds) (2001) *Palliative Care in Europe: Concepts and Policies.* Amsterdam: IOS Press.

PART I

Concepts and models of care

Introduction to Part I

In this first part of the book we present three chapters which contain important information about the current state of palliative care development in Europe. We set out material which outlines key phases in the historical development of palliative care. We also provide a detailed commentary on how, by 1999, palliative care services had developed in seven European countries. At the same time, our analysis of this pattern of institutional formation is part of a process whereby the philosophy and concepts of palliative care are developed and clarified. So we provide a chapter devoted to these issues. The three chapters which make up Part I of the book should therefore allow readers to make sense of how the early pioneers of palliative care first set about improving the care of dying and chronically ill people from the mid-twentieth century onwards; how their ideas worked into programmes of care; and some of the conceptual problems which underpin these.

In Chapter 1 Diego Gracia offers a less familiar view of the historical factors which shaped the origins of modern palliative care. He reminds us that until recently the subject of 'care' has been largely ignored by historians and ethicists. Yet palliative care is part of a wider history, whereby women, families and certain institutions have given succour and support to the most dependent members of society. Such caring is related to, but has different purposes from, the medical goal of cure. One interesting place where 'caring' and 'curing' have the potential to meet is in relation to the problem of pain. Gracia's chapter shows us something of the history of pain in the twentieth century and the way in which Cicely Saunders, in working through her ideas about hospice care, concentrated on and also expanded our view of pain, taking it from something solely physical, into aspects of social, mental and spiritual suffering. So it was that palliative care was able to draw on a wide set of influences, some located within long-established traditions of care, and others originating from major innovations in twentieth-century medicine. Gracia therefore suggests that the modern palliative care unit is the analogue of the intensive care unit. In the first, intensive efforts are made to provide complex and sophisticated care for the person known to be dying. In the second, complexity and sophistication of a different sort are harnessed to the goal of saving life. It is a striking parallel.

Thus conceived, how have palliative care developments been proceeding across Europe? In Chapter 2 David Clark, Henk ten Have and Rien Janssens provide a detailed analysis of the growth of palliative care services in seven countries of western Europe. They show marked variations in timing, formation and availability. Taking the 1967 opening of St Christopher's Hospice in south London as a benchmark for the start of modern palliative (then still called 'terminal') care, they show how developments occurred subsequently in Sweden followed by Italy (both home care), Germany (inpatient unit), Spain (hospital palliative care unit), Belgium (inpatient unit) and the Netherlands (inpatient hospice). These authors also point out that such a narrative history has its pitfalls, for in any given country the way in which palliative care developments in the past are portrayed will be influenced by current preoccupations and agendas. Notwithstanding, this chapter shows a pattern of dramatic growth over a short period of time. It also demonstrates that the continuing potential for service expansion seems to rely on the extent to which palliative care can find a degree of integration within the structures of the formal healthcare system in any given setting. Certainly, part of the history of palliative care in some countries is bound up with the work of independent, charitable or not-for-profit organizations which subsidize their costs through the work of volunteers, through fund-raising and alternative sources of income generation. These groups may well continue to function in future. But in a context where palliative care is seen as a service to be provided to the population of a country, and therefore funded through the mechanisms of its healthcare system, clearly palliative care must be deemed adequate by the criteria which apply to all systems of healthcare provision. This represents a strong challenge to a social movement which has taken a pride in its reformist and innovative ideals. By the same token, if palliative care is to be recognized in this way, then governments, healthcare planners and policy-makers must give due weight to its concerns and ensure the means for its support and development. At the end of the twentieth century, as Chapter 2 shows, this did not add up to an equitable state of affairs, even within the seven European countries described here. Across Europe, citizens of different countries can expect dramatically different levels of palliative care provision, nationally and locally. It does not appear that the interests of distributive justice are well served by the current situation.

The picture of institutional heterogeneity presented in Chapter 2 is echoed at least to some extent in the discussion of concepts of palliative care outlined by Clark, ten Have and Janssens in Chapter 3. This chapter asks: What are the goals of palliative care? At first sight this seems a simple question which should not detain us too long. Unlike other clinical specialties, however, palliative care is not concerned either with a particular organ of the body or with a specific disease. It does not seek to bring about a cure for the patient, nor is it solely concerned with rehabilitation. It occupies an unusual space, as the authors suggest, somewhere between the hope of cure and the fear of dying. Moreover it has explicitly gone beyond physical and even mental problems to address a level of suffering which might also encompass social, moral and spiritual concerns. In short it appears ambitious in its orientations. The authors suggest that palliative care has four goals, relating to quality of life, relief of suffering, the 'good death' and the prevention of euthanasia. On analysis, the coherence of all of these is found wanting. This may partly explain why, as palliative care grows, some attention is diverting away from its primary goals (especially relating to 'good death' and the prevention of euthanasia) and instead attention is focusing on what the authors call 'secondary purposes' – the day-to-day problems and activities encountered by palliative care practitioners and those involved in the promotion and expansion of their work.

Part I of the book thereby serves as an introduction to some of the models and concepts found in European palliative care. It provides some historical background, an assessment of patterns of growth and a critical review of key conceptual ideas. The contributors to its chapters have expertise, variously in ethics, the history of medicine, theology and sociology. The materials they present set the scene for the more detailed consideration of moral values underpinning palliative care, which is developed in Part II.

1 Palliative care and the historical background

DIEGO GRACIA

As we shall see throughout this book, palliative care is a *type* of care. It is therefore best understood as part of the general history of care. This at once poses a problem, for much of the general history of care is yet to be written, in particular that care which pertains to a so-called 'little history', the history of ordinary people, the history of everyday life; not the history of great discoveries, successes or persons. There is a little history and a big history of medicine. For instance, the history of curing technologies belongs to the big history and it has been written about extensively. Cure has its history, but care does not.

Historical interest in mentalities in the work of authors such as Philippe Ariès and Jean Delumeau is changing this situation. We are now beginning to understand the history of daily life, the history of the little things, of the ordinary people, the people without great power or social relevance. Accordingly, there has been growing interest in the study of the history of childhood, the history of women, the history of private life, the history of the elderly, the history of pregnancy, the history of family life, and so on. The history of *care* must be placed in this context, and is closely related to the history of women, the history of pain and the history of death and dying.

The same can be said for other dimensions of care, such as ethical issues. Only very recently has the ethics of care begun its development. Care has been forgotten not only by history, but also by ethics. It has been the feminist movement on one side, and the development of the nursing profession on the other – two of the most important groups in the little history of our society – which have begun and developed the ethics of care. Indeed, the ethics of care is now generally recognized as one of the most important parts of the general movement of bioethics.

In this chapter I first of all analyse the relations between care and cure. I then consider the historical development of palliative care in relation to the care system.

The social logic of care: curing and caring

Care and cure have the same origin, the Latin verb *curo*, which at the beginning meant caring, with no more precise specification. The verb *curo* was used in many different contexts, meaning sometimes the family care of parents for their children, or the spiritual care given by priests, as well as the medical care of physicians for their patients. Medical care is therefore only one dimension of a wider notion of caring in general. Within the generic semantic field of care there exist various types of care, such as spiritual care, familial care, medical care and nursing care. This can be seen in Figure 1.1.

So we see that there are different types of care, different specifications of the wide semantic genre covered by this term. The form that defines the specific care proper to medicine is 'somatic cure'. When cure is not somatic but spiritual, then the professional role defined is not that of the physician but of the priest. These are the roles of cure, at the same time there are others specifically related to care. One is the care given by relatives, which

Figure 1.1   Four types of care

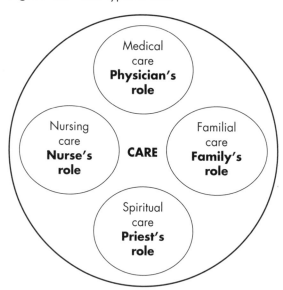

specifies the specific care of family members; the other is technical bodily care, specific to the role of nursing.

Thus we have the social and linguistic logic of care. There are different types of care: family care, nursing care, spiritual or religious care, and medical care. The latter coincides in western medicine with the promotion of health and the cure of diseases; in other words, medical care consists in prevention and cure. Both are medical interventions, but the latter is more characteristic of medicine. Consequently, it can be said that the type of care specific to medicine is cure.

The consequence of this analysis of the social and linguistic logic of care is that medicine has not considered care as its goal, if care is understood as being responsible for the patient and all their needs 24 hours a day. By contrast, the care of the physician is purely technical, and related to the prevention of disease and the cure of the body – no more. An old aphorism, wrongly attributed to the Hippocratic authors, states that 'The first duty of medicine is to cure sometimes, to relieve often, and to comfort always'. Helping and consoling are duties of the physician, but only as a complement to the direct goal, which is the cure of patients. Helping and consoling are complements of curing, but not caring in itself. The true goal of medicine has always been curing, rather than taking care of the patient. Caring has never been the goal of medicine.

In this context, an interesting question becomes where to place 'palliative care' in the logical structure of caring. And if Cicely Saunders' idea of 'total care', in the sense of care for all aspects of the person, is to mean something, then the answer must be that palliative care is related to all these specifications of care. Of course, it is related to familial care, to medical care, to nursing care and to spiritual care. Nobody challenges the relationship of palliative care to nursing, familial and spiritual care. The key question however is whether palliative care is related to medical care, that is if palliation begins when cure is no longer possible. Thus, if the type of care specific to medicine is curing, then palliative care has nothing to do with medicine. But medicine is the technical use of hygiene, drugs and surgery in order to improve human well-being. And palliation is, in one of its dimensions, the pharmacological and surgical control of symptoms, and especially of pain. This is a typical goal of medicine and therefore palliation is related to the four types of care specified in Figure 1.1.

In this way, palliative care has opened up a new field in the general domain of caring. This field does not coincide with that defined previously, yet at the same time it is not a completely new and independent one. On the contrary, it is an integration, at least a partial integration of the other four sets. Therefore, palliative care integrates some parts of nursing care, of family care, of medical care and of spiritual care. Consequently, palliative care has influenced the old roles of all those types of care, leading unavoidably to their redefinition. For instance, it has stimulated a redefinition of the role of care in medicine, stressing the importance of symptomatic control, on the one hand, and also the need to attend to other dimensions of caring.

Keeping in mind this analysis of the logic of caring, let us now turn to the general history of care in western culture as it relates in particular to the care of the chronic sick and the dying, dividing it into three different periods, each rather different in length. The first is the period of intuitive and empirical care of the impaired. The second begins with the birth of technical care. The third sees the rise of modern palliative care.

Stages in the history of care

Intuitive and empirical care

Care is among the most ancient behaviours of humankind. Caring is one of the typical characteristics of humanity. Humans are beings specially comprised in taking care of themselves and of others. Animals certainly take care of their offspring, but human caring is fundamentally different because it is an intellectual and moral enterprise. In this context the family has always been the primary site of caring. As T.S. Eliot wrote in *Four Quartets*, 'Home is where one starts from. As we grow older, the world becomes stranger, the pattern more complicated'. Home is the primary place for caring, the main and oldest institution for caring. This continues today, even in the era of the 'nuclear family', but it was only when the wider family network decreased in social importance that technical caring became necessary. Nowadays family care must be, at least, complemented and integrated with another more technical and institutionalized care.

The activity of curing has been, throughout history, a positively privileged social role, and caring, by contrast has been negatively privileged. This is the traditional difference between professions and occupations. Medicine, traditionally, has had the status of a male profession, while caring as a female occupation has been assigned a lower social value. We have here the classic distinction between cure as a *productive* activity, and care as a *reproductive* one. This permits us to understand why the goal of medicine has always been curing, not caring. Only in this way can the history of medicine be understood, as well as the lack of attention of medicine to care. In traditional societies curing has been the goal of medicine, leaving care to the traditional institutions, especially the family. Other institutions of caring apart from families, such as hospices and hospitals were founded in order to take care of those without families or those whose family was incapable of taking care of them. Hospices and hospitals were not originally curing centres, but caring institutions. Of course, curing and caring are not always divisible because caring includes curing, when possible. This is the reason why physicians had a place in hospitals, but physicians did not like caring. Their focus was upon curing, but because curing was in many cases not completely different to caring, they accepted caring as a related occupation.

Traditionally, caring was understood as a work of beneficence or charity but not of justice, hence its close association with families and churches, rather than the state. Hospices and hospitals were in general religious foundations, engaged in the so-called works of mercy, especially consoling the afflicted and visiting the sick. This was the particular goal of religious orders, some of which were especially founded for this purpose. Thus St Benedict writes in his *Rule* (Regula 36: 1): 'Before all, and above all, attention shall be paid to the care of the sick, so that they shall be served as if they were Christ Himself' (Colombas and Aranguren 1979: 132).

Things began to change only when the traditional society of agricultural production and the extended family as a reproductive and caring unit were gradually substituted by another system in which production came to be industrial, and the unit of reproduction became the so-called nuclear family. This change began in the seventeenth century, and was well underway in the eighteenth. Only then did physicians medicalize hospitals, making them centres of curing more than of caring. At the same time, hospital caring led to the birth of technical nursing with Florence Nightingale, in the nineteenth century. Hospitals became centres of curing, with caring as a subordinate activity (Núñez Olarte 1999).

Meanwhile, the family lost its old capacity of being the only unit of caring. This was the result of the turn from the extended family to the nuclear family, a consequence of the industrial revolution and the division of labour. By the term nuclear family we understand the society of parents and their children. It is therefore smaller than the corporate and extended family, living in smaller groups with both parents working and both taking care of the children. The capacity of the nuclear family to take care of its sick and dependent members is generally considered to be small. Caring by young parents of their older kin becomes practically impossible.

Most affected by this change have been elderly people and those with chronic diseases. These often cannot be cared for in families, but require care in hospitals or other institutions. At the same time, the increasingly technical orientation of hospitals, and not least the capacity to manipulate death and dying, has made hospitalized death much more common, even when curing strategies become ineffective and irrational. This, indeed, is the framework in which the new strategies of managing terminal patients acquire part of their meaning. There are, also, other frameworks, developed as social and cultural attitudes towards death have themselves changed. As families could no longer take care of terminally ill patients, and when hospitals progressively became specialized in tertiary and intensive care, the need for new ideas became necessary. The two most important were the pain units and hospice care. This is the second part of our history.

The technical care of terminally ill patients: from the 'management of pain' to 'total pain' and 'total care' in the hospice movement

During the Second World War ideas about the treatment of pain were markedly altered. Traditionally, pain was poor and incorrectly treated. Western culture, due to the influence of Stoicism, considered the resistance to pain as the highest virtue and saw pusillanimity or the fear of pain as a vice. The stoic maxim of conduct was *sustine et abstine*, 'fortitude and abstinence'. But this was not the only reason to consider the relief of pain as a negative moral behaviour. Christian theology developed the redemptive character of pain. Saint Paul wrote to the Colossians (Col: 1, 24): 'I fill up that which is behind of the afflictions of Christ in my flesh' (Saint Paul 1991: 1051). The relief of pain was thought of, therefore, as philosophically and theologically inconvenient and incorrect (Donovan 1989).

Medicine in turn assumed these points of view, adding medical reasons against pain control. The first and most important medical reason was that physicians conceived pain as the most important sign of disease and there-fore thought that silencing pain was inappropriate, likely to confuse the physician and mislead the treatment of the patient. Traditionally medicine has assumed that pain reveals illnesses, that it is a defence mechanism, a welcome warning which alerts us to danger of impending illness and is therefore useful and necessary. Silencing pain should therefore be considered as one of the most dangerous things a physician might undertake.

Yet many thinkers accepted, for humanitarian reasons, the need to re-lieve pain. There is a classical maxim that says *divinum opus sedare dolorem*, 'the relief of pain is a divine work'. This relief was to some extent possible, because the ancients knew the so-called narcotic analgesics, all opium deriv-atives of the poppy *Papaver somniferum*, a plant native to Asia Minor, and known throughout the history of western culture. The Greeks also knew other analgesic natural substances, such as willow bark, which was used to relieve pain and fever. Its effectiveness as an analgesic was due to one of its components, salicin, the most important mild analgesic from 1874 onwards. From 1803, when pure narcotine was first obtained from opium, many other analgesic products were developed, including morphine. But narcotic analgesics were not widely used by physicians, due (among other reasons) to the physical dependence they produced, and the wider fear of drug addic-tion. A convergence of philosophical, theological and medical reasons there-fore meant that the relief of pain was not adequate.

Between the two world wars, 'dolorism' emerged as a movement (see Rey 1995: 318–19 for a full account). It was founded by the French writer and journalist Julien Teppe, who published two books in rapid succession, first *Apologie pour l'anormal* or the 'Dolorist manifesto' in 1935, and *Dictature de la douleur* in 1937. During the same period, Julien Teppe launched the *Revue doloriste*, an episodic publication which struggled to survive after the war but managed to include such prestigious writers as Gide and Valéry, and other celebrated names such as Benda, Colette, Léautaud and Daniel-Rops. The main idea of dolorism was that pain represents a means of self-discovery and a way to understand basic truth in relation to oneself: 'I am suffering, therefore I am', said Teppe, who saw in pain a type of catharsis, a means of purification from non-essentials, incidentals and falsehoods. Thus:

> Pain, of all the psychological states, is the one which takes over the entire being, both the flesh and the spirit, with the greatest urgency and force. It is a disposition which sweeps away, blots out, and annihilates all the rest. It does not allow for cheating or compromise. It is there and is enough to eliminate all the rest . . . I consider extreme anguish, particularly that of somatic origin, as the perfect incitement for developing pure idealism, created anew in each individual.
>
> (quoted in Rey 1995: 318)

Teppe and the French dolorists were not alone. In fact, they were reformulating the ideas proclaimed some years before by German philosophers such as Karl Jaspers and Martin Heidegger. Jaspers described suffering as an exceptional and privileged situation in human life, one of the 'limit-situations', in which human beings can experience the most profound dimensions of existence, touching what he calls 'transcendence'. Martin Heidegger centred all his philosophy on the experience of anguish. Between the two world wars, dolorism was well accepted by European culture, due, perhaps, to the increased importance of neo-romanticism.

But dolorism also provoked a strong reaction. The leader of this in France was the surgeon René Leriche. A disciple of the physiologist Claude Bernard, Leriche had gained surgical experience in the First World War during which he became interested in the surgical treatment of pain associated with battlefield injuries. His book, *La Chirurgie de la douleur* (Leriche 1937) immediately became a classic in the treatment of 'pain disorders'. Leriche's central idea is that surgery performed on the sympathetic system is the most powerful and physiological means of relieving pain because by acting on vasomotricity, it influences the internal environment which is responsible for many such disorders. In fact, in his final texts, Leriche increasingly suggested substituting chemical means by surgical means (Rey 1995: 317).

Perhaps because he was so often confronted with pain in his daily practice, and also because early in his career he had tried to relieve the pain of a young man suffering from neuralgia who had attempted suicide several times, Leriche was more than a great 'pain surgeon', he was also a militant humanist, fighting every kind of 'dolorist' tendency which attempted to exalt the value of pain. He was violently opposed to the notion of beneficial or useful pain, no matter what it represented and pain had little value in his eyes, either from a diagnostic standpoint or a prognostic one:

It reveals only a minute proportion of illnesses and often, when it is one of their accompaniments, it is misleading. On the other hand, in certain chronic cases it seems to be the entire disorder which, without it, would not exist. Despite this harsh reality, doctors readily state that pain is a defence mechanism, a welcome warning which cautions us about the danger of impending illness, that it is useful, and, I was about to add, necessary . . . My belief is entirely different . . . Defence mechanism? Welcome warning? In actual fact, most illnesses even the most severe, take hold without giving any warning. Sickness is generally a drama, which unfolds in two acts: the first one appears stealthily and plays its part in the dark, in the drab silence of our tissues . . . When the pain does arrive, it is already too late. The outcome has already been decided; it is imminent. The pain has only made the whole battle, lost early on in the game, sadder and more unbearable . . . Pain is always a sinister bequest which diminishes the individual, making him sicker than he would have been without it, and a doctor's most pressing duty is to do his utmost to suppress it if he can – always.

(Leriche 1937: 27–8, quoted in Rey 1995: 322 ff)

Pain surgery presumes an ethical stance regarding pain, and represents a vibrant plea in favour of living a full life under the best possible circumstances.

It is also a resolute indictment against the practices Leriche witnessed around him, against the hypocrisy of all those who speak of 'handling' pain when they have never experienced it, against those who are not driven by the impatience of fight, to answer the challenge presented by pain, that unspeakable experience above all.

(Rey 1995: 323)

Leriche's work did not pay attention to the pharmacological treatment of pain. In fact, he assumed the traditional idea that morphine should not be used as a normal treatment, due to the dependence it caused. This was the unquestionable idea until the Second World War. For instance, in 1941, the highly reputed French physiologist, Jean L'hermitte, participated in a debate about pain entitled *Qu'est-ce que la douleur?* (see Rey 1995: 319). After assuming the Hippocratic precept, 'the first duty of medicine is to heal when it can, to relieve often, and to comfort always', he adds that pain has a highly physiological importance, and notes: 'From this we may conclude that pain is a necessary evil.' He thinks that morphine can in some circumstances be an effective means of avoiding potential suicides among sufferers of causalgia, cancer or neuralgia. But immediately after that he adds: 'I insist strongly on this particular point, as it seems so essential to me: some physicians give out morphine too freely; morphine should only be injected if one is quite certain a patient is suffering a great deal. Morphine should not be given out lightly.' After quoting this paragraph, Roselyne Rey concludes:

> How much suffering has been endured by patients in the name of this therapeutic conservatism, in the name of this ambiguous reticence to alleviate the suffering of others? How many deaf ears have been turned to patients' complaints of pain, how much misunderstanding and suspicion has confronted those who say 'I am in pain'?
>
> (Rey 1995: 319–20)

It was only during the Second World War that this view began to change. The architect of the new approach was John J. Bonica. His thesis was that the treatment of pain was not a clear competence of a concrete speciality, as anaesthetics or general medicine. No one believed themselves to have the responsibility of patients' pain, and as a consequence pain was generally incorrectly treated. Lack of due knowledge, absence of adequate skills and a large amount of anxiety and fear were the causes of this untenable situation. Bonica, an anaesthesiologist, attempted to address the situation, turning the management of pain into an organic body of knowledge and skills, as well as ascribing this new activity to anaesthesiology as a speciality. His book *The Management of Pain* (Loeser 2000) has become a classic source of reference for the treatment of pain. Bonica thought that pain should be treated in hospitals, in new units called 'pain units' or 'pain clinics'. Immediately, others such as Beecher, Dundee, Lasagna and LeShan began to work in the same way as Bonica. The Pain Clinic of the University of Washington in Seattle was opened in 1961, and in 1973 an International Symposium on pain management took place in the same university. Finally, in 1974, the International Society for the Study of Pain was founded. During the 1970s the movement of pain control spread all over the world, and pain units became a normal aspect of the tertiary care hospital.

Bonica was not the only one who took an interest in the treatment of pain during these years. In an autobiographical essay, published in 1996 in the *British Medical Journal* and entitled 'A personal therapeutic journey', Cicely Saunders (1996) describes her beginnings in this way:

> I began training as a ward nurse in 1941 at St Thomas's Hospital . . . Young patients dying of tuberculosis and septicaemia from war wounds begged us to save them somehow, but we had little to offer except devoted nursing. Osteomyelitis led to amputation and gastric ulcers to a milk diet. Penicillin appeared after D Day, when soldiers arrived saying that they could not face another blunt needle. We had morphine by injection but used it sparingly . . . In March 1948 I began working as a volunteer nurse once or twice a week in one of the early homes for 'terminal care'. St Luke's Hospital had 48 beds for patients with advanced cancer. Here I met the regular administration of a modified

'Brompton cocktail' every four hours. The St Luke's version omitted the cannabis and, I think, the cocaine. They adjusted the morphine dose to the patient's need; if more than 60 mg was required the route was changed to injection. Hyoscine was used with morphine for terminal restlessness.

(Saunders 1996: 1599–601, passim)

From 1951 to 1957, Cicely Saunders was a medical student, again at St Thomas's. On qualifying she arrived at St Joseph's Hospice in October 1958. Here a clinical research fellowship from the Department of Pharmacology at St Mary's Hospital Medical School under Professor Harold Stewart enabled her to begin working to investigate terminal pain and its relief. The results of the work carried out by the Department of Pharmacology, but with St Joseph's patients, were presented to the Royal Society of Medicine in 1963, and published the same year in a comprehensively famous paper (Saunders 1963). The paper analyses the problems and treatments in some 900 patients at St Joseph's Hospice. It concentrates not on the drugs used with these patients, but rather on the method of their deployment. The 'cardinal rules' are set out: careful assessment of the symptoms that trouble the patient; assessment of the nature and severity of pain; the regular giving of drugs. Where opiates are used over a long period, amiphenazole may also be combined. Diamorphine finds particular favour: 'In the doses we use, it does not cause changes in personality, frank euphoria or a "could not care less" attitude' (Saunders 1963: 196). It may however be short-lived in effect, and require more frequent administration. The paper concludes with a discussion of mental distress – 'perhaps the most intractable pain of all' (Saunders 1963: 197) – and the appropriate drug treatments which may be used, as well as the importance of listening.

This paper was particularly relevant because it affirmed strongly the importance of using opiates in terminally ill patients without the fear of provoking dependence. It showed that the pains of these patients were incorrectly treated, due to the prejudices of physicians and also restrictive rules regulating the prescription of relevant drugs (see also Rey 1995: 336). As a result of the work of Cicely Saunders, the management of pain began to change at St Joseph's Hospice and therapeutic advances transformed the wards.

The best control of physical pain also permitted better management of other difficulties. This was the great work of Cicely Saunders after 1963, when as David Clark (1999) has shown, she crystallized out the full-blown concept of 'total pain', to include physical, social, spiritual and psychological problems. The argument thus became that 'The last stages of life should not be seen as defeat, but rather as life's fulfilment' (Saunders 1965: 70). Working in this way:

It soon became clear that each death was as individual as the life that preceded it and that the whole experience of that life was reflected in a patient's dying. This led to the concept of 'total pain', which was presented as a complex of physical, emotional, social, and spiritual elements. The whole experience for a patient includes anxiety, depression, and fear; concern for the family who will become bereaved; and often a need to find some meaning in the situation, some deeper reality in which to trust. This became the major emphasis of much lecturing and writing on subjects such as the nature and management of terminal pain and the family as the unit of care.

(Saunders 1996: 1660)

From physical pain to total pain, and from total pain to 'total care': this was the shift in Cicely Saunders' thinking from the 1940s to the 1960s. In the specific case of terminally ill and dying patients, her idea was that this total care is in need of more special units, particularly for those patients who did not need the resources of a large hospital and who could not be cared for at home. Accordingly,

The provision of an institution primarily devoted to what is often called terminal care should not be thought of as a separate and essentially negative part of the attack on cancer. This is not merely the phase of defeat, hard to contemplate and unrewarding to carry out. In many ways its principles are fundamentally the same as those which underlay all the other stages of care and treatment although its rewards are different.

(Saunders 1964: 1)

Hospices should be these new institutions, which she defined as 'something between a hospital and a home' (Saunders 1964: 1).

This description of the work of Cicely Saunders permits an understanding of her contribution to the development and enhancement of technical care. She worked, like others during these decades, towards a better management of pain. Bonica, an anaesthesiologist, tried to perfect the treatment of pain through an improved use of anaesthetic and analgesic drugs in hospitals. His contribution was a better pharmacological treatment of pain. Cicely Saunders, who had trained as a social worker, a nurse and a physician, was also concerned about pain management, but did not reduce it to largely somatic dimensions. From this perspective, the correct management of terminally ill patients called for an integrated approach, which could not be achieved adequately in the tertiary care hospital, with its largely curative orientation. A new caring strategy was therefore necessary and this was the origin of the modern hospice movement. Hospices were conceived as the new institutions for the total care of dying patients.

Cicely Saunders stressed especially the need to take into account the spiritual dimensions of pain and death and saw the need for a new *ars moriendi*. Dying is an exceptional and privileged situation in human life. In the second half of the twentieth century it acquired a metaphysical dimension. Karl Jaspers (1932), for example, described dying as a privileged existential situation, and centred all his philosophy on the fact of human mortality. Many others have been convinced of the need of a new culture of death and dying in the modern world.

From 'total care' to 'palliative care': the birth of a specialty

The term palliation has been used in medicine for centuries. When medicine could only control symptoms, and was unable to reverse the situation by eradicating the cause of the disease, then the term used was palliation. Medicine has been for centuries, therefore, curative (when curing etiologically) and palliative (when controlling symptoms). As Clark and Seymour (1999) show, the medical use of the term 'palliation' dates at least to the seventeenth and eighteenth centuries and there are absolutely clear and concrete references in the nineteenth century. Cicely Saunders summarizes the history of the medical use of this word from the end of the nineteenth century in the following terms:

> In 1890, Dr Herbert Snow, Surgeon to the Cancer Hospital, Brompton, London, published a book on *The Palliative Treatment of Incurable Cancer, with an Appendix on the use of the Opium Pipe*. He also published an article in the *British Medical Journal* on 'Opium and cocaine in the treatment of cancerous disease'. The Cancer Hospital (now the Royal Marsden Hospital) was next door to the Brompton Hospital for Diseases of the Chest. Perhaps the pharmacists were in touch when the latter hospital produced the Brompton Cocktail in the early 1930s, with its main ingredients of morphine and/or diamorphine and cocaine. Its regular, four-hourly use in St Luke's Hospital, London can be traced back to 1935, through the memories of a former Matron. The Cancer Hospital was committed to patients with advanced disease. In 1909, a Dr Horder was allocated 19 beds for such patients and in 1964 a ward was reopened with 16 beds in Dr Horder's name. I can find no record of what happened in the interim period.
>
> (Saunders 1998: vii)

It is interesting that in the earlier writings of Cicely Saunders, palliation is understood in this classical sense, as a merely symptomatic treatment, and not as the search for the total comfort of the patient. This allows us to understand why during this time she does not consider palliation a correct word to express the hospice philosophy. Rather, she considers that the 'terminal stage' begins 'when all curative and palliative measures have been exhausted' (Saunders 1960: 16). The same point is echoed in another paper from 1966, which begins by defining 'terminal illness' as 'a claim for comfort rather than curative or even palliative procedures' (Saunders 1966:

225). Likewise in another article published a year later, in 1967, when she writes: 'Care for the dying person should be directed no longer towards his cure, rehabilitation or even palliation but primarily at his comfort' (Saunders 1967: 385). All these texts emphasize the same idea: that cure and palliation are correct measures in treatable patients, but not in terminally ill patients, for whom only comfort is a correct goal.

This permits an understanding of why the expression 'palliative care' was coined neither by Cicely Saunders, nor by her most closely related associates. Instead, the phrase was used for the first time in Canada in 1975, when Balfour Mount opened the Palliative Care Service in the Royal Victoria Hospital, Montreal (Hamilton 1995). Palliative care, like intensive care, began in the tertiary hospital setting, and not in hospices. 'Hospice' was an inappropriate name for a ward or service of a tertiary care hospital. The new nomenclature marked a sea-change in thinking: the ideas and practices, first developed in inpatient hospices, could now, under a new name, be promulgated in a variety of care settings, including the acute hospital itself. Clearly, palliative care is not just about hospices. Acknowledging the same point, Cicely Saunders has written: 'These developments demonstrated that hospice care did not have to be limited to a separate building, but that the new attitudes and skills could be practised in a variety of settings' (1998: vii).

One view of this development is to see it as a consequence of the increasing importance of 'intensive' treatments which arose in the 1970s. Seen in this way, palliative care becomes a corollary of intensive care. That is to say, there are situations in which intensive treatments are indicated, but others in which they can be considered as harmful, or contra-indicated. In oncology, for instance, there are therapies of intensification and therapies of palliation, and the birth of the first and the second was simultaneous.

Yet the dialectics of intensification-palliation, or intensive care versus palliative care were not primarily related to the idea of intensification in oncology, but rather to the growth of new life support techniques. During the 1970s, a new strategy of management for critically ill patients began to appear. It was called 'intensive support' or 'intensive care', and it was placed in new units opened in tertiary care hospitals, called 'intensive care units' or 'intensive therapy units'. At the very beginning, it was thought that intensive care should be the final way for all diseased human beings, either critically or terminally ill. At the end, all patients are in a critical situation. The consequence of this strategy was over-treatment, a phenomenon that began to be known as 'therapeutic furor'. Palliative care was the answer to this situation. Only critically ill patients should be treated in the intensive care units. Terminally ill patients were in need not of intensive care but of palliative care; not of intensification but of palliation, that is, not of cure but of care. So palliative care can be seen as a response by the healthcare community to the 'fallout' generated from life-prolonging medical interventions.

From this premise, certain consequences flow directly. First, there is the idea that palliative care cannot be understood as a 'soft' type of management of terminally ill patients, in the hands of families, volunteers and nurses. This means that palliation becomes a body of specific medical knowledge and skills and should be understood as a type of therapy or medicine. In the preface to her book *Living with Dying: A Guide to Palliative Care*, Cicely Saunders has written:

> When St Christopher's Hospice opened in 1967 as the first research and teaching hospice, its main aim was that tested knowledge should flow back into all branches of the National Health Service, as well as to the older homes and hospices to which it owed so great a debt. Earlier links with workers overseas had also encouraged hopes of extending even more widely, and these have been fulfilled. That there should now be specialist wards in general hospitals, and home and hospital teams working in consultation with the patient's own doctors, are in many ways more important developments than the growth of special units. Most important of all has been the general change of attitude to a more analytical and positive approach to the needs of a dying patient and his family. Anecdotal evidence is replaced increasingly by objective data as the scientific foundation of *this branch of medicine* are laid. The essentials of good management at this stage have been clarified and are now being widely discussed. Advances in this area of *treatment (and it is still 'treatment', not some kind of soft option labelled 'care')* [our italics] are now likely to come from the traditional hospital setting as well as from the special units or teams.
>
> (Saunders 1995: vii–viii)

The second consequence of this new approach has been the necessity to define with precision parameters of a new speciality, which now begins to be called 'palliative medicine'. Chapter 3 will explore in detail some of the problems associated with this. Palliative care is a wide and interdisciplinary field, within it is contained palliative medicine as a medical speciality. It is not accidental that the most important book written in this field is entitled the *Oxford Textbook of Palliative Medicine*. This book makes a distinction between palliative medicine and palliative care. It defines palliative medicine as 'the [medical] speciality practised by doctors', and palliative care as 'the care offered by a [multidisciplinary] team of doctors, nurses, therapists, social workers, clergy, and volunteers' (Doyle et al. 1998: 3). Palliative care is looking for 'total comfort', and palliative medicine is also a specific part of the whole strategy for achieving this goal. This distinction between palliative care and palliative medicine is especially clear after 1987, when palliative medicine was recognized as a medical speciality in the United Kingdom.

Palliative care is the active total care of terminally ill patients in an era of life support technologies and intensive care strategies. Intensive care and palliative care are deemed necessary for the same reasons. This has been the philosophy developed by the World Health Organization in its Expert Committee Report entitled *Cancer Pain Relief and Palliative Care* (WHO 1990). The WHO defines palliative care in the following terms:

> Palliative care is the active total care of patients whose disease is not responsive to curative treatment. Control of pain, of other symptoms and of psychological, social and spiritual problems is paramount. The goal of palliative care is achievement of the best possible quality of life for patients and their families. Many aspects of palliative care are also applicable earlier in the course of the illness in conjunction with anticancer treatment.
>
> (WHO 1990: 11)

The palliative care movement emphasizes that the practice of medicine includes more than specific treatments. Advances in pharmacology and the new technologies are not the whole story, as Cicely Saunders has said many times. Palliative care physicians should not be 'merely symptomologists' (a theme explored further in Chapter 3). Caregivers are hosts to their patients and their visiting families and should be aware of the human and spiritual needs. The whole approach of palliative care has been based on the understanding that a person is an indivisible entity, a physical and a spiritual being. Palliative care thus becomes akin to a complete philosophy of life, rather than simply a system of caring. This is the reason why palliative care is compatible with many different types of organization and why in Chapter 2 we are able to show the varied forms it has taken in the countries of Europe, taking root in different settings, but apparently espousing a common purpose and set of aims.

Conclusion

From Hippocratic medicine onwards, diseases have been divided in two different categories: 'acute' and 'chronic'. The first set has, among other characteristics, that of ending through 'crisis' or 'resolution', while the second generally ends by 'lysis' or 'dissolution'. *Critical care medicine* is the strategy of management of the 'critical' and 'reversible' patients, and *palliative medicine* was born as a new strategy of management for those patients whose illness is 'chronic' and who are in the last stages of life, that is the terminally ill patients. How to treat correctly these terminally ill patients from the biological, psychological, social and spiritual point of view: that is the question. Palliative care is the more creative, complete and efficient answer we have been capable of imagining and implementing so far: no more, no less.

References

Clark, D. (1999) 'Total pain', disciplinary power and the body in the work of Cicely Saunders, 1958–67, *Social Science and Medicine*, 49: 727–36.

Clark, D. and Seymour, J. (1999) *Reflections on Palliative Care*. Buckingham: Open University Press.

Colombas, G.M. and Aranguren, I. (eds) (1979) *La Regla de San Benito*. Madrid: Biblioteca de Autores Cristianos.

Donovan, M.I. (1989) An historical view of pain management: how to get where we are!, *Cancer Nursing*, 12(4): 257–61.

Doyle, D., Hanks, G.W.C. and MacDonald, N. (eds) (1998) *Oxford Textbook of Palliative Medicine*, 2nd edn. Oxford: Oxford University Press.

Hamilton, J. (1995) Dr. Balfour Mount and the cruel irony of our care for the dying, *Canadian Medical Association Journal*, 153(3): 334–6.

Jaspers, K. (1932) *Philosophie*. Vol. 1: *Philosophische Weltorientierung*. Vol. 2: *Existenzerhellung*. Vol. 3: *Metaphysik*. Berlin-Göttingen-Heidelberg: Springer.

Leriche, R. (1937) *La Chirurgie de la douleur*. Paris: Masson.

Loeser, J.D. (2000) *Bonica's Management of Pain*. Philadelphia, PA: Lippincott Williams and Wilkins.

Núñez Olarte, J.M. (1999) Care of the dying in 18th century Spain – the non hospice tradition, *European Journal of Palliative Care*, 6(1): 23–7.

Rey, R. (1995) *History of Pain*. Cambridge, MA: Harvard University Press.

Saint Paul (1991) Colossians, *The Holy Bible* (King James Version). New York: Ivy.

Saunders, C. (1960) Drug treatment of patients in the terminal stages of cancer, *Current Medicine and Drugs*, 1: 16–28.

Saunders, C. (1963) The treatment of intractable pain in terminal cancer, *Proceedings of the Royal Society of Medicine*, 56: 195–7.

Saunders, C. (1964) The need for institutional care for the patient with advanced cancer, *Anniversary Volume, Cancer Institute, Madras*, 1–8.

Saunders, C. (1965) The last stages of life, *American Journal of Nursing*, 65: 70–5.

Saunders, C. (1966) The management of terminal illness, *British Journal of Hospital Medicine*, December: 225–8.

Saunders, C. (1967) The care of the dying, *Gerontologica Clinica*, 9(4–6): 385–90.

Saunders, C. (1995) Preface, in C. Saunders, M. Baines and R. Dunlop, *Living with Dying: A Guide to Palliative Care*, 3rd edn. Oxford: Oxford University Press.

Saunders, C. (1996) A personal therapeutic journey, *British Medical Journal*, 313: 1599–601.

Saunders, C. (1998) Foreword, in D. Doyle, G.W.C. Hanks and N. MacDonald (eds) *Oxford Textbook of Palliative Medicine*, 2nd edn. Oxford: Oxford University Press.

World Health Organization (WHO) (1990) *Cancer Pain Relief and Palliative Care*. Geneva: WHO.

2 Palliative care service developments in seven European countries

DAVID CLARK, HENK TEN HAVE
AND RIEN JANSSENS

Shaped by the historical developments described in Chapter 1, the rapid expansion of specialist palliative care services has been a notable achievement of healthcare development across Europe in recent years. In an era of medical modernization, exponential growth in curative and rehabilitative treatments and soaring healthcare spending, the attention of European health policy-makers has also begun to turn to questions of end-of-life care. Indeed, in June 1999 the Council of Europe adopted a resolution on the protection of the human rights and dignity of terminally ill and dying patients and called for a legal entitlement to palliative care for all individuals (Watson 1999). Across western Europe, particularly since the late 1960s, we have seen first the germinating seeds of new terminal and palliative care services, followed in the 1990s by significant innovations in almost every country. Similar patterns are emerging, albeit slightly later, in the countries of central and eastern Europe and of the former Soviet Union. While our knowledge of palliative care developments in individual countries has begun to improve, with a few exceptions (Hockley 1997), we still lack much in the way of a comparative perspective. This chapter seeks to shed light on the problem through the examination of palliative care service developments in seven western European countries: Germany, Sweden, Italy, the Netherlands, Belgium, Spain and the United Kingdom. The chapter describes how palliative care initiatives came into being in the different settings, together with variations in their mode of organization. This is linked to a discussion of the balance of provision in each country as at the end of 1999, and in particular the degree of linkage with the formal healthcare system. By setting out a detailed analysis of the organization of palliative care in various European countries, we hope to provide a platform, later in the book, for a detailed analysis of ethical issues in palliative care practice. At the same time, the differential provision of palliative care in the seven countries we describe is itself a matter for ethical comment and reflection.

Aims, methods and problems of comparability

The chapter has two aims. First, to offer a comparative analysis of palliative care development in a number of western European countries. Second, to pave the way for a deeper understanding, to be addressed in subsequent chapters, of variations in the *concepts* of palliative care which prevail across Europe. To achieve the first aim, members of the core group of the *Pallium* project, representing each of the seven countries, produced a detailed report on their own local context. These 'country reports', which we draw on throughout this chapter, covered the following themes: population structure; the wider healthcare system; the development of palliative care services with particular reference to inpatient facilities, home care, hospital and nursing home care; palliative care education; specialization and academic development; relevant policy documents. Production of the country reports built on a wide range of documentary sources, including national and regional statistics relating to populations, healthcare and service provision; published work on palliative care services in each country; 'grey' literature and reports on palliative care; as well as information collected and published by specialist palliative care umbrella and non-government organizations.

This proved to be a complex task. Although such information was available to varying degrees in all seven countries, it was often presented in forms which made comparison difficult. Also, while some countries had extensive documentation, even a secondary literature, on the growth of local palliative care provision, in others this information had to be obtained *de novo*. Accordingly, comparisons within our data sometimes proved difficult and it was not always possible to present information which compares one country with another at the same time. To document and assess the development of palliative care across countries is to focus on a moving target, and one which in some cases is moving very quickly indeed. Keeping this in mind we have sought in this chapter to present the best evidence available to us at the end of 1999. We believe it provides the first detailed comparison of how palliative care was developing in Europe during the closing decades of the twentieth century. It provides also some guide to decision-making processes which will influence palliative care development in Europe in the new century. Our experience in gathering this information has confirmed the well-known sociological maxim that official statistics are social constructions, serving particular organizational, political and strategic purposes. We have strived for objectivity but in each country we studied forces at work which have vested interests in how the figures should be presented and interpreted. In particular the figures on service provision which we present should be viewed with a cautious eye: depending on the purpose to be served they may be seen as either an over- or under-estimation of the 'true' picture.

Early origins

Within the seven countries studied, the 'founding' specialist hospice or palliative care initiatives took place over a period of almost a quarter century, from 1967 to 1991 (Table 2.1). Nor were the initiatives of uniform character in each country, so that a first step on the palliative care path might take the form of an inpatient hospice, a hospital-based service, or a home care programme. At the beginning of the period the influences of St Christopher's Hospice in south London and of its founder, Cicely Saunders, were widely felt. In these early years, it had become apparent that St Christopher's was not simply going to be a lone example of high quality care for the dying, but was also to serve as the wellspring for a much wider movement capable of crossing national borders (Clark 1998). In some cases this led to examples of hospice pioneers in other countries seeking to transplant the St Christopher's concept, more or less intact, to other settings. Conversely, others, while impressed with the model, saw its limitations and sought to refine it in ways more closely tailored to local problems. In Germany, for example, a 1971 television broadcast on the work of St Christopher's seems

Table 2.1   'Founding' specialist hospice/palliative care services in seven European countries

Country	Date	Type of service	Name of service
United Kingdom	1967	Inpatient hospice	St Christopher's Hospice
Sweden	1977	Home care service	Motala Hospital-based Home Care
Italy	1980	Home care programme	Pain Therapy Division of National Cancer Institute of Milan and Floriani Foundation
Germany	1983	Hospital inpatient unit	Palliative Care Unit, University Clinic, Cologne
Spain	1984	Palliative care unit within hospital medical oncology department	Medical Oncology Department, Valdicella Hospital, Santander
Belgium	1985	Palliative care unit; home care service	Unité de Soins Continus St Luc *and* Continuing Care, Brussels
The Netherlands	1991	Inpatient hospice	Johannes Hospice, Vleuten

to have been a source of inspiration for some early hospices. In Spain however, while the work of the UK founding hospices was studied with interest, it was not charitable innovation, but rather a public health model, rational planning and a powerful emphasis upon coverage and equity of access which fuelled developments (Gómez-Batiste 1994a,b).

It was a full ten years after the opening of St Christopher's Hospice that the first specialized palliative care service began elsewhere in Europe, in Sweden. Located in the south of the country, the Motala Hospital-based Home Care Service was designed to provide 'a hospital bed in the patient's own home' on a 24-hour basis (Beck-Friis and Strang 1993). It was intended as an *alternative*, rather than a *complement*, to hospital care, in a context where 85 per cent of deaths take place in institutional settings, but where a preference for home care persists, subject to the availability of appropriate practical help. At first the service operated on only a small scale, predominantly for geriatric patients, and with a provision in the first year of 10,000 bed days. Later a total of five teams covered the whole county of Ostergotland (Beck-Friis 1997). By 1979 a national report had appeared in Sweden, promoting such developments, but explicitly rejecting the 'hospice' model of free-standing institutions for the care of the dying.

In 1980, the first palliative home care service appeared in Italy, based on a collaboration between the Pain Therapy Division of the National Cancer Institute of Milan, the Floriani Foundation and the Italian League Against Cancer. Following discharge from hospital, terminally ill cancer patients were followed up in their own homes by a multidisciplinary team which comprised doctors, nurses, psychologists, social workers and volunteers (Ferrario and Saita 1998). It too became a model for later home care services in other Italian regions (De Conno and Martini 1997; De Conno et al. 1996).

In Germany, a cluster of developments inspired by various approaches to palliative care first appeared between 1983 and 1987 (Albrecht 1990). In Cologne a five-bed inpatient unit was opened as part of the University Hospital (1983); in Aachen, the 'Haus Hörn', a purpose-built 63-bed accommodation, began operation, in close association with a neighbouring nursing home (1985); and in Reckinghausen the St Elizabeth Hospital began to make available seven rooms in a nearby apartment house, which could be rented by terminally ill patients and their families (1987). The different financial arrangements underpinning each of these, as we shall observe, had implications for the direction of future development.

Almost contiguous with the German developments, new services began to appear in Spain (Gracia and Núñez Olarte 1999). Following several years in which a group of Spanish physicians had sought information and received training abroad (in the United Kingdom, Italy and Canada), the first Spanish palliative care service was begun in 1984 in the medical oncology unit of Valdicella Hospital, Santander. In 1987 palliative care services were begun in chronic care hospitals in Vic (Catalonia) and in Las Palmas (Canary Islands), where a home care service was also developed. Spain's largest cancer centre, the Gregorio Marañón tertiary care hospital, in Madrid, opened a palliative care unit in 1990.

In Belgium also, the mid-1980s was the time in which developing palliative care aspirations began to come to fruition (Broeckaert 1999). Here an early advocate of terminal care was the British woman Joan Jordan, who had experienced the final illness of her Belgian husband and who, together with a community nurse, Lisette Custermans, established an organization called Continuing Care, in 1981, the purpose of which was to promote hospice care. It was in 1985, however, that the first palliative care services in Belgium became operational when Continuing Care started its specialized home care service in Brussels and when, also in Brussels, an eight-bed unit opened, Unité de Soins Continus St Luc. Other palliative care units followed with Foyer St François in Namur (1989) and the Sint-Jan Hospital, in Brussels (1990). Belgium's second home care service was Intensieve Zorg Thuis ('intensive care at home'), later Palliatieve Zorg Thuis ('palliative care at home'), which began in West-Vlaanderen in 1987.

In the Netherlands the precise character of the early period of sensitization and gestation, together with the timing of the first palliative care services, is itself a matter of dispute (Janssens 1999). Some commentators (for example Zylicz 1993) take the view that the Netherlands is a late arrival at the European palliative care table. Others (for example Keizer 1999) argue that in Dutch nursing homes, over a period of 30 years from the late 1960s, physicians had been developing and disseminating palliative care skills and practice. It is clear in this context that the account of palliative care development in any given country has the potential to become a disputed ideological terrain, in which the 'history' of palliative care can be written and rewritten in relation to the prevailing goals, intentions and claims of the key actors involved. We return to this theme in the context of the goals of palliative care, in Chapter 3. As Janssens (1999) points out, in the Dutch case, the implications highlight 'whether palliative care in the Netherlands should be conceived of as a young and largely underestimated area of expertise in Dutch society or whether the Netherlands should be seen as one of the first countries to have explicitly adopted palliative care'. As early as 1972 a Dutch organization Voorbij de Laatste Stad (Beyond the Last City) had been formed to promote the improvement of terminal care in the Netherlands. In 1975 it gave support to the Antonius IJsselmonde nursing home in Rotterdam which was seeking to enhance the quality of its terminal care provision. Various issues were investigated by the project, including the patient's transition from hospital to nursing home, nursing care in the terminal phase, and bereavement support. In the late 1970s the project made contacts with St Christopher's and St Luke's Hospices in the United Kingdom. When the project ended in 1985, those involved could acknowledge a growing interest in terminal care in the Netherlands, particularly among voluntary groups influenced by the work of Elisabeth Kübler-Ross, as well as in nursing homes, hospitals and other institutions; and so the claim was made that care of the dying had ceased to be a 'taboo' issue within Dutch society (Bruning and Klein Hesselink 1985). Despite this it was not until the early 1990s that full specialist palliative care services appeared in the Netherlands. In 1991 the first high care hospice, the Johannes Hospice in Vleuten, began its work; in 1993 the Antonius-IJsselmonde nursing home itself in Rotterdam opened a palliative care unit (Baar 1999); and in 1994 Hospice Rozenheuvel commenced in Rozendaal.

By the late 1990s, palliative care services in these seven European countries were at various stages of development. In some countries, particularly the United Kingdom, a phase of maturation had been reached in which the establishment of a critical mass of palliative care provision had generated other consequences: recognition as a healthcare specialty, extensive education programmes, together with a growing culture of research and academic inquiry (Clark and Seymour 1999). In all seven countries the provision of palliative care had moved beyond (in some examples, well beyond) isolated examples of pioneering services run by enthusiastic founders. In this context it becomes possible to compare and contrast the level and type of palliative care provision in each country before moving on to consider how such provision relates to wider questions of health policy in the European context.

Service provision by the late 1990s

In reviewing recent palliative care provision in the seven countries, two forms of variation become clear (Table 2.2). First, we can see that palliative care is being delivered in a variety of settings: domiciliary, quasi-domiciliary and institutional. Second, it is apparent that these are not prioritized uniformly in each country. In examining this we should also keep in mind the significant variations in population size across the seven countries, with a tenfold difference, for example, between Sweden and Germany.

Inpatient hospices and palliative care units

Inpatient provision constituted the foundational palliative care service in five of the seven countries (Sweden and Italy were exceptions), suggesting from the outset a strong medical orientation to service development. In the United Kingdom the first inpatient hospices to be developed from the late 1960s were independent, charitable institutions. Despite the existence of the welfare state, which promised care 'from the cradle to the grave', policy

Table 2.2   Palliative care services in seven European countries (1999)

	Belgium	Germany	Italy	The Netherlands	Spain	Sweden	United Kingdom
Population	10.1 m	81.9 m	57.4 m	15.6 m	40.0 m	8.8 m	57.1 m
Inpatient hospice	1	64	3	16	1	69	219
Inpatient palliative care unit	49	50	0	2	23		
Hospital (and nursing home) teams	55	1	0	34	45	41	336
Home care	45	582	88	286	75	67	355
Day care	2	9	0	0	0	13	248

indifference to terminal care provision created a vacuum, which independent charitable endeavour was able to fill (Clark 1999). Continuing care units (as they were then called) within the National Health Service (NHS) first appeared in the mid-1970s, usually as purpose-built facilities within the curtilage of acute hospitals. By the mid-1990s such units accounted for around one-quarter of inpatient palliative care provision in the United Kingdom.

In Germany, inpatient provision of palliative care in the late 1990s was perceived to be inadequate and it was estimated that just 1–2 per cent of patients dying from cancer were able to be looked after in a palliative care unit or hospice (Nauck and Klaschik 1998). Only three such units had been established in German universities by 1998, in Cologne, Berlin and Göttingen. Although Spain has the lowest number of *hospital* beds per inhabitant of any country in Europe, the hospital context has been the engine room for much initial palliative care development. By 1999 there were 23 palliative care units in acute hospitals; interestingly, Spain had just one independent hospice, CUDECA, in Malaga, which emerged from and seeks to serve the expatriate community in the Costa del Sol (Hunt and Martin 1997). In Belgium the provision of hospital beds for palliative care was determined by a royal decree of 1997, which following a careful calculation of need (Leontine 1992), set a figure of 360 beds for the whole country, located in departments of 6–12 beds each, to be spread out evenly over the Belgian territory (Wouters 1998; Broeckaert 1999). Efforts in the Netherlands focused on establishing six academic centres of palliative care, part of a wider set of reforms seeking to integrate Dutch hospice provision within the formal healthcare system. Dutch hospices however vary significantly in character; in 1999 of the 12 which offered low intensity care, all

Table 2.3   Ratio of inpatient hospice and palliative care beds to population in
seven European countries (1999)

Country	Beds	Ratio of beds to population
United Kingdom	3196	1 : 17,866
Belgium	358	1 : 28,212
Sweden	298	1 : 29,530
Spain	812	1 : 49,261
Germany	989	1 : 82,812
The Netherlands	119	1 : 131,092
Italy	30	1 : 1,913,333

were independent organizations and five of them were explicitly Christian. In addition the country had four 'high care' hospices, all of which relied upon charitable support and were likewise Christian in orientation. Finally, there were just two inpatient palliative care units in hospitals (Janssens and ten Have 1999). In Sweden, also in 1999, 32 of the 69 inpatient units had seven or more beds, and 12 of these units adopted the 'hospice' name. Some 37 units offered more modest facilities, where a small number of palliative care beds were secondary to the provision of generic or geriatric care. Approximately one-half of Swedish palliative care units had either an associated advanced home care service, or palliative care consulting service, or both (Valverius 1999).

The total provision of palliative care beds across the seven countries in 1999 proved difficult to calculate. Table 2.3 shows the best available figures, based on extensive consultation and inquiries. The United Kingdom had the largest absolute number of beds, with substantial numbers also in Germany and Spain. The provision of palliative care beds across any country must however be seen in relation to the total population and we present this calculation in Table 2.3. Both practitioners and policy-makers may wish to reflect on the significance of this 'league table', which is headed by the UK and in which Italy is in a very distant seventh place. Certainly it raises questions about the equity of palliative care provision available to European citizens in the seven countries studied.

Other hospital-based and nursing home services

The notion that teams of professionals in hospitals and nursing homes can offer palliative care to patients in the care of other medical specialties has been explored in several European countries. In Britain the first team of this type to be established was at St Thomas's Hospital, London, in 1976; by 1990 there were 40 such teams and by 1999 this had risen to around 336 (from a total of about 1900 hospitals in the country as a whole). However, most of these do not have the full multidisciplinary make-up of the specialist palliative care teams in the inpatient units and in 1999 some 117 of these UK teams were made up of one or two specialist nurses only (Clark and Seymour 1999). Nevertheless, such numbers are not found elsewhere in Europe and indeed the *total* number of hospital support teams in the other six countries covered by our review is considerably less than the number for the UK only. Despite this the coverage of palliative care support teams in UK hospitals does remain uneven. In Spain there is evidence that these teams may be highly concentrated in particular areas, such as Catalonia (Gómez-Batiste et al. 1997). Seeking to address this kind of problem, Belgium's royal decree on palliative care of 1997 required *every* hospital (217) and recognized residential or nursing home (446) to have its own multidisciplinary palliative care support team, making a total of 663 teams. By 1999 only a small minority of these were operational: the membership lists of the Belgian palliative care federations contained the names of 55 such teams. Coverage in the Netherlands amounted to a palliative care service in only 2 per cent of its nursing homes and rest homes; three out of nine regional cancer centres (Integrale Kankercentra) had a consultant in palliative medicine, though all had specialist nurses; and there were just seven acute hospital palliative care teams in a country of 144 hospitals. Sweden had a total of 41 consulting teams for palliative care in 1999, working in a variety of different ways. Some were cancer-only; some (for example Linköping) dealt with other conditions; about one-fifth also provided home care; some were located with inpatient palliative care units, others were not. The model of consulting to other service providers in the county councils or municipalities expanded rapidly in Sweden at this time.

Home care

Care in the home was the first form of palliative care provision to be developed in two of the seven European countries: Sweden and Italy. In 1999 Sweden's 67 specialized palliative home care teams took various organizational forms. For example, Linköping had a large palliative care department with several specialized home care units, inpatient beds and consultant teams; whereas Uppsala began with a service inside a district nurse unit. Here it was not uncommon for the home care teams to be based in hospital, and also in general practice. Italy is another country which has made considerable progress in home care, where it is perceived to be an affordable means of meeting the country's palliative care needs (De Conno and Martini 1997); nevertheless such services are much more developed in the north of the country than further south (Ferrario and Saita 1998). Palliative home care first began in the UK in 1969 and some 355 home care teams were in operation by late 1999 (Clark and Seymour 1999). About one-third of these were attached to hospice inpatient units and the remainder were mainly organized by NHS community healthcare trusts. It is estimated that 90,000 new patients per year are seen by home care nurses and that 40 per cent of those dying of cancer are cared for by home care teams. Home care services in the UK offer a variety of provision (Clark and Seymour 1999): clinical nurse specialists who work in a consulting/advisory capacity; extended home nursing (often provided by the charity Marie Curie Cancer Care); respite for informal carers; 'hospice at home'; and crisis intervention services.

Despite its relatively low levels of inpatient provision, Germany appears to have been more successful in establishing palliative home care services, but Sabatowski et al. (1998) suggest that only a minority of this provision is specialist and multidisciplinary. In 1999, 28 of Spain's 75 home care programmes were run by the Spanish Cancer League through agreements with the public healthcare system. As in Germany, links between such teams and inpatient palliative care units were seen as a way of reducing isolation and the risk of failure (Gómez-Batiste et al. 1992). In Belgium, some early home support services were forced out of existence by cuts in resources (Wouters 1998); by 1999 provision had been made for 30 multidisciplinary palliative home care teams, each responsible for about 300,000 people. The teams were intended to inform, support and advise, but not take over from, general home care. In the Netherlands, 46 professional initiatives for palliative home care could be identified in 1999; again some specialize in psychosocial support, others are nurse-led, some seek to provide advanced medical care at home. Beyond these were some 240 voluntary home care services, affiliated to the Network for the Palliative Care of Terminal Patients in the Netherlands.

Structural and policy development

The diversity of palliative care service provision in the seven countries does of course relate in part to differences in the structure of health policy, as well as variations in preferences for particular models of care in each setting. In considering palliative care development in the wider policy context it is helpful to examine the extent to which palliative care services are *integral* to, *symbiotic* with or *separate* from the formal healthcare system. We should note of course that these relationships may change over time.

Integration, symbiosis, separation?

Among the seven countries studied, Spain and Sweden are the paradigm cases from the outset of high order integration with the formal healthcare system. For example, in Catalonia collaboration between local physicians, regional politicians and the World Health Organization led to the formation of a five-year plan for palliative care development, begun in 1990 (Gómez-Batiste 1994a,b). The project covered several key components including assessment of needs; the introduction of specific services; measures to improve generic provision; education and training; models of finance; and the evaluation of results, incorporating public coverage, equity, quality, and satisfaction with care (Gómez-Batiste et al. 1992, 1997). We see here a powerful reaction against other models of palliative care development based on demands and emotive pleas and leading to an uneven patchwork of services. Instead the Catalan experiment has sought on the basis of calculated need to insert properly organized teams of palliative care providers within acute hospitals, long-stay facilities, and community services. Its ability to do so has been in part due to the fact that full responsibility for the funding and organization of *both* health and social services rests with the autonomous community of Catalonia itself (the Canary Islands is another example where palliative care development has been assisted in this way). In 1999 this situation applied however to only 7 of the 17 autonomous communities in Spain. Yet, as Gracia and Núñez Olarte (1999) point out, this is not the sole determinant of successful palliative care development. Madrid, for instance, has made considerable strides in palliative care without regional autonomy, whereas the Basque country has a less developed palliative care system, despite controlling its own health and social care destiny. Two demographic factors are also important when considering the close integration of palliative and mainstream healthcare in Spain. First, this is a society in which 80 per cent of deaths take place in hospital. Rejecting the idea of independent hospices, Spanish policy is to provide palliative care where the population in need is already to be found, hence the heavy orientation to hospital care. Second, Spain has the lowest birth rate in Europe; this together with increasing female participation in the labour market is bringing about a change in family life which calls into question the long-term viability of extensive palliative home care. Coupled with less developed generic community services, the implication again is that palliative care is most likely to be delivered in healthcare institutions of one sort or another. In this sense Spain can be contrasted, for example, with the United Kingdom and Belgium, where a reduction in hospital deaths is often seen as one of the longer term goals of palliative care and where wider health policy in recent years has been seeking to expand primary and community care (Van Orshoven 1996; Clark and Seymour 1999).

In Sweden we see some similar echoes. As early as 1979 a government report took a stand against the opening of hospices as the solution to improving care for the dying; and there was also scepticism among Swedish doctors about the emphasis on religious values to be found in the British hospice movement. Instead a multidisciplinary model of palliative care has been preferred, with the emphasis initially upon care at home, and consulting teams. By 1995 a government commission had allocated to palliative care the same level of priority as life-threatening acute illness, since when a rapid expansion of palliative care services has resulted (Valverius 1999).

The Italian case poses problems in terms of any assessment of the degree of integration with the formal healthcare system. Shaping any consideration here is the enormous north–south divide which exists in the provision of all healthcare in Italy. Inadequate resources, dilapidated facilities, individual orientations among staff which militate against teamwork, and a lack of any research evidence upon which to base a strategy for improvement, all serve to isolate the south of Italy from its more prosperous counterpart to the north. Such inadequacies within the formal healthcare system have created opportunities for private and charitable foundations to promote palliative care development. This has not led, however, to the proliferation of charitable and religious hospices. Rather the development of palliative care has taken place in close conjunction with oncology. It is a situation in which recent commentators in the late 1990s could observe that Italian palliative care development

> is completely dependent on local and individual initiatives and relies on the goodwill of hospital directors and financial support provided by the Floriana Foundation and the Italian League Against Cancer . . . national legislation is still lacking in this area and many health providers carry on with only local support.
>
> (Ferrario and Saita 1998: 254)

So Italy appears more as an example of relative separation from the formal healthcare system and where until recently governmental support at the policy level has been lacking.

In Belgium, Germany and the Netherlands we have examples of greater symbiosis between the healthcare system and other initiatives. It appears that Belgium has been a country in which some scope has existed for charismatic and innovative individuals to initiate new service developments which have, quite quickly, influenced the mainstream (Broeckaert 1999). Here royal decrees set out a comprehensive organizational framework for palliative care and formalized the principles for which the early founders sought recognition. Palliative home care is seen as the first and most important palliative care institution, and the object of policy is to add a palliative dimension to general healthcare rather than to supplant the mainstream in the final stages of life with palliative care delivered by specialist services. The vehicle for achieving this is the palliative care networks or cooperatives which have been established in every part of the country and whose purpose is to support specific palliative care initiatives (home care, hospitals, nursing homes, palliative care units) in each region. In short, palliative care organizations and government are seen to have entered into a fruitful cooperation which, underpinned by a robust legal and organizational framework, seeks to ensure the satisfactory delivery and funding of palliative care across the country, and the full integration of palliative care within the mainstream system.

Germany, however, seems yet to have resolved some inherent tensions (Nauck and Klaschik 1998). Here there appears to be substantial evidence of lay organizations and groups of various kinds concerned with the improvement of care for dying people and promoting some amelioration in societal attitudes to suffering, death and dying. There is little sense of a productive coalition between this group however and those elements of academic medicine concerned with palliative care development. The latter concentrated their efforts upon the development of hospital and university centres, an endeavour in which they were often frustrated. In consequence commentators in the 1990s could describe Germany as 'still only a developing country in the field of palliative care' (Klaschik and Nauck 1998: 203). Even more graphically a 1998 report from the German Cancer Society condemned the situation of palliative medicine in the country as 'miserable and extremely bad', lacking in academic leadership, without provision of adequate education for medical students, in a system exclusively oriented to curative medicine. The result is an uneven array of services and relatively low coverage of palliative care *vis-à-vis* the seven countries.

The Netherlands has some similar problems, albeit further complicated by debates surrounding the ethics and practice of euthanasia (Janssens and ten Have 1999). Here hospice provision has largely been led by organizations outside the formal healthcare system. One group of physicians, in nursing homes, claims a long-standing commitment to sound principles of terminal care. Yet mainstream provision of hospital and community palliative care services is not well developed and it was only in the late 1990s that significant interest in palliative care appeared in academic centres. Certainly it would seem that the independent, Christian hospice sector used publicity about euthanasia in Holland, promulgated abroad, to create a lobbying platform inside the Netherlands. This appears to have created a two-edged sword for Dutch hospices. It stiffened government resolve to support palliative care on the one hand. But no new money was found for the free-standing hospices, which were then required to become more closely integrated with mainstream systems.

The United Kingdom, often regarded as further advanced in its palliative care development than other countries, displays almost all of the tensions and dynamics found elsewhere (Clark and Seymour 1999). Here charismatic innovation and charitable development were the wellspring of the early hospice movement. Within a short time however, indeed as early as 1980, there was official concern about the unregulated proliferation of hospices. Palliative care services began to develop in the NHS, sometimes with pump-priming from charitable sources. Meanwhile public enthusiasm for the hospices continued to grow, while between 1989 and 1995 special government monies were made available to them, and NHS providers often felt the poor relations. The Conservative government's changes to the UK healthcare system introduced from the 1990s an internal market, with contractual links between purchasers and providers of care. Most evidence suggests that both NHS and charitable palliative care providers benefited under this system, though it was politically unpopular. After 1997 the New Labour government abolished the internal market, prioritized healthcare partnerships and placed greater emphasis upon fairness and quality of provision. The independent hospices are, once again, at a crossroads. Highly dependent upon mainstream funding and with increasingly symbiotic networks of service provision with the NHS, they must identify for themselves a future in which they can go on achieving the levels of charitable donations and voluntary support which are essential to their continuance (Clark and Seymour 2000).

Funding and reimbursement

Reimbursement of palliative care services across the seven countries is a common thread, with various manifestations. In Germany, rather like the United States, there has been considerable debate about whether health insurance companies will meet the costs of palliative care. The position of the insurance sector initially appeared to be one of refusal to pay for palliative care if the state is also contributing and also if palliative care is defined as anything more than simply the relief of cancer pain in the end stages of disease; however, after July 1998 a daily rate from the insurance companies was agreed for all hospices providing palliative care. Nevertheless, in such a situation, as Sabatowski et al. (1998) point out, palliative care services looked to financial subsidies from churches, private groups and charities, particularly the German Cancer Foundation. A similar situation prevails in Italy. This can be contrasted with Sweden, for example, where almost all palliative care is paid for by state funds, generated through the taxation system (Fürst et al. 1999).

In Belgium, as in the United Kingdom for a time, the government made available through the Busquin experiments of 1991–98, a specific funding stream for specified palliative care services, totalling BFr.412 million in 1997 (US$11.26 million) (Broeckaert 1999). This was then replaced by a broader framework which made provision for the funding of the totality of palliative care. Nevertheless, despite its well-developed organizational structure for palliative care, there are continuing funding problems to be resolved in Belgium. Similarly the Dutch Health Minister in 1996 dedicated modest monies to the further development of palliative care in existing institutions and the following year a major funding programme of some Dfl.35 million (US$18 million) was announced to promote regional academic centres for palliative care development. In a move akin to the incorporation of UK hospices into contracting arrangements, special funds of Dfl.2.35

million (US$1.2 million) were also set aside in the Netherlands to integrate the hospices into the formal healthcare system. Meanwhile in the United Kingdom, such 'integration' was achieved on the part of the independent charitable hospices at a funding level which still required them to raise two-thirds of revenue from charitable, that is non-governmental sources. Even within the mainstream of UK NHS palliative care services it remained usual for some form of charitable subvention to be in evidence.

Three key issues affect the funding of palliative care across the seven countries. First, there are structural divisions concerning where financial and planning responsibility may lie; for example between health authorit-ies, local authorities, districts, regions or central government. Second, there are questions about whether palliative care is seen as primarily a healthcare issue, to what extent it incorporates some aspects of social care, and the organizational manner in which these services are funded and delivered. Across Europe there is great diversity in these mechanisms, but on balance palliative care is seeking to define itself as a healthcare specialty, with fund-ing being derived accordingly. Third, there is the issue of balance between hospital-based and community services. Some countries still have only par-tially developed community care, but retain high investment in large hos-pitals. In others there has been disinvestment from the hospital sector and reinvestment in primary and community services. It follows that to attract and secure appropriate funding, palliative care may have to position itself in different ways according to prevailing norms. As we shall see in Chapter 3, this may in turn further stretch the definition of what constitutes palli-ative care. Despite a strong ideological compunction to define a core range of palliative care activities, it may be that the European palliative care community is already highly diverse in character, despite the 'shared goals' of a palliative care 'movement'.

Conclusion

The extent to which palliative care is developing as a specialty varies con-siderably between the seven countries studied here. Nor does this necessar-ily relate to the degree of palliative care service development or the relative affluence of each context. For example in Spain, where comprehensive palli-ative care planning is in evidence, the Spanish Association of Palliative Care (SECPAL) initiated discussions with the National Ministry of Health towards recognition as a new interspecialty medical discipline only in 1998. Whereas in one of Europe's most prosperous nations a commentator could observe in 1999: 'No university in Germany has a chair of palliative medicine, and this subject is not included in the curriculum' (Kreymann 1999: 785) – a matter addressed later that year, when the first Professor of Palliative Medicine was appointed, in Bonn. A chair of palliative medicine was also established in 1999 in Antwerp, Belgium and plans for a chair also existed in the Netherlands (where an earlier attempt had failed). The UK (with ten) and Sweden and Italy (each with one) had also established chairs in specialist academic departments of palliative medicine or palliative care in recent years. Palliative medicine has been a recognized specialty in the UK since 1987 and around 120 doctors are entered in a specialist training programme; more than double this number hold consultant positions in palliative medicine. Specialty status however is far from unproblematic. As Fordham et al. (1998) point out, there has 'been little discussion so far about how specialization in palliative medicine came about, whether it is the most appropriate way to address acknowledged deficiencies in care, or whether it can be sustained in the long term' (Fordham et al. 1998: 568). Moreover, the new specialty appears to be having particular difficulties in establishing an evidence-base for its activities (Higginson 1999).

Specialization per se has not been the driving force for palliative care service development in the seven European countries studied. Rather, debates about specialty status arise out of perceived gains in the development of services on the ground. As can be seen from the material presented here, palliative care services in most European countries have only reached an initial stage of integration with the formal healthcare system and its funding mechanisms. It is therefore a point of conjecture whether the process of specialization, not only for doctors, but also for nurses, social workers, counsellors and therapists of various kinds – all working within palliative care – can serve to consolidate these achievements and build a platform for future improvement.

Such an agenda will not however be under the sole control of those who work within palliative care. Political support at national and European level will be required and here palliative care will have to make its claims against many competing voices. The work of the World Health Organization has already done a great deal to draw attention to the issue (Stjernsward 1997), both in Europe and further afield. Declarations and consensus statements made at conferences (Barcelona Declaration on Palliative Care 1995; Poznań Declaration 1998) have also been published, together with exhortations from the editorial columns of professional journals (Roca 1995; Hoy 1996; Ventafridda 1998). The evidence presented here however suggests that the future security of palliative care will depend upon the extent to which it can embed itself within the wider structures of national and European health policy.

Note

This chapter is based on D. Clark et al. (2000) Common threads? Palliative care service developments in seven European countries, *Palliative Medicine*, 14(6): 470–90.

References

Albrecht, E. (1990) Palliative care in West Germany, *Palliative Medicine*, 4(4): 321–5.

Baar, F. (1999) Palliative care for the terminally ill in the Netherlands: the unique role of nursing homes, *European Journal of Palliative Care*, 6(5): 169–72.

Barcelona Declaration on Palliative Care (1995) *European Journal of Palliative Care*, 3(1): 15.

Beck-Friis, B. (1997) A Swedish model of home care, in D. Clark, J. Hockley and S. Ahmedzai (eds) *New Themes in Palliative Care*, pp. 142–7. Buckingham: Open University Press.

Beck-Friis, B. and Strang, P. (1993) The organization of hospital-based home care for terminally ill cancer patients: the Motala model, *Palliative Medicine*, 7(2): 93–100.

Broeckaert, B. (1999) Le cure palliative in Belgio, *Bioetica e Cultura*, 8: 45–54.

Bruning, H. and Klein Hesselink, J. (1985) Conclusies en suggesties van het projekt Antonius-IJsselmonde, in *Project Antonius IJsselmonde, Omgaan met sterven, deel IV. Symposium-verslagen*. Leiden: Zorn.

Clark, D. (1998) Originating a movement: Cicely Saunders and the development of St Christopher's Hospice, 1957–67, *Mortality*, 3(1): 43–63.

Clark, D. (1999) Cradled to the grave? Terminal care in the United Kingdom, 1948–67, *Mortality*, 4(3): 225–47.

Clark, D. and Seymour, J. (1999) *Reflections on Palliative Care: Sociological and Policy Perspectives*. Buckingham: Open University Press.

Clark, D. and Seymour, J. (2000) Changing times for the independent hospices, *British Journal of Health Care Management*, 6(2): 53–6.

De Conno, F. and Martini, C. (1997) Video communication and palliative care at home, *European Journal of Palliative Care*, 4(5): 174–7.

De Conno, F., Caraceni, A., Groff, L. et al. (1996) Effect of homecare on the place of death of advanced cancer patients, *European Journal of Cancer Care*, 32: 1142–7.

Ferrario, R. and Saita, L. (1998) Palliative care – 'the Italian reality', *International Journal of Palliative Nursing*, 4(5): 254.

Fordham, S., Dowrick, C. and May, C. (1998) Palliative medicine: is it really specialist territory?, *Journal of the Royal Society of Medicine*, 91: 568–72.

Fürst, C.J., Valverius, E. and Hjelmerus, L. (1999) Palliative care in Sweden, *European Journal of Palliative Care*, 6(5): 161–4.

Gómez-Batiste, X. (1994a) Catalonia's five year plan: basic principles, *European Journal of Palliative Care*, 1(1): 45–9.

Gómez-Batiste, X. (1994b) Catalonia's five year plan: preliminary results, *European Journal of Palliative Care*, 1(2): 98–101.

Gómez-Batiste, X., Borras, J.M., Fontanals, M.D., Stjernsward, J. and Trias, X. (1992) Palliative care in Catalonia 1990–95, *Palliative Medicine*, 6: 321–7.

Gómez-Batiste, X., Fontanals, M.D., Roca, J. et al. (1997) Rational planning and policy implementation in palliative care, in D. Clark, J. Hockley and S. Ahmedzai (eds) *New Themes in Palliative Care*. Buckingham: Open University Press.

Gracia, D. and Núñez Olarte, J.M. (1999) Le cure palliative in Spagna, *Bioetica e Cultura*, 16: 163–71.

Higginson, I. (1999) Evidence based palliative care (editorial), *British Medical Journal*, 319: 462–3.

Hockley, J. (1997) The evolution of the hospice approach, in D. Clark, J. Hockley and S. Ahmedzai (eds) *New Themes in Palliative Care*. Buckingham: Open University Press.

Hoy, A. (1996) Beyond our national boundaries – palliative care moves forward, *European Journal of Palliative Care*, 3(1): 4

Hunt, J. and Martin, M. (1997) Hospice in Spain, in C. Saunders and R. Kastenbaum (eds) *Hospice Care on the International Scene*, New York: Springer.

Janssens, R. (1999) *Report on Concepts of Palliative Care in the Netherlands*. Nijmegen: Pallium Project.

Janssens, R. and ten Have, H. (1999) Le cure palliative in Olanda, *Bioetica e Cultura*, 8: 23–32.

Keizer, B. (1999) Het regent in die hospices morfine, *Trouw* (Dutch newspaper), 22 April.

Klaschik, E. and Nauck, F. (1998) The German experience, *European Journal of Palliative Care*, 5(6): 203.

Kreymann, B. (1999) Dying patients need a good relationship with their doctor (letter), *British Medical Journal*, 319: 785.

Leontine, Zuster [Sister] (1992) *Menswaardig Sterven Palliatieve zorg . . . als een mantel om je heen* [Dignified Dying: Palliative care . . . as a cloak around you]. Leuven: Davidsfonds.

Nauck, F. and Klaschik, E. (1998) *The Role of Healthcare Policy in the Development and Organization of Palliative Medicine*. Nijmegen: Pallium Project.

Poznań Declaration (1998) *European Journal of Palliative Care*, 6(2): 61–5.

Roca, J. (1995) Towards Barcelona 95, *European Journal of Palliative Care*, 2(2): 50.

Sabatowski, R., Radbruch, L., Loick, G., Grond, S. and Petzke, F. (1998) Palliative care in Germany – 14 years on, *European Journal of Palliative Care*, 5(2): 52–5.

Stjernsward, J. (1997) The WHO cancer pain and palliative care programme, in D. Clark, J. Hockley and S. Ahmedzai (eds) *New Themes in Palliative Care*. Buckingham: Open University Press.

Valverius, E. (1999) Le cure palliative in Svezia, *Bioetica e Cultura*, 8: 33–44.

Van Orshoven, A. (1996) Inhoud en organisatie van de palliatieve hulp, in A. van Orshoven and J. Menten (eds) *Palliatieve zorg, stervensbegeleiding, rouwbegeleiding: Handboek voor deskundige hulpverlening in de thuiszorg en in het ziekenhuis*. Leuven: Acco.

Ventafridda, V. (1998) Ten years on, *European Journal of Palliative Care*, 5(5): 140.

Watson, R. (1999) Council of Europe urges better palliative care, *British Medical Journal*, 319: 146.

Wouters, B. (1998) Palliative care in Belgium, *European Journal of Palliative Care*, 5(6): 201–2.

Zylicz, Z. (1993) Hospice in Holland: the story behind the blank spot, *American Journal of Hospice and Palliative Care*, 4: 30–4.

3 Conceptual tensions in European palliative care

DAVID CLARK, HENK TEN HAVE
AND RIEN JANSSENS

In this chapter we move from the analysis of the provision of palliative care in Europe to some of the concepts which underpin it. We shall argue that the 'metanarrative' of palliative care across Europe consists of four specific goals: achievement of best quality of life for patients and families; relief of suffering; promotion of 'good death'; prevention of euthanasia. These appear to be the overarching goals, held in common across many settings. Within this metanarrative, however, the explicitness of each goal can be seen to vary, the goals do not appear to be given equal priority within the palliative care community and, when subject to critical analysis, they can appear a weak platform on which to build a new healthcare specialty. It will become clear also that the metanarrative of palliative care has been constructed through certain 'secondary purposes': by this we mean the day-to-day objectives which can preoccupy palliative care service providers as they go about their business, and which may at times require considerable attention. For example, it has been claimed (Fordham et al. 1998) that as an emerging field of healthcare specialization, palliative care relies on access to specific resources: a disease or a group of clinical problems upon which to focus; 'willing' patients; potentially innovative technologies of yet unproven worth; third party payments; a knowledge and/or evidence base; facilities in which to practise; a renewable labour force. While the four goals of palliative care make up its metanarrative, for those working in the field it is these 'secondary purposes' which consume much of the energy of daily life. To what extent is this a feature of what has been seen in Weberian terms as the 'routinization' or 'bureaucratization' of palliative care (Clark and Seymour 1999) or does it mask a real sense of division about the nature of the goals? Disagreement about the metanarrative should not be seen as necessarily problematic. Within the reflexive processes of late modernity it is to be expected that individuals, professions, organizations and social movements of all kinds will give regular attention to the renewal of their 'goals': indeed this becomes central to concepts of identity in late modern culture. At the organizational level however, the revision of goals cannot be allowed to destabilize daily activity and so we must ask whether the existence of a cohesive metanarrative is essential to the future well-being of palliative care and those it seeks to serve.

The goals of palliative care

David Barnard et al. (2000: 1) assert that 'the goals of palliative care are easy to state'. The claim seems unwarranted. Palliative care, as an emerging healthcare specialty, appears beset with problems of definition, boundaries and purpose. Much of this chapter will concentrate on a literature which demonstrates this. In print, in conferences and in their daily clinical work 'palliateurs' seem unclear, unsure and in difficulty when defining precisely what it is they do and how it differs from other forms of healthcare. A striking example of this has been the well-documented shift in terminology, from 'terminal care' to 'hospice care' to 'palliative care' and now, in some quarters to 'supportive care' (Clark and Seymour 1999).

In the year the specialty of palliative medicine was formally recognized in the United Kingdom, Cicely Saunders asked 'What's in a name?' and offered a careful analysis of several terms found within the palliative care lexicon: palliation, continuing care, support, hospice (Saunders 1987). In 1993 Derek Doyle considered several problems associated with the term palliative medicine and the accompanying definition which had been formulated through the process of obtaining specialty recognition. Part of the difficulty lay in a field which 'relates to a stage of a patient's condition, rather than its pathology' (Doyle 1993: 253); there was also the apparent euphemistic avoidance of death implied by the move away from the use of 'terminal care'; while another issue stemmed from the fact that many oncologists already saw themselves doing this work and questioned the need for separate specialty status. A major concern however was between 'palliative medicine and the palliative *approach*' (Doyle 1993: 254), the latter should be the responsibility of the total healthcare system, whereas the former constitutes a specialist activity. Girling et al. (1994) make a similar point:

> A potential source of confusion has arisen by the adoption of the terms 'palliative care' and 'palliative medicine' for the generic philosophy of this type of care and for the medical specialty which supports it, respectively.
>
> (Girling et al. 1994: 80)

It is interesting that in both cases there is room in the specialty only for the profession of medicine and not for those other members of the multidisciplinary team in which the rhetoric of palliative care takes such pride.

By the mid-1990s the confusion seemed unresolved, as one editorial writer and a Professor of Palliative Medicine could state:

> I am constantly reminded when I give lectures to doctors, nurses or other professionals and discuss my work with lay members of the public, that there is still much confusion, or at least uncertainty, about what palliative care is and does. The usual questions posed are: what does it do, who does it treat, when is it used and where is it done?
>
> (Ahmedzai 1996: 1)

For Ahmedzai, the trajectory from diagnosis to death should be seen more as an analogue than a digital progression, accordingly there is no discernible point of transition which marks the point of interface between curative, palliative and terminal care. Thus a more appropriate model is one that overarches this trajectory, unified by quality of life goals, rather than quantity of life goals. This model also creates conceptual problems, however, for the only definition of palliative care which it allows is *that which is delivered by a specialist in palliative care*; in other words it is difficult to demarcate specialist palliative care, delivered across the entire disease trajectory, from other palliative care delivered by any one of a range of specialists whenever their interventions are not focused on treatment of the primary disease. We are seeing here some of the problems in taking an essentialist view of palliative care. When we seek to do this, it becomes extremely difficult to define core goals and activities.

Randall and Downie (1999) have attempted to shed some light on these and related issues in their distinction between the 'intrinsic aim' of palliative care (which they define as 'the medical good') and the 'extrinsic aim' ('the psychological good'). Yet this seems a crude formulation which takes little account of the *embodied* aspects of suffering, so ably captured in ethnographic studies of palliative care (for example, Lawton 2000). Equally, it is at odds with the multiplex and dynamic viewpoint envisaged in Cicely Saunders' important concept of 'total pain' (Clark 1999). It seems unhelpful to follow Randall and Downie (1999: 18) in regarding the patient's 'primary problems' as 'medical problems' and in so doing to accept a rather rigid body–mind dualism in both the apprehension and relief of patients' problems.

In this chapter, rather than concentrate on the definition of palliative care, we proceed from the position that it is an activity which has four distinct goals. We examine each of these goals in turn and consider their implications for ethical and conceptual clarity.

Achieving the best quality of life for patients and families

At first sight this seems an unproblematic goal for palliative care. After all, it is enshrined in the World Health Organization definition of 1990 which states that 'The goal of palliative care is achievement of the best quality of life for patients and their families' (WHO 1990: 11). Also, as we shall see in Chapter 4, this definition is adhered to by almost seven out of ten palliative care practitioners across Europe. Among the same group there is also universal agreement (97 per cent) that quality of life is an important moral notion in palliative care. Indeed, promotion of quality of life can be found in the mission statements of countless European palliative care services. For example, following an extensive review in one country Sandman (2001) is able to state: 'The central, most dominating goal in the recent Swedish literature on palliative care is quality of life' (Sandman 2001: 73). It is also a commonly declared outcome measure for palliative interventions in many countries (Massaro and McMillan 2000). On this basis we might regard it as an *absolutely explicit* goal of palliative care.

Nevertheless, the adoption of 'quality of life' as a goal of palliative care conceals many problems. Clinch et al. (1998) review several of these, including competing definitions, cultural variation, instrument development and applications in research, use in clinical settings and the interpretation of evidence. Proponents seem reluctant to define what quality of life is at the end of life and there is a growing tendency to circumvent this problem by saying nothing or to allow 'quality of life' to be what a person defines it to be. In such ways, teleological thinking finds a comfortable niche in the world of palliative care. Although Sandman (2001) notes that Swedish writers on quality of life in palliative care appear to be unanimous in accepting it as a goal of care, they vary in their degree of ambition about what might be achieved. Thus for some it is making life *endurable*, for others it is something *higher than just survival*, or it may be the achievement of an *ordinary* life, or *quality in line with the patient's own condition* (Sandman 2001). Broeckaert and Schotsmans (2001) make similar points about Belgium, where since the healthcare system began to give serious attention to palliative care in the early 1990s, various usages of quality of life have appeared in official definitions. Thus the focus might be on *preservation of a certain quality of life* or, more strongly, it might relate to *guaranteeing an optimal quality of life*. We might conclude that the level of ambition surrounding this particular goal of palliative care has been increasing in recent years, yet there has been no commensurate increase in conceptual clarity on the subject.

Nor is it easy to see quality of life as a medical goal, since so many other factors affect it: wealth and poverty, gender, age, social class, locality. We might argue that quality of life is more about *social* capital than access to a particular medical service, even at the end of life. To some extent even *getting* palliative care is a product of the social capital which produces quality of life. Yet at the same time the assessment of quality of life has become something of an industry and even devotees have expressed concerns about it. As Nord et al. (2001) put it, 'the use of the term has gone too far', so much so that there is a sense in which quality of life research has become bogged down in narrowly technical debates and the competing claims of individual measures. Conceptually, few of these succeed in getting beyond Calman's (1984) succinctly stated 'gap' theory: quality of life is in inverse ratio to the gap between an individual's expectations and the perceived reality. Beyond this lies much psychometric obfuscation and little evidence of a pay-off in clinical practice. 'Ideally it should be discarded', Randall and Downie (1999: 301) say of the term.

Although the achievement of good quality of life may be retained as a goal for palliative care, it is one which will continue to lack precision. Nor is it going to be exclusive to the specialty: many in cognate areas of care such as geriatrics, rehabilitation or psychiatry can make a similar goal for their own interventions. The meaning of 'quality of life' will vary according to setting and the impact of palliative care on quality of life will remain difficult to ascribe. In the context of end-of-life care, when death is near, there is an acknowledgement too that measurable quality of life will in any event be on a downward trajectory; is it the role of palliative care to try to reverse this trajectory, or to slow-down the movement along it? Quality of life appears likely to obsolesce as a salient concept. It seems too tied up with a particular social and economic era, too much a part of the machinery of western capitalist ideology, too loaded with overtones of consumption and consumerism. Whatever it might mean, few will challenge the notion of 'improving', 'maximizing' or 'maintaining' good quality of life for dying people. Why this should be the overriding aim of any one field of healthcare specialization, however, seems less clear.

The relief of suffering

To attend to *suffering* rather than quality of life may therefore seem a more realistic goal for palliative care. Moreover, the language of suffering has formed part of the palliative care worldview from the early days (Saunders 1961). Palliative care can rightly claim an excellent record in appreciating the complexities and the subtleties of human suffering at the end of life. Although Cicely Saunders adopted the term 'total pain' to refer to the physical, emotional, spiritual and social distress of patients and those close to them, it is clear that she was using a familiar medical concept in order to get at something more multifaceted in character. Such an approach allowed the interest in 'holistic' care to flourish in palliative care circles, focused around two themes: the patient seen as a 'whole' person in social context and the deployment of all the skills of the multidisciplinary team in providing care. These are ideas which seem at least partly compatible with the wider goals of medicine.

Despite this, the nature of suffering has become a contested territory in which competing definitions and emphases are at work. Seeking to hold onto a wider sense of purpose, Michael Kearney, a palliative medicine consultant working in Ireland, has observed:

> if we sell out completely to the literalism of the medical model that such suffering is *only* a problem, we will be in danger of following a pattern which could significantly limit our scope for development and lead to our becoming 'symptomatologists', within just another specialty.
>
> (Kearney 1992: 41)

Certainly there is a tendency, as palliative care develops, for its medical attention to focus on pain and symptom management as a subset of problems within the relief of suffering. It is in this biomedical area too that some of the most measurable successes of palliative care are to be found, in the use of pain-relieving technologies and in the inventive use of antidepressants, antibiotics and anxiolitics. A paper by Cherny et al. (1994) seeks to encompass both arguments by proposing a clinically relevant taxonomy of suffering encompassing physical symptoms, psychological symptoms, existential concerns, empathic suffering with others, and distress related to healthcare services. Ahmedzai (1994) however has not only criticized the taxonomy for its failure to recognize the positive and creative elements of suffering and its tendency 'to reinforce the notion of suffering as *pathology*' (1994: 220, original emphasis), but also cautioned that 'Ultimately, suffering from losses, lack of love, existential doubts as well as from poverty and cruelty are not medical issues, and the response to them is not necessarily the responsibility of any healthcare discipline' (Ahmedzai 1997: 236). Interestingly, social workers, counsellors, volunteers and pastoral care workers who in their professional work do indeed respond to many such privations, may not set quite so narrowly the limits of the 'healthcare discipline' of which they are a part. Elsewhere Ahmedzai himself takes a more overtly biomedical line: 'As a physician working in palliative care, I feel justified in declaring that symptom analysis and management lies at the heart of the subject' (Ahmedzai 1997: 236). For such a new field, in which there are so few qualified specialists, palliative medicine appears remarkably unclear on its view of a central focus of its interventions: human suffering.

The good death

In Chapter 6 we have ample evidence that attempting to achieve the 'good death' is a shaky edifice upon which to build a goal of palliative care. Much of the problem here revolves around the question of cultural and moral relativism. How, in what ways, and for whom is any death 'good'? Macnamara (2001) argues that the 'good death' is an idealized concept which was central to modern hospice and palliative care philosophy in the first 30 years of their development. Its key elements have been open communication and acceptance of dying. She also recognizes that this is changing, that some patients will resist the imposition of a 'hospice ritual' surrounding their death, that sometimes 'bad deaths' may occur, even in hospices, and that an increasing emphasis on consumerism and patient choice make the concept less workable. We are beginning to get some evidence in the European context of what may constitute cultural variation in the good death. In Spain it is bound up in the *agonía*, the gradual slipping away of the senses when life is extinguishing gradually and somnolence is acceptable, even preferable (Núñez Olarte and Gracia 2001). In the northern countries it may be much more associated with an 'open awareness context', with the resolution of previously unfinished psychological 'business', and with some attention to spiritual or existential concerns. In some southern European countries a strong tradition of medical paternalism may accompany perceptions of the good death, whereas elsewhere the principle of 'autonomy' is given more cultural weight, at least in theory (Wilkinson 1999).

We might argue that the shift in orientation in western Europe from 'terminal' to 'palliative care' has brought about a diminished emphasis on the 'good death'. This is precisely the point made by Bronwen Biswas when she argued:

> Palliative care shifts the focus of attention away from death and there is a real danger that by talking about and focusing upon palliation, people may stop talking about and confronting the fact that the individual is going to die.
>
> (Biswas 1993: 135)

Within the diversifying field of palliative care, achieving the 'good death' has become a much less explicit goal. Some early founders may cling to it and resist what they perceive to be a denial of death through the adoption of a broader view of the specialty. Others may see the 'management' of the final days and hours of life as almost a sub-specialty of palliative care, something which is by implication a smaller task than the provision of good pain and symptom management or of 'supportive care' for a much longer period throughout the disease trajectory. It is no coincidence that it is nurses who tend to the former view and doctors to the latter.

We find that debates about the 'good death' figure little in the discourse of pain and symptom management. Two factors are reducing its saliency. First, the trend towards the integration or 'mainstreaming' of palliative care into the central functions of the healthcare system leads to a greater concentration on the problems of the living than of the dying. Second, as the boundaries of palliative care are moved 'upstream', to earlier stages in the disease process, and as they are extended to include chronic, life-limiting conditions, so the rhetoric of 'quality of life' tends to predominate over 'good death'. For example a paper based on an Italian study of quality of life (QoL) and outcomes in palliative care can make the following statement:

> Dying during the study period is a strong indicator of patients who entered the palliative care intervention in very poor health conditions. We expected and observed a worst QoL outcome for patients like these.
>
> (Paci et al. 2001: 186)

The authors could be forgiven for implying that the patients themselves had somehow got things wrong.

The notion of the 'good death' is increasingly abandoned as an orienting principle by the practitioners of modern palliative medicine. Content to discuss the sedation of patients with refractory symptoms, they show less willingness to engage with prescriptive arguments about the manner of a good ending to life. Some have seen in this evidence of the 'medicalization' of death (Field 1994). They are only partially correct. What we are seeing is the medicalization of *palliative care*, a specialty which has already opened up a space somewhere between the hope of cure and the acceptance of death. In doing so it makes appeals to what 'patients' want in a modern culture where they may not fear death but may well fear the process of dying. Who is writing about the 'good death' today? Not the 'palliateurs', but sociologists, anthropologists, historians and ethicists.

The prevention of euthanasia

In the United Kingdom the 'euthanasia movement' and the 'hospice move-ment' have an absolutely oppositional history. Indeed the second ever pub-lication from the pen of Cicely Saunders opposed euthanasia on both moral and practical grounds (Saunders 1959). Thirty-five years later, the first issue of the *European Journal of Palliative Care* contained an official statement on euthanasia from the European Association of Palliative Care. In this the authors concluded: 'We should maintain an uncompromising stand against a law that would permit the administration of death' (Roy and Rapin 1994: 59). The next two issues of the journal contained articles by Fiona Randall summarizing the recently concluded deliberations of the UK House of Lords Select Committee on Euthanasia and in particular the submission to the committee of evidence from the UK's National Council for Hospice and Specialist Palliative Care Services. The Council's evidence provides a clear illustration of the lack of dialogue between those supporting euthanasia and those supporting palliative care:

> The Council believes that the issue of active voluntary euthanasia with all the complex legal and ethical problems it presents is entirely separate from the provision of good palliative care . . . Council believes there is no place for the direct killing of patients at their own request.
>
> (quoted in Randall 1994: 103)

This lack of dialogue was highlighted in two subsequent articles by Giorgio Di Mola (1994a,b). In the first he drew attention to studies revealing variation in health professionals' attitudes to euthanasia. In the second he criticized the official statement of David Roy and Charles-Henri Rapin (1994) as 'an ideological crusade against the regulation of euthanasia' (Di Mola 1994b: 192).

There seems to be a good deal of evidence to support Di Mola's assertion, though in 2001 the European Association of Palliative Care did set up a task force to review its statement on euthanasia and its results are awaited. In Sweden, Sandman (2001) suggests that palliative care is seen as an alternative to euthanasia and even as something mutually exclusive to it. In Belgium and the Netherlands, the two countries within the *Pallium* project which have done most to legalize euthanasia, debates have become particularly heated, with fiery exchanges taking place in the press between the various proponents. In the Netherlands, Janssens and ten Have (2001) report that those who oppose euthanasia and support the development of palliative care have been criticized for an untenable and even hypocritical viewpoint. It is said that such a position diminishes the role which euthanasia-tolerant practitioners are already playing in the delivery of palliative care; it is also claimed that the heavy use of morphine in hospices is evidence that palliative care practices come close to the administration of euthanasia itself. In Belgium one of the influential pioneers of palliative care, Sister Leontine, produced a book in 1995 with the title *Why Euthanasia Still?* Her argument was clear: the demand for euthanasia will be abated by the provision of comprehensive palliative care. Yet some prominent supporters of palliative care in that country have also given public recognition to the argument for euthanasia, in so doing bringing down the opprobrium of those such as Sister Leontine, who argue that all official international declarations state that palliative care should neither lengthen nor shorten life (Broeckaert and Schotsmans 2001). Belgium may yet prove an important test case as it seeks to legislate in favour of euthanasia, for in that country palliative care has become well developed. Overall the situation seems to require some *rapprochement* in acknowledgement that neither palliative care nor euthanasia alone are capable of resolving all of the end-of-life problems which arise in the face of intractable suffering. However, if such dialogue *does* develop, then in turn it will pose problems for those who have seen one of the goals of palliative care as the prevention of euthanasia.

In Spain, the Catholic tradition rejects active euthanasia, but accepts the widespread use of pain relief to the point of sedation, even in cases where it may speed up death. Thus the Thomistic principle of 'double effect', broadly developed in the Salamanca School of the sixteenth century, is commonly used by physicians to support the use of analgesics and sedatives. In France the 'lytic cocktail' (containing a mixture of opiates, sedative and anti-emetic) has been widely used (and abused) as part of an acceptance between public and professionals that sedation for pain relief may accelerate dying (Meunier-Cartal et al. 1995). In the United Kingdom, Cicely Saunders' (1958) early writings did much to promote the use of the Brompton mixture, though the studies of Twycross went on to demonstrate that oral morphine alone had many advantages (see Twycross 1979). Modern palliative medicine seems to have usurped the role of such 'cocktails', which are now viewed as unsophisticated approaches to pain management; but it may simply have ushered in a new set of dilemmas based on the use of other combinations of drugs. As Núñez Olarte and Gracia (2001: 48) observe: 'the ethical dilemma is not "euthanasia – yes or no" but "sedation – when and how"'. At the same time they acknowledge that one of the reasons Spanish politicians and government at both national and regional level have supported palliative care is precisely to avoid the 'politically difficult and disturbing debate about active euthanasia' (2001: 49).

Hermsen and ten Have (2001) have shown that when articles appear on ethical issues within the palliative care literature, the most common topic of discussion is euthanasia. This issue has often been addressed as a demarcation instrument; it is easier to explain what palliative care involves by referring to what it is not. The problem with such a 'negative' approach generally is twofold. First, it is unclear how the concept of euthanasia is used (for sometimes it includes terminal sedation, withholding life-sustaining treatment, or advanced pain medication). This lack of conceptual clarity is also shown in the empirical survey conducted as part of the *Pallium* project (see Chapter 4, this volume). Second, the antagonism towards euthanasia may be complete or partial. Palliative care can be considered to take away all requests for euthanasia, so that palliation and euthanasia are synchronic activities in end-of-life care that are mutually incompatible. This is the view of many first-generation founders within the palliative care movement. However, an alternative argument is that even the best palliative care may not eliminate all euthanasia requests, though it may significantly reduce the number of these requests. Palliative care and euthanasia, seen in this way, are therefore diachronic activities; euthanasia should be considered as a last resort only when the full potential of palliative care has been explored.

It is hard not to see the prevention of euthanasia as at least an implicit goal of palliative care, and for some an explicit one. It remains to be seen how this can be maintained in the face of changes in public and professional attitudes and in legislation. We sense that the time is right for a new dialogue drawing together those who support the work of palliative care, but who also acknowledge the case for a more tolerant view of euthanasia.

Achievable goals and secondary purposes

Examining the goals of palliative care in this way, it appears that each can be found conceptually and practically wanting. The proponents of palliative care across Europe appear to lack internal unity and cohesion about the central purposes of their work. At the same time we can see that the goals vary in their degree of explicitness and also that they are susceptible to influence by forces which lie outside of the field of palliative care itself. This does not mean of course that in their public representations European palliative care practitioners appear disunited. On the contrary, the reforming purpose of palliative care has called for high levels of external cohesion in the face of wider indifference or even outright hostility. Paradoxically, this has been achieved by uniting around the very goals of palliative care described here: quality of life; the relief of suffering; the good death; opposition to euthanasia. But outward and inward unity are not the same thing. The first may be vital to achieving recognition and acquiring resources; the second may be difficult to sustain through the process of maturation in a new healthcare specialty. Either way they make for discomfort. In such a climate it may be tempting for 'palliateurs' in their daily work to allow these contradictions within the central goals to be eclipsed by other, more middle-range, concerns. We refer to these as the 'secondary purposes' of palliative care.

Secondary purposes are made up of phenomena which relate to the consolidation of palliative care within the mainstream. They include attention to funding streams within general healthcare budgets; the expansion of palliative care service delivery; the development of programmes of education and accreditation; the fostering of professional identities through conferences, journals and other publications; the creation of a so-called 'evidence base' to support the activity; and the work of national and international associations of various kinds. Within the internally referential system of a specialist field like palliative care, it is possible to give greater priority to these than to the primary goals. Clark and Seymour (1999) show how several commentators have adopted a Weberian perspective to explain this. Those who speak of the 'bureaucratization' or 'routinization' of palliative care suggest that an unintended consequence has taken place. Today's practitioners have become diverted from the goals of the founders. They have lost some of the early convictions and become caught up in bureaucratic battles and professional rivalries. As a result, it is argued, the original goals and concepts are subject to unwelcome modification. Such a viewpoint displays two weaknesses. First, it displays a poor understanding of the history of modern palliative care, in which it is possible to see that several of the current secondary purposes were eagerly anticipated by the founders who looked to them as evidence of progress and success. Second, it masks the subtle and nuanced differences of interpretation which surround key goals and concepts in palliative care.

According to Alasdair MacIntyre (1984) concepts derive their meaning from practices, and these involve a teleological structure. They are aimed at the realization of a goal that is internal to the practice. Institutions, by contrast, are instrumental in character and are aimed at the realization of external goals, such as money and status; institutions sustain and are the bearers of practices. Yet practices are exclusively aimed at goals internal to themselves. If we adopt this teleological line of thinking, it would follow that if there were to be consensus on the internal goal of the practice of palliative care, then we would be able to speak of one concept of palliative care. If however there is disagreement on the internal goals, then we would have to speak of the existence of differing *concepts* of palliative care. In this case palliative care is not one coherent practice but rather a set of overlapping, different practices. The evolution of palliative care across Europe seems to suggest that palliative care is developing within diverging practices: in hospices, hospital units, home care services and consultation teams (ten Have and Janssens 2001). These practices are characterized by 'family resemblance' rather than one basic unifying concept. We are suggesting here that there is no unanimity on the internal goals. Indeed, one reading of this chapter might suggest that the external goals of palliative care (the 'secondary purposes') are the subject of greater consensus, while the internal goal has become blurred. Critics of palliative medicine have observed that although 'specialists in palliative medicine frequently restate the philosophy of their field, they cannot be shown to base their practice on it' (Fordham et al. 1998: 569). This chapter provides some evidence of the problems which lie within the philosophy.

References

Ahmedzai, S. (1994) Suffering and the art of compassion and hope (editorial), *Progress in Palliative Care*, 2(6): 217–21.

Ahmedzai, S. (1996) Making a success out of life's failures (editorial), *Progress in Palliative Care*, 4(1): 1–3.

Ahmedzai, S. (1997) Five years, five threads (editorial), *Progress in Palliative Care*, 5(6): 235–7.

Barnard, D., Towers, A., Boston, P. and Lambrinidou, Y. (2000) *Crossing Over: Narratives of Palliative Care*. Oxford: Oxford University Press.

Biswas, B. (1993) The medicalization of dying: a nurse's view, in D. Clark (ed.) *The Future for Palliative Care*. Buckingham: Open University Press.

Broeckaert, B. and Schotsmans, P. (2001) Palliative care in Belgium, in H. ten Have and R. Janssens (eds) *Palliative Care in Europe: Concepts and Policies*. Amsterdam: IOS Press.

Calman, K.C. (1984) Quality of life in cancer patients – a hypothesis, *Journal of Medical Ethics*, 10: 124–7.

Cherny, N.I., Coyle, N. and Foley, K.M. (1994) Suffering in the advanced cancer patient: a definition and taxonomy, *Journal of Palliative Care*, 10(2): 57–70.

Clark, D. (1999) 'Total pain', disciplinary power and the body in the work of Cicely Saunders, 1958–67, *Social Science and Medicine*, 49(6): 727–36.

Clark, D. and Seymour, J. (1999) *Reflections on Palliative Care*. Buckingham: Open University Press.

Clinch, J.J., Dudgeon, D. and Schipper, H. (1998) Quality of life assessment in palliative care, in D. Doyle, G.W.C. Hanks and N. MacDonald (eds) *Oxford Textbook of Palliative Medicine*, 2nd edn. Oxford: Oxford University Press.

Di Mola, G. (1994a) Attitudes of healthcare professionals towards euthanasia, *European Journal of Palliative Care*, 1(3): 140–4.

Di Mola, G. (1994b) Euthanasia: another view, *European Journal of Palliative Care*, 1(4): 192–3.

Doyle, D. (1993) Palliative medicine – a time for definition?, *Palliative Medicine*, 7: 253–5.

Field, D. (1994) Palliative medicine and the medicalization of death, *European Journal of Cancer Care*, 3(2): 58–62.

Fordham, S., Dowrick, C. and May, C. (1998) Palliative medicine: is it really specialist territory?, *Journal of the Royal Society of Medicine*, 91 (November): 568–71.

Girling, D.J., Hopwood, P. and Ahmedzai, S. (1994) Assessing quality of life in palliative oncology, *Progress in Palliative Care*, 2(3): 80–6.

Hermsen, M. and ten Have, H. (2001) Moral problems in palliative care journals, *Palliative Medicine*, 15(5): 425–31.

Janssens, M.J.P.A. and ten Have, H.A.M.J. (2001) Palliative care in the Netherlands, in H. ten Have and R. Janssens (eds) *Palliative Care in Europe: Concepts and Policies*. Amsterdam: IOS Press.

Kearney, M. (1992) Palliative medicine – just another specialty?, *Palliative Medicine*, 6: 39–46.

Lawton, J. (2000) *The Dying Process*. London: Routledge.

MacIntyre, A. (1984) *After Virtue: A Study in Moral Theory*. Notre Dame, IN: University of Notre Dame Press.

Macnamara, B. (2001) *Fragile Lives*. Buckingham: Open University Press.

Massaro, T. and McMillan, S.C. (2000) Instruments for assessing quality of life in palliative care settings, *International Journal of Palliative Nursing*, 6(9): 429–33.

Meunier-Cartal, J., Souberbielle, J.C. and Boureau, F. (1995) Morphine and the 'lytic cocktail' for terminally ill patients in a French general hospital: evidence for an inverse relationship, *Journal of Pain and Symptom Management*, 10: 267–73.

Nord, E., Arnesen, T., Menzel, P. and Pinto, J-L. (2001) Towards a more restricted use of the term 'quality of life', *Quality of Life Newsletter*, 26: 3–4.

Núñez Olarte, J.M. and Gracia, D. (2001) Cultural issues and ethical dilemmas in palliative and end-of-life care in Spain, *Cancer Control*, 8(1): 46–54.

Paci, E., Miccinesi, G., Toscani, F. et al. (2001) Quality of life assessment and outcome of palliative care, *Journal of Pain and Symptom Management*, 21(3): 179–88.

Randall, F. (1994) Decisions on life and death, *European Journal of Palliative Care*, 1(2): 102–3.

Randall, F. and Downie, R.S. (1999) *Palliative Care Ethics: A Companion for All Specialties*, 2nd edn. Oxford: Oxford University Press.

Roy, D. and Rapin, C. (1994) Regarding euthanasia, *European Journal of Palliative Care*, 1(1): 57–9.

Sandman, L. (2001) Palliative care in Sweden, in H. ten Have and R. Janssens (eds) *Palliative Care in Europe: Concepts and Policies*. Amsterdam: IOS Press.

Saunders, C. (1958) Dying of cancer, *St Thomas's Hospital Gazette*, April: 37–47.

Saunders, C. (1959) Care of the dying 1: the problem of euthanasia, *Nursing Times*, 9 October: 960–1.

Saunders, C. (1961) *Why does God Allow Suffering?* London: Church Union.

Saunders, C. (1987) What's in a name?, *Palliative Medicine*, 1: 57–61.

Ten Have, H.A.M.J. and Janssens, M.J.P.A. (eds) (2001) *Palliative Care in Europe: Concepts and Policies*. Amsterdam: IOS Press.

Twycross, R. (1979) The Brompton Cocktail, in J.J. Bonica and V. Ventafridda (eds) *Advances in Pain Research and Therapy*, Vol. 2. New York: Raven.

Wilkinson, S. (1999) Palliative care in Europe: ethics and communication (editorial), *International Journal of Palliative Nursing*, 5(4): 160.

World Health Organization (1990) *Cancer Pain Relief and Palliative Care*. Geneva: WHO.

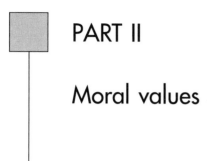

PART II

Moral values

Introduction to Part II

Having set out our analysis of models and concepts of palliative care in Part I of this book, we now turn in Part II to a consideration of some underlying moral values. The four chapters included here represent two distinct approaches to this problem, making use of both empirical data (from surveys and case presentations) and also deploying ethical reflection and argumentation. In this way we have sought to capture the views of palliative care workers in several European countries, to describe specific cases occurring in particular settings and to offer a number of theoretical perspectives, particularly from European philosophy, anthropology and sociology. This section of the book illustrates what may be termed the 'empirical turn' in bioethics – a concern to identify research evidence in support of argumentation. It also offers some alternative perspectives to the view of bioethics which prevails in the Anglo-American tradition and which is summed up in the notion that a given number of 'principles' can be identified as central to all problems of healthcare ethics.

In Chapter 4, which is authored by all the members of the *Pallium* project core group, we report on a major survey of European palliative care workers, conducted in 1999. Responses from almost 800 practitioners in 32 countries represent a substantial information base on how palliative care is viewed by those working within it. We highlight the varying terms which practitioners use to describe their work, the definitions they employ, the extent to which palliative care is thought to be integrated with the mainstream, or is becoming medicalized and bureaucratized. The survey reveals a continued opposition to euthanasia, but surprisingly, some endorsement of the intentional shortening of life within palliative care. It is also clear from the survey that notions such as quality of life, human dignity, the acceptance of human mortality and 'total care' are universally endorsed within palliative care, but far less evidence was found for the centrality of religious values, usually regarded as a powerful motivation to first-generation palliative care founders.

It is precisely this ethical transition which is at the heart of Chapter 5, in which Diego Gracia takes the work of Max Weber as his starting point in exploring the shift from 'conviction' to 'responsibility' ethics in palliative care. In doing this he draws on an extensive body of feminist literature concerned with the history of nursing and with the ethics of care. Kantian ethics are the paradigm for an ethics which gives priority to principles and intentions over facts, reality and consequences. By contrast a moral life is also one which is attentive to consequences. 'Responsibility ethics' seeks to take care not only of consequences, but also of principles and convictions. Bioethics, from its beginnings, is an ethics of responsibility, whereas the dominant ethics within nursing history has been one of conviction. Gracia shows how a tendency to responsibility ethics has developed in the work of Cicely Saunders over time and how responsibility ethics has come to the fore in major palliative care texts.

In Chapter 6, Wim Dekkers, Lars Sandman and Pat Webb combine perspectives from medicine, philosophy and nursing and from the Netherlands, Sweden and the United Kingdom, to return in detail to the moral notions underpinning ideas about the 'good death'. We saw in Chapter 3 that 'good death' is problematic as a goal of palliative care. In this chapter the proposition is deepened, first through the presentation of three contrasting cases and then through a process of philosophical reflection. Although the authors make no attempt to prescribe whether, or in what form, palliative care should seek to bring about the good death, they do demonstrate some of the complex questions and issues which surround it. The 'good death' may refer to the process of dying, to the event of death or to the state of death. The 'good death' also raises questions about the 'good life', a distinction made problematic by some philosophers, such as Heidegger, who see human existence as 'being-toward-death'. There is also the question of the 'good' death or life for whom? And here we see the role of judgement, evaluation, even ideology in shaping ideas and practices within the palliative care setting. Within palliative care literature the 'good death' seems to have many components, several of which are not mutually exclusive, leading to a sense of vagueness and ambiguity. The chapter serves as a call for further clarification by practitioners on this important goal within palliative care.

In Chapter 7, Paul Schotsmans, like others in this volume, is eager to stress alternative formulations to bioethics from those of the 'principlists' who concentrate exclusively upon autonomy, beneficence, non-maleficence and justice. This predominantly Anglo-American approach is seen to be one which gives little place for the analysis of the experience of giving and receiving care. It is therefore a 'relational model' which is examined here, again by using a single case as a starting point. This fascinating chapter introduces palliative care to the gaze of the late Emmanuel Levinas, a Jewish Lithuanian, who conducted most of his philosophical work while living in France. Levinas is preoccupied with the human 'other' and in the caring relationship we see something of the importance of this. For as Schotsmans states, the key ethical question for the carer becomes: 'To what extent do I permit myself to be appealed to by the patient who has become entrusted to my care?' In Schotsmans' analysis, this constitutes a major responsibility, but also a liberating one which can do much to enhance the quality of human experience at the end of life, for both 'patients' and 'carers' alike.

This second part of the book therefore provides us with empirical evidence and philosophical reflection on some of the key moral notions which pervade modern palliative care. It also shows that we are still at an early stage in articulating these rigorously and that much benefit can be gained from the introduction of ideas, theories and concepts which so far have remained outside of palliative care discourse, but which may yet help us to shed light on important issues.

4 Moral values in palliative care: a European comparison

RIEN JANSSENS, HENK TEN HAVE,
BERT BROECKAERT, DAVID CLARK,
DIEGO GRACIA, FRANZ-JOZEF ILLHARDT,
GÖRAN LANTZ, SALVATORE PRIVITERA
AND PAUL SCHOTSMANS

We saw in Chapter 3 some of the conceptual problems to which palliative care gives rise. The need for a critical analysis of such issues was one of the motives behind the European *Pallium* project on palliative care ethics. Our project was carried out at a time in which the understanding of the concept of palliative care seemed to be undergoing important changes. The concept has become increasingly associated with a variety of meanings. We thought it important to explicate these various meanings, especially those which might lay below the surface of the dominant rhetoric.

One source of ambiguity is the increasing integration of palliative care within the broader healthcare system. The more palliative care becomes a part of a variety of medical practices, the harder it becomes to demarcate it from these practices. The demarcation of palliative care can no longer be based on its institutionalization since palliative care is being developed in many different institutions. Nor can the patient category serve as a demarcating criterion since it is more and more acknowledged that palliative care is not only relevant for cancer patients but also for patients suffering from Alzheimer's disease, cardio-vascular, neurological, haematological and chronic diseases. A demarcation in time is also problematic since the association of palliative care with terminal care is not generally accepted.

In the course of the project, it became increasingly apparent that clarification and analysis of the concept of palliative care is an important ethical enterprise. The demarcation of palliative care from other medical practices requires ethical attention. Moral notions that are used in the debates are indicative of a certain specificity of palliative care, either because they differ from notions that are used in the context of curative medical practices, or because they are attributed a specific meaning within palliative care. However, if one follows the debates on palliative care, critical analysis of these notions remains absent. The notion of autonomy is adopted uncritically from its use in curative practices. The notion of pain is still approached with a medical gaze. It remains unclear what is meant by 'quality of life'. In other words, ethical analysis of palliative care should be based on conceptual clarification, and conceptual clarification in its turn is at least in part an ethical enterprise: the specificity of palliative care is to an extent a moral specificity.

The integration of palliative care is one aspect of a process of maturation. At the same time it makes conceptual clarification particularly urgent since palliative care runs the risk of continuing ambiguity. Moreover, the integration process of palliative care means that normative statements regarding the morality of medical decisions at the end of life no longer suffice if they are not based on sound ethical argument. The (im)morality of euthanasia, the moral relevance of the principle of double effect, indications of whether to withdraw or withhold medical treatment, all these require ethical justification in the midst of pluralistic debates where different opinions seem to coexist. Since palliative care is now being offered in a variety of institutions, it is more and more acknowledged that normative statements require arguments to sustain them.

As we saw in Chapter 3, one way to articulate the many-sided conceptual and ethical aspects of palliative care is through the literature produced by caregivers and protagonists of various kinds. This can provide an essential insight into practice and tends to form the main subject matter of ethics. At the same time, primary empirical research can also provide insight into the varied views of experts and practitioners in the field. As part of the *Pallium* project, we therefore conducted a survey in order to gain insight into the variety of views and opinions on conceptual, as well as ethical, aspects of palliative care. Conducted in 1999, the survey was sent to participants of the Congress of the European Association of Palliative Care (EAPC), held in Geneva. The survey results help both to articulate the ambiguous aspects of palliative care and to provide directions towards an articulation of the (moral) specificity of palliative care.

We describe here the methods of the survey, together with relevant demographic and professional data concerning the respondents. We then set out the results in three key areas: terminology, definitions, and the situation of palliative care in the context of medicine and society. Results relating to values and norms in palliative care are then described, followed by a broader discussion.

A survey of European palliative care workers

The survey sample was based on a mailing list of the European and Israeli delegates attending the sixth Congress of the EAPC, held in Geneva from 22 to 24 September 1999. A French version was sent to delegates from France and Switzerland and an English version went to all other participants. It was distributed to 2174 European and Israeli delegates of the conference at the beginning of November 1999. By mid-January 2000, 782 questionnaires were returned, of which 14 were unusable. This made a response rate of 35.3 per cent.

The questionnaire consisted of five sections, starting with questions relating to demographic and professional issues (age, profession, institutional setting, nationality, sex). Next came two questions concerning the definition of palliative care. Subsequently, the respondents were confronted with 25 statements to which they were asked to give their level of agreement/disagreement on a 5-point Likert scale. The fourth section presented 18 moral notions which respondents were invited to rank according to their perceived importance for palliative care. Finally, the questionnaire presented 14 morally relevant acts, which the respondents were invited to consider.

We present here the results from the total number of returned questionnaires, with occasional reference to responses from the seven *Pallium* project countries, considered as a separate group.

Questionnaires were mailed to 44 European countries and also to Israel (total 45). Questionnaires were returned by respondents from 32 countries. The majority of returned questionnaires represent a limited number of countries. Just over 56 per cent of the questionnaires were received from three countries: Switzerland (21.5 per cent), France (20.3 per cent) and the United Kingdom (14.3 per cent). Belgium, Sweden, Germany, Italy, Spain, the Netherlands, Poland, Israel and Ireland contributed together 23.2 per cent of all respondents. The *Pallium* countries represented one-third (33.9 per cent) of the respondents.

Two-thirds (66.3 per cent) of all the respondents were female. The age of most respondents (89.7 per cent) was between 30 and 60 and two-fifths (41.5 per cent) were between 40 and 50. Almost a half (46.7 per cent) of the respondents had a background in medicine, 31.6 per cent in nursing, 5.9 per cent in other healthcare practice, with 12.6 per cent unspecified.

Conceptual queries in palliative care

Terminology

Within our sample, respondents describe their daily work as 'palliative care' (43.1 per cent), 'palliative medicine' (17.7 per cent), 'supportive care' (10.3 per cent) and 'palliative terminal care' (3.9 per cent). Only 0.9 per cent use 'terminal care' to characterize what they do, while 18.9 per cent use different terms. Respondents from the *Pallium* countries have even more preference for the labels 'palliative care' (49.8 per cent) and 'palliative medicine' (24.2 per cent); indeed only one respondent from these seven countries adopted 'terminal care' (0.4 per cent).

It seems therefore, as argued in the literature (Ahmedzai 1993) that respondents agree with the view that the scope of their work is wider than the terminal phase alone. This is also shown by the fact that the majority of respondents concurred with the statement that palliative care begins from the time of diagnosis (59.8 per cent total; 67.2 per cent *Pallium* countries) and by the fact that a minority agreed with the statement that in palliative care nothing is done to prolong life (34.9 per cent total; 20.4 per cent *Pallium* countries). Just under a half (44.4 per cent) held that palliative care begins when cure is no longer possible.

Definitions of palliative care

In 1987, when palliative medicine was recognized as a medical specialty in the United Kingdom, the following definition was adopted: 'palliative medicine is the study and management of patients with active, progressive, far-advanced disease for whom the prognosis is limited and the focus of care is the quality of life' (Doyle et al. 1996: 3). Three years later, the World Health Organization developed a definition of palliative care, meant not only for medical doctors but also for other members of the caregiving team:

> palliative care is the active, total care of patients whose disease is not responsive to curative treatment. Control of pain, of other symptoms, and of psychological, social, and spiritual problems is paramount. The goal of palliative care is achievement of the best quality of life for patients and their families.
>
> (WHO 1990: 11)

In our survey respondents were invited to identify the definition they used most commonly, with the two definitions quoted here provided in a footnote to the questionnaire. The majority (67.2 per cent) of those responding used the WHO definition of palliative care, 15.8 per cent used the UK definition of palliative medicine and 14.5 per cent used other definitions.

Palliative care in the context of medicine and society

The survey then invited respondents to consider 24 conceptual statements. These were ordered randomly, though our analysis here structures them into three domains: integration, medicalization and bureaucratization.

Integration

The statement that palliative care should be fully integrated within main-stream healthcare was accepted by most respondents, with 84.3 per cent agreeing or strongly agreeing. At the same time, over a half (53.4 per cent) disagreed about whether palliative care should be an alternative to main-stream healthcare, with almost one-third (31.6 per cent) agreeing or strongly agreeing. A variety of views existed about whether palliative care should retain a degree of independence from the healthcare system (6.4 per cent strongly agree; 27.7 per cent agree; 28.8 per cent disagree; 18.4 per cent strongly disagree). At the same time, more than half of the respondents (52.7 per cent) accepted that palliative care entails specific values, other than mainstream healthcare.

Medicalization

During the 1990s several publications addressed the issue of medicalization in palliative care (Field 1994; Bradshaw 1996; Clark and Seymour 1999). Do practitioners in the field also have the idea that palliative care is trans-forming into a medical discipline in which multifaceted problems of pati-ents are approached within a medical paradigm? Around one-half (51.9 per cent) of our respondents agreed that palliative care is becoming medicalized in his or her country, with just 15.6 per cent disagreeing. We are unable to say definitely whether this was seen as a positive or negative tendency, but the likelihood of the latter is suggested by the fact that one-half (50.5 per cent) also agreed that the role of the nursing profession is generally underestimated in palliative care, whereas less than one-third (30.4 per cent) disagreed. The idea that the autonomy of professionals other than medical doctors is threatened in palliative care has been observed by James and Field (1996). Despite the fact that only a minority of our respondents (31.6 per cent) had a professional background in nursing, only 18.7 per cent of the total agreed with the statement that the role of the medical profession is overestimated, whereas 55.0 per cent disagreed or strongly disagreed. The belief that the primary goal of palliative care is the achieve-ment of the best quality of life for the patient was almost universal in our sample (97.8 per cent) as was the belief that medical, psychological, social and spiritual care are of equal importance (92.4 per cent). Both of these sets of responses are indicative of a resistance to processes of medicalization, seen negatively.

Bureaucratization

Another theme in palliative care commentary has been the potential danger of bureaucratization – the process of transforming individual action into rational, administrative and hierarchical institutions (James and Field 1992). Only a minority (21.4 per cent) agreed with the statement that palliative care is increasingly bureaucratized due to regulations from the healthcare system, whereas 37.8 per cent disagreed or strongly disagreed, with 39.2 per cent who 'didn't know'. Apparently, bureaucratization and medicalization do not go hand in hand.

Values and norms in palliative care

As we have seen, the majority of our respondents took the view that palliative care implies a specific set of values, different from other healthcare practices (52.7 per cent). Yet only 13 per cent agreed with the statement that palliative care entails a religious set of values, though 14.3 per cent stated that palliative care *should* do so. A rather larger minority (30.6 per cent) held that palliative care has a surplus value compared to mainstream healthcare. It seems that, for most respondents, the specificity of the values of palliative care is not based on religious beliefs, nor can it claim a moral surplus.

In addition we presented respondents with 18 moral notions and asked them to rank their importance. The notions were selected because of their prevalence in the literature on palliative care as well as in the wider medical ethics literature. Notions with connotations of communitarianism (for instance sympathy, solidarity and compassion) were combined with notions that are often used in the libertarian tradition (for instance autonomy and non-maleficence). Respondents were invited to indicate whether they thought the notions were extremely important, important, quite important or not important for palliative care practice. The majority of notions were considered extremely important or important but as Table 4.1 shows, the ranking of the notions according to the degree of importance was different.

Finally, we presented respondents with 14 acts and asked whether or not each of these acts could be a component of palliative care. It was noted on the questionnaire that even if an act might be conceived of as a means of last resort, to be used in exceptional circumstances only, it should still be considered.

Active euthanasia

Only 5.3 per cent of the respondents could conceive of situations in which euthanasia might be performed in palliative care. Interestingly, 15.4 per cent agreed that the intentional shortening of life by raising opioid doses could form a part of palliative care, whereas 36.5 per cent of respondents accepted that the intentional shortening of a patient's life by withdrawing treatment might be a part of such care (Figure 4.1).

Table 4.1 The importance of moral notions in palliative care

Ranking of moral notions as important and extremely important (percentage of respondents)

Quality of life (97.5)
Human dignity (96.2)
Acceptance of human mortality (92.7)
Total care (91.3)
Non-maleficence/to do no harm (84.3)
Authenticity (84.1)
Autonomy (81.0)
Empathy (80.7)
Beneficence/to do good (78.2)
Hope (74.7)
Solidarity (64.9)
Compassion (64.7)
Prudence (64.2)
Holism (63.1)
Justice (61.9)
Love (50.7)
Sympathy (40.8)
Sanctity of life (30.8)

Figure 4.1 Life-shortening medical decisions

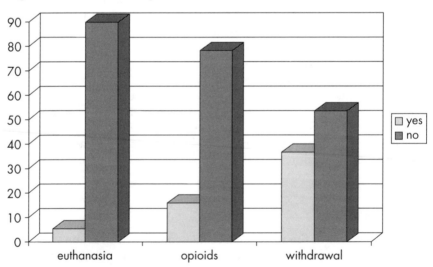

Note: Percentage of respondents agreeing or disagreeing that life-shortening medical decisions are a part of palliative care (euthanasia = active euthanasia; opioids = intentional shortening of life by raising opioid doses; withdrawal = intentional shortening of life by withdrawing treatment).

Figure 4.2   Terminal sedation

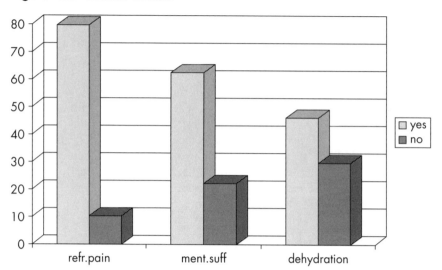

Note: Percentage of respondents agreeing or disagreeing that terminal sedation is a part of palliative care (refr.pain = terminal sedation for refractory pain; ment.suff = terminal sedation for relief of mental suffering; dehydration = dehydration in the heavily sedated patient).

Terminal sedation

Some important distinctions have been made between terminal sedation for refractory pain, terminal sedation for the relief of mental suffering, and dehydration in the heavily sedated patient (see Chapter 7). Terminal sedation for refractory pain can be part of palliative care according to 79.3 per cent of the respondents. Approval of terminal sedation for relief of mental suffering is less marked however, accounting for 62.9 per cent, whereas dehydration in the heavily sedated patient was approved of by 46.0 per cent with 28.8 per cent disapproving of this practice within palliative care (19.5 per cent did not know with 5.7 per cent missing, see Figure 4.2).

Withholding and withdrawing treatment

The vast majority of our respondents could make no moral distinction between withholding treatment and withdrawing treatment. The difference between the respondents who do not consider the withdrawal of life-prolonging treatment without the consent of the competent patient a part of palliative care and the respondents rejecting the withholding of life-prolonging treatment without the consent of the competent patient was a mere 1.6 per cent. Only a minority agreed that life-prolonging treatment can be withheld or withdrawn without the consent of the competent patient (7.6 per cent; 8.3 per cent). More respondents (19.4 per cent) could conceive of situations in which life-prolonging treatment is withheld without the knowledge of the incompetent patient's family. These findings indicate the importance of autonomy in palliative care (the notion of autonomy itself was considered extremely important or important by 81.0 per cent of respondents). To the statement that in palliative care, it is sometimes necessary to overrule the patient's autonomy in the patient's own interest, 60.8 per cent disagreed or strongly disagreed, whereas 18.9 per cent agreed or strongly agreed. For the *Pallium* countries, disagreement with this statement was lower (47.6 per cent) and agreement was higher (29.8 per cent), whereas withholding treatment without proxy consent was considered a potential part of palliative care by one-quarter (29.4 per cent) of the respondents from *Pallium* countries. Interestingly, respondents from the *Pallium* countries were also more likely to accept situations in which treatment is withheld or withdrawn without the consent of the competent patient (11.3 per cent; 11.7 per cent). It is remarkable that over 20 per cent of all respondents accepted that dehydration, withdrawing the ventilator and withholding the ventilator should not be part of palliative care. For the *Pallium* countries these three percentages are respectively 20.5 per cent, 13.6 per cent and 15.5 per cent (Figure 4.3).

Discussion

For many respondents in our European survey, palliative care is now the term of preference to denote their professional realm. Palliative medicine, denoting the medical specialty, and not so much the multidisciplinarity of palliative care (Doyle 1993), appears mostly used by the medical profession. Nevertheless, taking the 46.7 per cent of respondents with a medical background into consideration, the term palliative medicine is still used by only a minority of medical doctors working in the field.

The vast majority of respondents took the view that palliative care should be integrated within mainstream healthcare structures. Palliative care should, in other words, be delivered in the context of hospital wards, nursing homes, general practice, home care services and so on. Paradoxically, according to a substantial number of respondents, the integration of palliative care does not mean that it should become an alternative to mainstream healthcare. Nor does integration mean that palliative care would not entail specific moral values, other than the values of mainstream healthcare. Apparently, adherence to a specific set of values of palliative care can go together with integration in the mainstream healthcare system. In this respect, notions such as authenticity and hope have been proposed (Janssens et al. 1999), as concepts which may be useful in the moral landscape of palliative care. Of course, it can be argued that (re-)integration of palliative care has been a

Figure 4.3 Withholding/withdrawing treatment

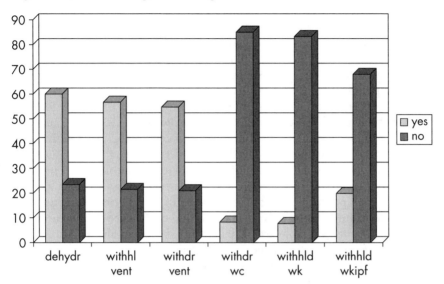

Note: Percentage of respondents agreeing or disagreeing that withholding/withdrawing treatment is a part of palliative care (dehydr = dehydration; withhl vent = withholding the ventilator; withdr vent = withdrawing the ventilator; withdr wc = withdrawal of life-prolonging treatment without the consent of the competent patient; withhld wk = withholding life-prolonging treatment without the knowledge of the competent patient; withhld wkipf = withholding life-prolonging treatment without the knowledge of the incompetent patient's family).

goal of the hospice movement from the beginning. Indeed, from 1967 (when Cicely Saunders established St Christopher's Hospice in London), an important aspiration has been to transfer hospice philosophy back into the wider healthcare system (Saunders et al. 1981).

Adherence to specific values within palliative care was demonstrated in our survey. Notions such as quality of life, acceptance of human mortality and total care were considered important or extremely important by over 90 per cent of the respondents, whereas for instance the four general moral principles of biomedical ethics (autonomy, beneficence, non-maleficence and justice) all ranked considerably lower. Three out of the four notions which were evaluated as most important (quality of life, total care, acceptance of human mortality) all refer to the WHO (1990) definition of palliative care. For the majority of our respondents, however, the specificity of palliative care does not imply a moral surplus in comparison to the values that pre- vail in the context of mainstream healthcare – a finding that has been argued for by others (Randall and Downie 1996).

Lower ranked notions in the survey reflected more general views of good medical practice. Notions that were considered less important (lower than

60 per cent) reflected either emotions with connotations of the private sphere (love, sympathy) or notions with explicit connotations of the Christian tradition (sanctity of life) (Hamel and Lysaught 1994). Notions with less strong, perhaps implicit connotations of the Christian tradition (human dignity, hope, prudence) were rated variably. This finding is corroborated by the small percentage of respondents who believed that palliative care implies an explicitly religious set of values.

Wider concerns within palliative care were expressed in the survey through the fact that many believe their field to be medicalizing (51.9 per cent) and that the role of the nursing profession is underestimated in palliative care (50.5 per cent). When we consider that 97.8 per cent see the best quality of life for the patient as the primary goal of palliative care, that 92.4 per cent think that medical, psychological, social and spiritual care are of equal importance, and 97.5 per cent think that the notion of quality of life is important or extremely important, it becomes clear that the supposed process of medicalization touches at the heart of palliative care. After all, medicalization implies an overestimation of the medical realm at the cost of other realms included in the concept of total care and in the idea of quality of life.

With regard to moral norms in palliative care, it is striking that for a substantial number of respondents, intentional life shortening decisions can be part of palliative care. According to the majority of the group we surveyed, active euthanasia is not one of these. However, at the same time, slightly more than 10 per cent of our respondents agreed that there is a crucial moral difference between active euthanasia and the intentional shortening of life by raising opioid doses, a difference that is refuted in the literature (Crul 1999). More than 30 per cent perceived a crucial moral difference between active euthanasia and the withdrawal of medical treatment with the intention to shorten the life of the patient. The question here is on what moral basis can specific life shortening decisions be included in palliative care, whereas active euthanasia is excluded?

With regard to terminal sedation, refractory pain is a more acceptable motive for its use than mental suffering. Dehydration in terminal sedation is common practice in some countries, but less common in others. No less than 28.8 per cent of our respondents indicated that, even in the most extreme circumstances, dehydrating the terminally sedated patient cannot be part of palliative care, an issue that was extensively discussed in the mid-1990s (Craig 1994; Ashby and Stoffell 1995; Craig 1996). An underlying argument may be that the practice seems hard to justify with the principle of double effect; it carries at least the suspicion of resembling 'slow euthanasia'. A similar argument can be raised against terminal sedation for relief of mental suffering. If we assume that it is difficult to assess refractory mental suffering, terminal sedation may easily be considered a disproportionate treatment, also not defensible by the principle of double effect (Billings and Block 1996; Mount 1996; Portenoy 1996).

Withdrawal and withholding of medical treatment, whatever the nature of the treatment, were reconsidered to be a potential part of palliative care by the majority. Yet, it is remarkable that a substantial 20 per cent of the respondents did not consider the withdrawal/withholding of the ventilator and of nutrition and hydration a part of palliative care. Perhaps, withdrawal of these medical treatments is associated with an inhumane death, even though in the literature, little support can be found for this association (Andrews et al. 1993; Brody et al. 1997). Another possibility is that hydration and nutrition are considered as components of essential care and not as medical treatment.

Withdrawal/withholding of these treatments may thus be considered as causing death in a manner which, according to some, might from a moral point of view be identical to euthanasia.

The patient's informed consent and the incompetent patient's proxy consent are for most respondents conditional upon the morality of withholding/withdrawing treatment, even though absence of proxy consent (if the patient is incompetent) is considered a possible part of palliative care by more respondents than absence of the competent patient's consent; this is in agreement with the literature (Farsides 1998; Osuna 1998; Scott 1999). Moral differences between withholding and withdrawing of treatment are negligible. However, more respondents from the *Pallium* countries could conceive of situations in which the autonomy of patients and their proxies is overruled, even though there is no significant difference regarding the importance of the notion of autonomy as such. It is possible that the moral significance of autonomy and informed consent is different between the southern and northern *Pallium* countries (Gracia and Núñez Olarte 1999; Privitera 1999). If not, the unlikely conclusion must be that, considering the nationality of the respondents, autonomy is of special moral significance in France and Switzerland.

Conclusion

This European survey identified diverging views on concepts of palliative care. Consensus exists on rather few issues. Nor is there a great deal of clarity about the scope of palliative care (when does palliative care begin?) Issues such as the medicalization of palliative care require further attention. There is also a lack of clarity with regard to the moral norms in palliative care. Though it seems easy to draw the line between active euthanasia, increasing pain medication and withdrawal of treatment, further analysis is necessary to unveil and weigh the intuitions and arguments that underlie the perceived different moral evaluations of these practices. What is the moral relevance of intention for the morality of these acts? What does the passive–active distinction amount to in practice and what are its moral implications? Fundamental ethical debates on medical decisions at the end of life can potentially create more clarity in such issues than is currently the case.

Autonomy is a moral notion that is widely adhered to in palliative care, but more research into the relevance of autonomy as a guiding principle in everyday practice is necessary. Important differences seem to exist across Europe. The question is whether informed consent is as fundamental for practice as it seems to be in theory. Do patients have to be informed that the treatment they receive is palliative? Should 'false hope' be eliminated from palliative care? Is there a duty to know? Such questions are only examples of those that should receive more attention.

In many countries palliative care was initially developed through individual action, inspired by religious commitment, outside the context of mainstream healthcare (Clark 1997, 1998). Even though, as we have seen, there was an idea of reintegrating the hospice concept into mainstream healthcare from the beginning, relations to mainstream healthcare were mainly antithetical. The hospice concept therefore implied a criticism of the values of mainstream healthcare. From the results of our survey here, it has once again become clear that palliative care is changing. Most respondents feel that palliative care should be fully integrated into mainstream healthcare. The religious commitment, so pervasively present in the beginning, is important only for a minority of present-day practitioners. Yet most respondents do adhere to a specific set of values for palliative care. Integration of palliative care does not, it seems, mean that the hospice philosophy is going to be neutralized. In many countries, caregivers in palliative care will have to find a way to keep doing justice to their innermost motivations in the context of institutions that are a part of mainstream healthcare systems. The traditional axiology of the hospice concept is increasingly subject to debate. Unequivocal, religiously inspired norms and values can and should no longer be taken for granted. Instead they require critical ethical analysis to sustain them. Be that as it may, the results of this questionnaire survey provide clues to argue that 'hospice', conceived of as a specific philosophy of care, should for many maintain its moral framework, not only for palliative care practice but also for healthcare in general.

References

Ahmedzai, S. (1993) The medicalization of dying – a doctor's view, in D. Clark (ed.) *The Future for Palliative Care: Issues of Policy and Practice*. Buckingham: Open University Press.

Andrews, M., Bell, E., Smith, S., Tischler, J. and Veglia J. (1993) Dehydration in terminally ill patients: is it appropriate palliative care?, *Postgraduate Medicine*, 93: 201–6.

Ashby, M. and Stoffell, B. (1995) Artificial hydration and alimentation at the end of life: a reply to Craig, *Journal of Medical Ethics*, 21: 135–40.

Billings, J.A. and Block, S.D. (1996) Slow euthanasia, *Journal of Palliative Care*, 12: 21–30.

Bradshaw, A. (1996) The spiritual dimension of hospice: the secularization of an ideal, *Social Science and Medicine*, 43: 409–19.

Brody, H., Campbell, M., Faber-Langendoen, K. and Ogle, K. (1997) Withdrawing intensive life-sustaining treatment: recommendations for compassionate clinical management, *New England Journal of Medicine*, 336: 652–7.

Clark, D. (1997) Someone to watch over me, *Nursing Times*, 93: 50–2.

Clark, D. (1998) Originating a movement: Cicely Saunders and the development of St Christopher's Hospice, 1957–1967, *Mortality*, 3: 43–63.

Clark, D. and Seymour, J. (1999) *Reflections on Palliative Care*. Buckingham: Open University Press.

Craig, G.M. (1994) On withholding nutrition and hydration in the terminally ill: has palliative medicine gone too far?, *Journal of Medical Ethics*, 20: 139–43.

Craig, G.M. (1996) On withholding artificial hydration and nutrition from the terminally ill: the debate continues, *Journal of Medical Ethics*, 22: 147–53.

Crul, B.J.P. (1999) *Mens en pijn: achtergronden en mogelijkheden van pijnbestrijding*. Nijmegen: Valkhof pers.

Doyle, D. (1993) Palliative medicine: a time for definition?, *Palliative Medicine*, 7: 253–5.

Doyle, D., Hanks, G.W.C. and MacDonald, N. (1996) Introduction, in D. Doyle, G.W.C. Hanks and N. MacDonald (eds) *Oxford Textbook of Palliative Medicine*. Oxford: Oxford University Press.

Farsides, C. (1998) Autonomy and its implications for palliative care: a Northern European perspective, *Palliative Medicine*, 12: 147–51.

Field, D. (1994) Palliative medicine and the medicalization of death, *European Journal of Cancer Care*, 3: 58–62.

Gracia, D. and Núñez Olarte, J.M. (1999) Le cure palliative in Spagna, *Bioetica e Cultura*, 8: 163–72.

Hamel, R. and Lysaught, T. (1994) Choosing palliative care: do religious beliefs make a difference?, *Journal of Palliative Care*, 10: 61–6.

James, N. and Field, D. (1992) The routinization of hospice: charisma and bureaucratization, *Social Science and Medicine*, 34: 1363–75.

James, V. and Field, D. (1996) Who has the power? Some problems and issues affecting the nursing care of dying patients, *European Journal of Cancer Care*, 5: 73–80.

Janssens, M.J.P.A., ten Have, H.A.M.J. and Zylicz, Z. (1999) Articulating the concept of palliative care: philosophical and theological perspectives, *Journal of Palliative Care*, 15: 38–44.

Mount, B. (1996) Morphine drips, terminal sedation, and slow euthanasia: definitions and facts, not anecdotes, *Journal of Palliative Care*, 12: 31–7.

Osuna, E. (1998) The right to information for the terminally ill patient, *Journal of Medical Ethics*, 24: 106–9.

Portenoy, R. (1996) Morphine infusions at the end of life: the pitfalls of reasoning from anecdote, *Journal of Palliative Care*, 12: 44–6.

Privitera, S. (1999) Accezioni semantiche e prassi medica in Italia, in S. Privitera (ed.) *Vivere bene nonostante tutto: le cure palliative in Europa e in Italia.* Acireale: Istituto Siciliana di Bioetica.

Randall, F. and Downie, R.S. (1996) *Palliative Care Ethics: A Good Companion.* Oxford: Oxford Medical Publications.

Saunders, C., Summers, D. and Teller, N. (1981) *Hospice: The Living Idea.* Leeds: Edward Arnold.

Scott, P.A. (1999) Autonomy, power, and control in palliative care, *Cambridge Quarterly of Healthcare Ethics*, 8: 139–47.

World Health Organization (1990) *Cancer Pain Relief and Palliative Care.* Geneva: WHO.

5 From conviction to responsibility in palliative care ethics

DIEGO GRACIA

Palliative care is quite new. It first began to develop out of 'terminal care' in the 1970s and so it has been influenced from the very beginning by certain new ideologies about care and caring, including the new feminist ethics and the recent ethics of nursing. At the same time it has been affected by earlier influences and paradigms. The thesis of this chapter is that in palliative care, as in other care-related activities, there is – and especially there was – what in the terms of Max Weber can be called 'conviction traits', more evident during the first decades of the movement than now. This chapter emphasizes the importance of promoting an 'ethics of responsibility' in this field, promoting personal autonomy and avoiding the old ideas of subservience and blind obedience.

Conviction and responsibility in ethics

Max Weber and the three ideal ethical types

Max Weber developed the concept of 'ethics of responsibility' at the beginning of the twentieth century. The concept must be seen as part of Weber's broader thinking on vocations and bureaucracy, but particularly in relation to Neo-Kantian philosophy. Neo-Kantianism was a particular interpretation of the philosophy of Kant, which emerged immediately after the crisis of the Idealistic movement. As with the other Idealist philosophers, such as Fichte, Schelling and Hegel, Kant thought that human reason is capable, especially throughout morality, of thinking and deciphering reality. In the *Critique of Pure Reason* Kant affirmed that scientific knowledge is incapable of knowing reality as such, other than as phenomenon; the fact of morality, more specifically, the fact of duty, induced him to think that human reason can penetrate the essence of reality. This was Kant's aim in his *Critique of Practical Reason*.

This last belief disappeared after the death of Hegel. The absolutely unrealistic systems constructed by the great thinkers of the Idealistic movement convinced philosophers that reason does not have the capacity to know reality as such, in its essence. This came to be known as 'the crisis of reason', one of the most important philosophical phenomena of the nineteenth century (Gracia 1996: 39–51). Reason is incapable of deciphering reality as such. Therefore, the knowledge of essences is impossible. The goal of reason is not theoretical and speculative, but principally positive and practical. This is the origin of Positivism and Pragmatism as philosophical movements. We do not know reality; we can only work with it.

Neo-Kantianism appeared in this context. Its main idea is that the best work of Kant was not the *Critique of Practical Reason* but the *Critique of Pure Reason*. This is the book in which Kant defended the incapacity of the human mind adequately to know reality. The problem is that Kant tried to correct this statement in the *Critique of Practical Reason*, analysing the fact of morality. Neo-Kantians considered that Kant's ethical system was wrongly constructed, because moral reason works exactly in the same way as described in the first *Critique*. Therefore, it is necessary to reconstruct the building of morality, or also to construct a new ethics, more adapted to the real data than the ethics elaborated by Kant.

In order to affirm absolute moral duties, Kant was compelled to avoid the empirical content of moral facts, stressing only formality and intention. Kantian ethics is therefore an ethics of intention. Kant did not take into account empirical facts, but only intentions. That is why Max Weber, like many other Neo-Kantians, used the term, an 'ethics of intention' (*Gesinnungsethik*). The word *Gesinnung* has here, to some extent, a negative meaning. Intentions are important, but so too are the empirical content of moral acts. Therefore, moral understanding must be understood as synthetic and a priori, exactly as other human judgements, for instance, scientific ones. Moral judgements are a synthesis of the empirical data and the moral categories of understanding. These categories are universal, but the empirical data are particular, and the consequence is that human understanding can elaborate universal moral categories but, when taking concrete decisions, these categories are not completely adequate to reality, or to empirical data, because they describe only the 'phenomenon', not the 'noumenon' of reality. Weber takes the view that there is an unavoidable tension between the universal concepts of understanding and concrete and particular facts. Accordingly, because moral decisions are always particular, they cannot be completely fitted to universal categories.

People who act morally, following only intentions and universal concepts, belong to the ideal type called by Weber *Gesinnungsethik*. On the contrary, when a person attempts to balance universal principles with concrete facts, that is, with the circumstances and consequences of the decision, then he or she is following the ideal type called *Verantwortungsethik*. Weber described these two types in different writings, especially in a conference in 1919 called *Politik als Beruf* (*Politics as a vocation*). There are, according to Weber, two types of politicians, those who have a true vocation, and those who come to politics with the only goal of increasing their power and particular interest. For Weber, the latter do not have a real political vocation, but merely a perverted one. As such, they do not have a true ethics. Weber considered that ethics and true vocation are directly related. Those who understand politics only as a means for increasing their particular interests and personal wealth are the opposite of true politicians. They are looking only for personal benefits, and not for the public and common good. They misunderstand their real goals. What must be thought only as a means, the use of power, is converted here into an end of political life. So they convert means into ends, and their ethics is the ethics of the use of means as ends. That is what Weber called *Erfolgesethik*, the ethic of the conversion of means into ultimate ends. These politicians do not live 'for' politics but only 'off' politics (Weber 1958: 84f).

The ethic of the use of means as ultimate means ('Erfolgesethik')

This is the typical ethics of the person who lives 'off' politics. Politics is turned into an economic enterprise, and the politician is conceived as an entrepreneur. Weber writes:

> He may assume the character of an 'entrepreneur', like the *condottiere* or the holder of a farmed-out or purchased office, or like the American boss who considers his costs a capital investment which he brings to fruition through exploitation of his influence.
>
> (Weber 1958: 86)

Weber specially describes the figure of the American boss, who does not have real political vocation, but only the desire for economic and political power. The boss works in politics like an administrator or a manager. The consequence is the conversion of politics into administration:

> the typical boss is an absolutely sober man . . . He seeks power alone, power as a source of money, but also power for power's sake . . . The boss has no firm political 'principles'; he is completely unprincipled in attitude and asks merely: What will capture votes?
>
> (Weber 1958: 109)

This description of Weber has also been used by some members of the 'Frankfurt School' to define a rationality called 'strategic' and 'instrumental' (Cortina 1985: 79–88; Habermas 1987, 1990; Serrano 1994).

The ethic of ultimate ends without any attention to means ('Gesinnungsethik')

The opposite of the 'unprincipled man' is the 'man with convictions' or the 'man with principles'. Weber opposes the one to the other. The first has no real political vocation, even though they have become a professional of politics. According to Weber, this is the tragedy of modern political life. The person with principles thinks that moral life consists in the realization of principles, and that therefore principles always have priority over reality. This is an idealistic conception of life, and of ethics also. Its classical expression is the Latin phrase *fiat iustitia pereat mundus*. Consequences are not important; only unconditional principles and intentions must guide moral action. A paradigmatic example is Kantian ethics. Principles and intentions must have priority over facts and reality. Weber analyses as an example of the ethics of intention or of the ethics of ultimate ends, the absolute ethic of the gospel, as expressed by the Sermon on the Mount:

> By the Sermon on the Mount, we mean the absolute ethic of the gospel, which is a more serious matter than those who are fond of quoting these commandments today believe. This ethic is no joking matter . . . it is not a cab, which one can have stopped at one's pleasure; it is all or nothing. This is precisely the meaning of the gospel, if trivialities are not to result. Hence, for instance, it was said of the wealthy young man, 'He went away sorrowful: for he had great possessions.' The evangelist commandment, however, is unconditional and unambiguous: give what thou hast – absolutely everything . . . Or, take the example, 'turn the other cheek': This command is unconditional and does not question the source of the other's authority to strike. Except for a saint it is an ethic of indignity. This is it: one must be saintly in everything; at least in intention, one must live like Jesus, the apostles, St Francis, and their like. *Then* this ethic makes sense and expresses a kind of dignity; otherwise it does not . . . The absolute ethic just does not *ask* for 'consequences.' That is the decisive point.
>
> (Weber 1958: 119f)

The ethic of responsibility ('Verantwortungsethik')

The absolute ethic does not ask for consequences. This is the decisive point for Weber. Consequences are important in moral life, and therefore it is necessary to balance principles and consequences. Aristotle called this *phrónesis*, practical wisdom, prudence. Human reason is not completely adequate to reality, and therefore our concepts and ideas, including moral ones, are not absolutely adequate to real facts. That is why it is necessary to analyse the circumstances and consequences of every specific situation, looking for a right and prudent decision. An ethics that does not take care of consequences is not responsible. We are responsible only for the future. As Weber puts it, 'one has to give an account of the foreseeable results of one's action' (Weber 1958: 120).

Responsibility ethics takes care not only of consequences, but also of principles and convictions. Weber says that in some ways both the ethics of conviction and the ethics of responsibility are opposite and irreconcilable:

> We must be clear – he says – about the fact that all ethically oriented conduct may be guided by one of two fundamentally differing and irreconcilably opposed maxims: conduct can be oriented to an 'ethic of ultimate end' or to an 'ethic of responsibility'.
>
> (Weber 1958: 120)

But in another way these categories are also complementary. There is no responsibility without convictions. What Weber calls responsibility can also be called responsible conviction or convictions with responsibility. Weber thus describes the balance between the respect for ultimate ends and the account of consequences:

> It is immensely moving when a *mature* man – no matter whether old or young in years – is aware of a responsibility for the consequences of his conduct and really feels such responsibility with heart and soul. He then acts by following an ethic of responsibility and somewhere he reaches the point where he says: 'Here I stand; I can do no other.' That is something genuinely human and moving. And every one of us who is not spiritually dead must realize the possibility of finding himself at some time in that position. In so far as this is true, an ethic of ultimate ends and an ethic of responsibility are not absolute contrasts but rather supplements, which only in unison constitute a genuine man.
>
> (Weber 1958: 127)

The development of the concept of responsibility ethics

From Max Weber onwards, the influence of the ethics of responsibility has been growing continuously. It is perhaps the most typical approach to ethics in the twentieth century. The reason for this is twofold. First, we are confronted with the crisis of reason, that is, the fact that philosophy does not believe today in the possibility of formulating deontological norms and principles completely adequate to reality. *Realitas semper maior*. There is a necessary inadequacy between our concepts and things, and therefore we must make our moral decisions taking into account not only the general criteria expressed by the moral principles, but also the analysis and evaluation of the specific circumstances and consequences which occur in a certain situation. Deciding only by means of principles is irresponsible. Our responsibility is always to the future, and therefore *consequences* must be taken into account, as an integral part of moral judgement. In the process of taking the right moral decisions, principles without consequences are blind, and consequences without principles are merely vain. The phenomenon of the 'crisis of reason' which took place immediately after the death of Hegel, addressed by authors such as Friedrich Nietzsche and Soren Kierkegaard, obliges us to shift from the ethics of conviction to the ethics of responsibility.

There is also a second reason for this change. Science and technology increased their power during the twentieth century to such an extent, that today they can put at stake the future of life in general, and of human life, in particular. This is why the evaluation of the consequences of our actions is now, from the moral point of view, more important than ever before. The argument is developed by Hans Jonas (1984) in his well-known book *The Imperative of Responsibility*.

A typical objection to the ethics of responsibility however is that it is relativistic, because it does not consider deontological principles as absolute and without any exceptions. But this is an important philosophical mistake. First, because 'relative' is the opposite to 'absolute' in metaphysics, but not in ethics. Here the opposite of 'absolute' is not relative but 'proportionate', and moral absolutism is not the contrary of moral relativism but of moral proportionalism (Finnis 1991).

The second reason why responsibility ethics theories are not relativistic is that they, certainly, deny the possibility of establishing absolute and exceptionless deontological mandates. But at the same time they assume that certain structures, which are the condition of possibility of the formulation of deontological propositions, are essential and constitutive to human beings, and therefore they work as absolute. In many cases, this absolute is an ontological property. It occurs in Heidegger's notion of the responsibility towards the Being, or the care of the Being (Heidegger 1972: 180–230). It can be found in Sartre's (1943) idea of the human being as an 'in-self' which is responsible for its 'by-itself'. It is revealed in Levinas's (1978) responsibility towards the Other. In other cases, the absolute is procedural, for example in Habermas where the principle of universalization constrains *all* those affected by the norm of assuming the perspectives of *all others* in the balance of interests (Habermas 1990: 65). It also occurs in Apel (1989) through the ideal community of communication and in Rawls (1999a) in the agreements assumed by all in 'the original position'. The consequence is always the same: human beings affected by a decision must be capable of participating in the process of deliberation, and therefore they are affirmed and accepted as moral agents, as subjects with dignity which must be respected. This is the canonical principle that the ethics of responsibility affirms as absolute. The point is that this principle is asserted as absolute only as formal and canonical, and not as material and deontological. This means we know *that* we must respect all human beings, but not *how* to do so. This last kind of judgement can only be approximate and prudential, due to its empirical and synthetic character. Therefore, it is individually, socially and historically determined. During the twentieth century, many attempts were made to manage correctly the complexity of this kind of judgement. Situationism, contextualism, hermeneutics, new casuistry, communitarianism, deliberationism, among others, are all examples of correctly performing concrete moral judgements. All these procedures share a quite similar view: assuming that reality is much more complex than our ideas about it, and that all those affected by a decision must have the possibility of participating in the process of deliberation, reasoning from their own points of view; in this way they are enriching the final decision, which must be freely assumed by all participants.

Bioethics is from its very beginning an ethics of responsibility. This is why it has developed out of the work of committees and commissions (Bulger et al. 1995). It also explains why the four principles that have become canonical, define only the prima facie duties (Beauchamp and Childress 1994), which make the evaluation of circumstances and consequences so necessary (Ross 1930). This evaluation is always and necessarily individually, socially and historically situated. For here and now, an absolute and overreaching perspective is not possible, it is rather a divine attribute.

In summary, it can be said that the ethics of responsibility assumes respect for all human beings as absolute, in the sense that all are entitled to participate in a free and equitable process of deliberation. The plurality of perspectives and values is not viewed as a difficulty but instead as the means of reaching more nuanced and enriched agreements. These cannot pretend to be completely rational but only reasonable; that is, practically wise or morally prudent. Accordingly, they are not absolute and must be continuously revised. Responsibility is always open to the future.

Conviction ethics and (palliative) care

Care ethics has traditionally been conceived as more emotional than rational, based in submission, confidence, faith, hope and love, and especially in obedience to authority. It has not been an autonomous ethics but a heteronomous one. The person with authority, the leader is the only one with the capacity to think and decide, and servants should therefore obey with faith, hope and love. This paradigm has been most frequently found in the groups and teams traditionally concerned with care: religious congregations of sisters, women, army servants and nurses. And this has also been the style and mentality proper to some kinds of palliative care.

The ethics based on submission and obedience is quite the opposite to the ethics of responsibility. It reduces autonomy and promotes heteronomy. As Nel Noddings says, it is necessary to have military goals in battle situations, 'but it tends to reduce individual responsibility'; the consequence is that 'one is at the mercy of an "ethical" elite' (Noddings 1984: 116). This ethical elite can be an individual, but can also take the form of an institution, such as a union, political party, fraternity, religious organization, and so on. The thesis of Noddings is that 'the frequent insistence on obedience to rules and adherence to ritual contributes to the erosion of genuine caring' (Noddings 1984: 117). In a genuine caring ethics, she continues, 'I must remain open to guidance and correction, but I am and remain responsible' (Noddings 1984: 117).

This description by Noddings of the ethics of obedience and conviction versus the ethics of responsibility can be applied to classical theories about women's ethics, the ethics of nursing, and the ethics of caring. Gender studies have stressed during the 1980s and 1990s how, traditionally, woman's role has been characterized by being passive (versus active), obedient (versus leading), private (versus public) (Elshtain 1981; Guerra 1998), reproductive (versus productive), emotional (versus rational) and care centred (versus cure centred) (Benhabib and Cornella 1987). It has been a role of subordination and subservience. Motherhood has been its paradigm. This is absolutely evident in the case of nursing. For many centuries the care of the sick in hospitals was in the hands of religious congregations of sisters (also called mothers). Florence Nightingale called them 'old-fashioned hospital "sisters"' (Nightingale 1969: 113, 127). The archetype of maternity has always been present and dominant in the care of the sick. For instance, the term 'nurse', which was introduced during the nineteenth century, comes from the Latin word *nutrire*, which means 'to nourish or suckle'. The paradigm of nursing is 'the mother-care of the young', and has been continuously stressed throughout history (Kuhse 1997: 14).

Florence Nightingale, the founder of the new nursing style, referred to 'nurses' instead of 'sisters' or 'mothers' (Nightingale 1969: 8). She wrote that she used this word due to the lack of a better one. In fact, before her the word 'nurse' was used to define the role of some women that Nightingale considered more harmful than beneficent (Nightingale 1969: 9). All Florence Nightingale's work deals with the duality of 'caring–poisoning' or 'caring–harming'. To reach this goal she used the old Hippocratic doctrine of the *vis medicatrix naturae* and the need to take account of the so-called *sex res non naturales* in order to promote health and prevent disease. She believed in the typical categories of the Neo-Hippocratic movement of the mid-nineteenth century. Her idea was that care is prior to cure, and that therefore the 'regime' of the body (Nightingale 1969: 33) has priority over drugs and surgery. Confounding this order is unnatural and harmful. Here Florence Nightingale reflected exactly the Hippocratic *oath* and the script entitled *On Airs, Waters and Places*. When drugs are necessary, she stressed the importance of homeopathy (Nightingale 1969: 131f), that is, of using the Hippocratic principle *similia similibus curantur*. Only when this strategy did not work, did she accept the necessity to begin with the opposite Hippocratic therapeutic principle, *contraria contrariis curantur*, which is specific to physicians. It is not a coincidence that homeopathy as a movement began during the first decades of the nineteenth century. All this is also closely linked with the Neo-Hippocratic movement of the nineteenth century, which coined the expression *primum non nocere* (Sharpe and Faden 1998: 36–42). Florence Nightingale was not completely 'nihilistic' in therapeutics, but she thought, as the nihilists, that the first duty is to care for the body and to prevent disease with well-tested measures, instead of giving drugs of completely unknown or dubious effect (Nightingale 1969: 9, 52). This is also the reason why she was so interested in observation and statistics, exactly as Pierre Louis in France. Instead of the 'scientific knowledge' of the internal causes of diseases, proper to physicians, she stressed the importance of 'experience' and 'observation' of the external factors that maintain health and bring about illness, proper to nurses. The first attitude is typical of the physician, while the second is specific to the professional nurse (Nightingale 1969: 122–5, 131f).

Florence Nightingale therefore considered the problem of 'poisoning' or 'harming' instead of 'caring' or 'nursing' as 'an ethical question' (Nightingale 1969: 125). Her ethics is therefore the ethics of *do no harm*. Sharpe and Faden have written that Florence Nightingale assumed

> that disease was the result of moral turpitude and could best be treated through a regimen focusing on the moral as well as the physical health of the patient . . . In her view, disease associated with hospitals could be prevented only by responsible, broad-based efforts at sanitation and hygiene.
>
> (Sharpe and Faden 1998: 157)

Florence Nightingale explains this idea at the beginning of her *Notes on Hospitals* with the following words:

> It may seem a strange principle to enunciate as the very first requirement in a Hospital that it should do the sick no harm. It is quite necessary, nevertheless, to lay down such a principle, because the actual mortality *in* hospitals, especially in those of large crowded cities, is very much higher than any calculation founded on the mortality of the same class of diseases among patients treated *out of* hospital would lead us to expect.
>
> (Nightingale 1863: 1)

She thought that a revolution, a moral and healthcare revolution, based on the principle of non-maleficence, *do no harm*, was necessary. The main point of this revolution is 'nursing', and the moral attitude to be stressed, 'responsibility' (Nightingale 1969: 25). She speaks of responsibility and not of accountability, perhaps because many of these things cannot be legally accounted; therefore, they are more moral than legal. This is why Nightingale was so interested in ethics. This ethics, she said, cannot be based in pure 'obedience', but in a different virtue, which she called 'trust-worthiness' (Nightingale 1969: 41; Kuhse 1997: 22). The ethics of pure obedience and subservience were typical of nursing both before and after Nightingale, but these were not her authentic beliefs. The ethics of Nightingale was not an ethics of conviction, or at least it was not under the traditional form of pure obedience and subservience. For this reason, what Helga Kuhse has called 'a history of subservience' (Kuhse 1997: 13), valid for a large part of the history of nursing, is not valid for Nightingale. In any case, 'until the 1960s, nurses saw themselves largely as helpmates to doctors and medicine, and echoes of the metaphors of subservience could still be heard in the 1965 version of the *International Code of Nursing Ethics*' (Kuhse 1997: 32).

Throughout its history, nursing has assumed more an ethics of conviction than an ethics of responsibility. And the same can be said, to some extent, about palliative care. The founder of this movement, Cicely Saunders, began her work as a nurse. Certainly, she was a nurse with a mentality closer to Florence Nightingale than to the typical ethics of subservience. She gave more importance to responsibility than to obedience. But like Nightingale, she also had some typical traits proper to the ethics of conviction. A common trait in both women is the idea that religious faith is necessary, or at least very important, in order to care adequately. Florence Nightingale asserted: 'she must be a religious and devoted woman' (Nightingale 1969: 126). Among many members of the early palliative care movement there was the belief that only with religious convictions can a right palliative care ethics be executed. This is what Randall and Downie (1996: 23) call the 'hidden agenda' of some professionals engaged in palliative care. These authors consider religious beliefs an 'extrinsic aim' to palliative care but not an 'intrinsic' one; they argue that 'there can be a pathological side to deeply held personal aims, especially the religious ones', and also that 'the dying patient is highly vulnerable to those who believe they have the truth about life and death' (Randall and Downie 1996: 23). We can see from the *Pallium* European survey described in Chapter 4 that this idea is present and actual in 15 per cent of those responding (see also Janssens et al. 2001: 7).

Another trait of conviction ethics in this field is the confusion between palliative care and the fight against euthanasia (see Chapter 3). This is also evident in some texts of Cicely Saunders herself. Especially at the beginning, the 'hospice movement' seemed to be a kind of 'anti-hemlock' movement. When Cicely Saunders writes: 'The doctor may not embark on any conduct with the primary intention of causing the patient's death' (Saunders et al. 1995: 6), she is expressing her personal belief and not an intrinsic criterion of palliative care.

In the 1960s Cicely Saunders was influenced by the North American civil rights movement and the emancipation and autonomy of women and patients. One consequence was an increasing respect for the autonomous decisions of patients when deciding about their lives and deaths; it marked, therefore, the moment of a shift from conviction ethics to another ethics more respectful of autonomy and patients' values. This shift is also evident in the fact that the hospice movement became more and more independent from the authority of physicians. Caring became an autonomous domain, and caring for terminally ill patients did so in particular.

The literature of bioethics and palliative care includes some papers clearly oriented towards conviction ethics. One of the most evident examples is the chapter on ethics and palliative care, written by J.D. Muñoz Sánchez and M. González Barón in the Spanish *Treatise of Palliative Medicine*, published in 1996. The authors oppose what they call 'principled ethics' with a 'personalist ethics'. They consider the first 'insufficient', because it does not identify human life or human beings with persons. On the contrary, so-called personalist bioethics affirms 'the duty of respect for all human life in all its manifestations, from the moment of conception (the fecundation) to the last instant (the total brain death)' (González Barón et al. 1996: 1222). They not only are convinced of these ideas, but also consider morally acceptable 'the attempt to *impose* their moral ideas on others' (González Barón et al. 1996: 1223). 'Respect for human life, its defence and promotion, as much the other's life as one's own, represents the first ethical imperative, the fundamental and first ethical principle'; therefore, 'the right to life is prior to the right to freedom. It must not be forgotten that to be free it is necessary to be alive, because life is the indispensable requisite for the exercise of freedom' (González Barón et al. 1996: 1223). In the next section of this chapter we analyse the work of other authors, who have developed palliative care ethics in a significantly different way.

Responsibility ethics and (palliative) care

In recent decades, studies in gender ethics and in the new nursing ethics have introduced a particular style of thinking to ethics, directly related to the idea of responsibility. One of the first authors to stress the importance of responsibility in care was Carol Gilligan. Her idea is that women were traditionally reduced to the role of obedience, because men were imbued by conviction ethics. Men are closer to conviction ethics, while the ethics specific to women is that of responsibility. For instance, studying only male samples, Kohlberg conceived 'the highest stages of moral development as deriving from a reflective understanding of human rights' (Gilligan 1982: 19), therefore, oriented by abstract and universal principles and norms, to universal human rights. Thinking this way, women are described as less morally developed than men, reaching only the middle stages of moral development, the so-called 'conventional' stage, instead of the 'post-conventional' one. Post-conventional morality is defined as that governed by the primacy and universality of individual rights, and not of being responsible to real facts in specific contexts. The new female morality, in the words of Gilligan, takes the view that

> the moral problem arises from conflicting responsibilities rather than from competing rights and requires for its resolution a mode of thinking that is contextual and narrative rather than formal and abstract. This conception of morality as concerned with the activity of care centers moral development around the understanding of responsibility and relationships, just as the conception of morality as fairness ties moral development to the understanding of rights and rules.
>
> (Gilligan 1982: 19)

For Gilligan 'conviction ethics' is closer to the male conception of the world, and to the contrary, therefore, women have more sensitivity for 'responsibility ethics': 'From a male perspective, a morality of responsibility appears inconclusive and diffuse, given its insistent contextual relativism' (Gilligan 1982: 20). Conversely, when women are claiming rights, they understand rights as the capacity of being responsible for themselves, in order 'to address issues of responsibility in social relationship' (Gilligan 1982: 129).

The idea of Gilligan is therefore that only through responsibility can a new ethics of care be developed:

> The morality of rights is predicated on equality and centered on the understanding of fairness, while the ethic of responsibility relies on the concept of equity, the recognition of differences in need. While the ethic of rights is a manifestation of equal respect, balancing the claims of other and self, the ethic of responsibility rests on an understanding that gives rise to compassion and care.
>
> (Gilligan 1982: 165)

And she concludes that 'yet in the different voice of women lays the truth of an ethic of care, the tie between relationship and responsibility' (Gilligan 1982: 173).

From this it might be argued that the ethics of care is less universal and geometric than the ethics of principles, and that the latter is closer to males and physicians, while the former is more related to females and nurses. As Noddings states:

> Moral decisions are, after all, made in situation; they are qualitatively different from the solution of geometry problems. Women, like act-deontologists in general, give reasons for their acts, but their reasons

point to feelings, needs, situational conditions, and their sense of personal ideal rather than universal principles and their application.

(Noddings 1984: 96)

A very important question is whether these differences between man and woman are natural or cultural, or perhaps both. For much of history the most accepted answer has been that these differences are natural, that is, biologically grounded. Today, on the contrary, the importance of sociocultural factors is given much greater emphasis. This is the reason why the old idea that the behavioural and moral differences are the consequence of sex has turned to another one in which these differences are now considered to be related to 'gender'. Gender is a sociocultural construct, while sex is a biological difference. Therefore, the moral differences between man and woman are more cultural than natural, and are closely related to the political structures of society. Here studies like the ones of Seyla Benhabib have opened new perspectives (Benhabib and Cornella 1987).

The thesis of Gilligan that women tend to be more relational and thus emphasize responsibility and mutuality, whereas men tend to be more competitive and thus give more importance to individual rights, can in fact be interpreted in both directions, as sexually grounded or as based on gender. Sociological studies show that there are no significant differences between men and women in how they resolve conflicts between the person's rights and their responsibilities to others (Wuthnow 1995: 164). Indeed in one study of the trade-off between rights and responsibilities it has been shown that 'despite the large number of cases in the study, the differences were too small to be statistically significant' (Wuthnow 1995: 165). According to Deborah Tannen (1990), the differences between men and women are more related to the linguistic construction of reality, and therefore to a different use of language, which is indicative of a deeper contrast in the way women and men perceive themselves, than to biological factors. Women approach conversation as 'negotiations for closeness in which people try to seek and give confirmation and support, and to reach consensus' (Tannen 1990: 25). On the contrary, 'men use language in a way that discloses their orientation toward accomplishment, their concern with achieving goals, their desire for status, and their proclivity to compete and oppose' (Wuthnow 1995: 166).

Differences in language are clearly gender related and they have moral significance, because they constitute, as Bellah has suggested, 'modes of moral discourse that include distinct vocabularies and characteristic patterns of moral reasoning' (Bellah et al. 1985: 334). These differences permit us to conclude that men as well as women perceive caring as morally important, but that they understand its moral relevance differently: 'Women are more likely to regard caring as an expression of their selfhood, whereas men are more likely to associate caring with the specific roles they may play' (Wuthnow 1995: 166). Consequently:

women think of themselves as being invested in their caring relationships and use words that signal this involvement. Men, in contrast, are
more likely to use words that distance themselves from their caring,
showing instead that it is defined by the roles they play and is thus
governed by norms of goal attainment, competition, and status.

(Wuthnow 1995: 166)

The differences stressed by Gilligan seem to be more cultural than natural.
As María José Guerra has pointed out, 'care is not feminine, it has been
"feminized"; and justice is not masculine, but it has been "masculinized"'
(Guerra 1998: 261). In any case, the differences exist, both in caring and in
ethics. What perhaps is excessive is the dichotomy between the principle-
based approach of the masculine ethical approach and the feminine care
approach, as suggested by Noddings. This antinomy has played an important role in the development of the new nursing ethics of care, in the hands
of Patricia Benner (Benner and Wrubel 1989) and Sara Fry (1990), among
others. Kuhse has strongly criticized this approach, saying 'Yes to Caring,
but No to a Nursing Ethics of Care' (Kuhse 1997: 142). Her thesis is that
care is not sufficient, because not all caring is good, it can be arbitrary, and
especially because care knows no limits, no fairness and equality. She
concludes:

> If nurses eschew all universal principles and norms they will not be
> able to participate in ethical discourse. They will not be able to speak
> on behalf of the patients for whom they care, nor will they be able to
> defend their own legitimate claims.

(Kuhse 1997: 166)

This is why one of the most important topics of the new gender ethics
is how 'care-relatedness-trust' can be meshed with 'justice-equality-rights-
obligations' (Held 1995: 2).

The solution to this problem can once more be found in the idea of
responsibility. Responsibility takes into account moral principles and norms,
but also circumstances and consequences. Responsibility looks for universality but also for context. This balance is particularly important in nursing
ethics. Two splendid examples of the application of the responsibility
approach to nursing ethics are Verena Tschudin's (1992) book *Ethics in
Nursing* and *Ethical Decision Making in Nursing* (Husted and Husted 1991).
Just as Tschudin has applied to ethics the ideas of responsibility developed
by H. Richard Niebuhr, the French ethicist Bruno Cadoré (1994) has worked
with Emmanuel Levinas's idea of responsibility, stressing the importance of
vocation for caring, and so has Peta Bowden (1997) with the philosophical
ideas of the second Wittgenstein.

The importance of responsibility ethics has grown in the work of Cicely
Saunders from the very beginning until recent years. In any case, the

progression has not been continuous or without crisis. There was an inflection point during the 1970s. From the 1970s until now, the principle of respect for the autonomy of patients has become more important, and at the same time the religious zeal for saving souls and converting people to true faith has been tempered.

The responsibility approach is evident in many of the followers of Saunders, and especially in those who have applied the common bioethical topics to the analysis of ethical problems. This is obvious in the work of Randall and Downie (1996). Here is a good example of an analysis of the ethical problems raised by palliative care from the point of view of the ethics of responsibility. The same can be said about the chapter on 'Ethical issues in palliative care', by Roy and MacDonald (1998) for the second edition of the *Oxford Textbook of Palliative Medicine*. Randall and Downie's book is particularly responsibility orientated. It begins by avoiding euthanasia as the main and quite the only moral topic: 'Euthanasia is not part of palliative care, although the subject may sometimes arise in that context' (Randall and Downie 1996: xi). If palliative care is important, it is so by itself, and not as a means of avoiding euthanasia. Randall and Downie (1996: xii) then try to analyse the moral problems of palliative care using what they call 'balanced judgments'. This expression brings to mind the criterion of 'balancing principles and reasons' used by Beauchamp and Childress (1994: 28–38), and also the 'reflective equilibrium' of John Rawls (1999a: 18f, 42–6; 1999b: 288ff). There are no absolute judgments in ethics, but decisions that will be necessarily uncertain and at the same time reflective, balanced or prudent. It is no accident that Randall and Downie begin the first chapter quoting the text of Aristotle in the *Nicomachean Ethics*, which says:

> Nothing is fixed in matters of conduct and of what is useful, any more than in matters of health. Since even the general account is like this, the account of particular cases is still less exact. The cases do not fall under any art or precept. Instead the agents themselves must all the time consider what is appropriate to the particular occasion, just as in medicine or navigation.
>
> (Aristotle 1995: 285)

That is the object of what Aristotle called *phrónesis* or practical wisdom, which the authors consider 'the central concept in palliative care or indeed in all healthcare' (Randall and Downie 1996: 17).

These 'balanced judgments' must take into account two general ethical principles which are relevant but at the same time opposite, those of utility and justice (Randall and Downie 1996: 9). Randall and Downie think these are 'first-order moral principles', that is, prima facie principles, which must be weighed against each other in order to take a wise decision. The *art* of palliative care 'is concerned with particularities and is based on practical wisdom or *phrónesis*' (Randall and Downie 1996: 77).

The approach of Roy and MacDonald (1998) is also typical of a responsibility approach to ethics. The task of ethics, they say, is not that of 'constructing arguments' but of 'constructing practical judgments' about what must be done:

> Ethics in palliative care is a matter of practical reasoning about individual patients, specific cases, and unique situations. Attention to this unique nature, and respect for it, may lead to decisions that we cannot always show to be consistent with either widely accepted principles or decisions taken earlier in similar situations. The starting point of clinical ethics, as also of clinical practice, is the consideration of a patient as a person like any other, what Charles Fried has called the principle of personal care.
>
> (Roy and MacDonald 1998: 99)

The bedside norm is 'the patient's body and biography'. This kind of ethics is not, therefore, deductive but inductive:

> We cannot simply pass each individual case through a grid of philosophical and religious moral principles to reach a clinical ethical conclusion. We simultaneously have to pass these principles through the grid of individual cases to arrive inductively at a reconstruction of these traditions.
>
> (Roy and MacDonald 1998: 99)

Clinical ethics, then, is not the direct application of principles; therefore, it 'is not applied philosophy or theology', but an original work which obliges us in every situation to look for the right decision; that is, which obliges us to develop a continuous exercise of responsibility.

These two texts, of Randall and Downie and of Roy and MacDonald, are good examples of how the ethics of palliative care is changing from a conviction perspective to one based on responsibility. Certainly, conviction ethics was important at the beginning of the palliative care movement, and it still is important today in some members or groups within the movement. This explains the findings of the empirical survey among the European delegates of the sixth Congress of the EAPC in Geneva in 1999 (see Chapter 4). In the commentary to the survey it is stated that there is a majority who believe that palliative care entails a specific set of values, different from other healthcare practices (52.7 per cent). To the statement however, that palliative care entails a religious set of values, only 13.0 per cent agree or strongly agree whereas only 14.3 per cent think that palliative care *should* entail a set of religious values. Likewise a minority hold that palliative care has a surplus value compared to mainstream healthcare (30.6 per cent versus 37.1 per cent who disagree or strongly disagree) (Janssens et al. 2001). The idea that palliative care entails a religious set of values, like for example the opposition to euthanasia (Janssens et al. 2001: 8), and the promotion of the idea of 'quality of life' (Janssens et al. 2001: 10) are typical of the 'conviction approach' to palliative care ethics. The suggestion that the 'percentage of respondents holding that palliative care entails an explicitly religious set of values' (Janssens et al. 2001: 10) is diminishing, confirms the hypothesis that conviction ethics is being substituted in the palliative care movement by an ethics of responsibility.

Conclusion

From Piaget and Kohlberg onwards it is well known that there is an evolution of the moral conscience. Kohlberg thought that this development goes from conventional norms to universal rules and principles. This assumption has been strongly criticized, as we have seen in this chapter. Moral development does not usually go from conventions to universal rules, but from heteronomy to autonomy, or from conviction and a priori moral criteria to other more complex judgments, based on the balance between principles and consequences.

These kinds of judgments require a great psychological and moral maturity. This is one of the reasons why they need time, being less frequent but more difficult during the first phases of the development of individuals and institutions. In some specific fields, like gender ethics, nursing ethics and care ethics, as in the female and care roles, the responsibility approach is quite new. These roles have traditionally been more influenced by conviction ethics than by the ethics of responsibility. This framework can be useful in order to understand the historical evolution and the present situation of ethics in palliative care. In this movement, like in many others, conviction ethics has been influential throughout its longer history, but especially during the early decades. Today, the idea of responsibility is growing in importance. The thesis of this chapter is that this idea is essential in order to develop a genuine care ethics, and more precisely, an ethics of palliative care.

References

Apel, K-O. (1989) *Diskurs und Verantwortung*. Frankfurt: Suhrkamp.
Aristotle (1995) *Nicomachean Ethics*, in S.M. Cahn (ed.) *Classics of Western Philosophy*. Indianapolis and Cambridge: Hackett.
Beauchamp, T.L. and Childress, J.F. (1994) *Principles of Biomedical Ethics*, 4th edn. New York: Oxford University Press.
Bellah, R.N., Madsen, R., Sullivan, W.M., Swidler, A. and Tipton, S.M. (1985) *Habits of the Heart: Individualism and Commitment in American Life*. Berkeley, CA: University of California Press.

Benhabib, S. and Cornella, D. (eds) (1987) *Feminism as Critique: Essays on the Politics of Gender in Late-Capitalists Societies*. London: Blackwell.

Benner, P. and Wrubel, J. (1989) *The Primacy of Caring: Stress and Coping in Health and Illness*. Menlo Park, CA: Addison Wesley.

Bowden, P. (1997) *Caring: Gender-Sensitive Ethics*. London: Routledge.

Bulger, R.H., Bobby, E.M. and Fineberg, H.V. (eds) (1995) *Society's Choices: Social and Ethical Decision Making in Biomedicine*. Washington, DC: National Academy Press.

Cadoré, B. (1994) *L'Expérience bioéthique de la responsabilité*. Lille: Université Catholique de Lille.

Cortina, A. (1985) *Crítica y Utopía: La Escuela de Francfort*. Madrid: Cincel.

Elshtain, J. (1981) *Public Man, Private Woman*. Princeton, NJ: Princeton University Press.

Finnis, J. (1991) *Moral Absolutes*. Washington, DC: Catholic University of America Press.

Fry, S.T. (1990) The philosophical foundation of caring, in M.M. Leininger (ed.) *Ethical and Moral Dimensions of Care*. Detroit, MI: Wayne State University Press.

Gilligan, C. (1982) *In a Different Voice*. Cambridge, MA: Harvard University Press.

González Barón, M., Ordóñez, A., Feliu, J., Zamora, P. and Espinosa, E. (1996) *Tratado de Medicina Paliativa*. Madrid: Editorial Médica Panamericana.

Gracia, D. (1996) Zubiri y la crisis de la razón, in A.A. Gómez and R. Rafael Martínez (dir.) *La filosofía de Zubiri en el contexto de la crisis europea*. Santiago de Compostela: Universidad de Santiago de Compostela.

Guerra, M.J. (1998) *Mujer, Identidad y Reconocimiento: Habermas y la crítica feminista*. La Laguna: Centro de Estudios de la Mujer.

Habermas, J. (1987) *Theorie des kommunikativen Handelns*, 4th edn. Frankfurt am Main: Suhrkamp.

Habermas, J. (1990) *Moral Consciousness and Communicative Action*. Cambridge, MA: MIT Press.

Heidegger, M. (1972) *Sein und Zeit*, 12th edn. Tübingen: Max Niemeyer.

Held, V. (ed.) (1995) *Justice and Care: Essential Readings in Feminist Ethics*. Boulder, CO: Westview.

Husted, G.L. and Husted, J.H. (1991) *Ethical Decision Making in Nursing*. St Louis, MO: Mosby.

Janssens, R., ten Have, H., Clark, D. et al. (2001) Palliative care in Europe: towards a more comprehensive understanding, *European Journal of Palliative Care*, 8(1): 20–3.

Jonas, H. (1984) *The Imperative of Responsibility: In Search of an Ethics for the Technological Age*. Chicago: University of Chicago Press.

Kuhse, H. (1997) *Caring: Nurses, Women and Ethics*. Oxford: Blackwell.

Levinas, E. (1978) *Autrement qu'être ou au-delà de l'essence*. The Hague: Martinus Nijhoff.

Nightingale, F. (1863) *Notes on Hospitals*, 3rd edn. London: Longman, Green.

Nightingale, F. (1969) *Notes on Nursing*. New York: Dover.

Noddings, N. (1984) *Caring: A Feminine Approach to Ethics and Moral Education*. Berkeley, CA: University of California Press.

Randall, F. and Downie, R.S. (1996) *Palliative Care Ethics: A Good Companion.* Oxford: Oxford University Press.

Rawls, J. (1999a) *A Theory of Justice*, rev. edn. Cambridge, MA: Belknap Press of Harvard University Press.

Rawls, J. (1999b) The independence of moral theory, in S. Freeman (ed.) *John Rawls: Collected Papers.* Cambridge, MA: Harvard University Press.

Ross, D. (1930) *The Right and the Good.* Oxford: Clarendon.

Roy, D.J. and MacDonald, N. (1998) Ethical issues in palliative care, in D. Doyle, G.W.C. Hanks and N. MacDonald (eds) *Oxford Textbook of Palliative Medicine*, 2nd edn. Oxford: Oxford University Press.

Sartre, J-P. (1943) *L'Etre et le néant: Essai d'ontologie phénomenologique.* Paris: Gallimard.

Saunders, C., Baines, M. and Dunlop, R. (1995) *Living with Dying: A Guide to Palliative Care*, 3rd edn. Oxford: Oxford University Press.

Serrano, E. (1994) *Legitimación y racionalización: Weber y Habermas: la dimensión normativa de un orden secularizado.* Barcelona: Anthropos.

Sharpe, V.A. and Faden, A.I. (1998) *Medical Harm: Historical, Conceptual, and Ethical Dimensions of Iatrogenic Illness.* Cambridge: Cambridge University Press.

Tannen, D. (1990) *You Just Don't Understand: Women and Men in Conversation.* New York: Ballantine.

Tschudin, V. (1992) *Ethics in Nursing.* Oxford: Butterworth-Heinemann.

Weber, M. (1958) Politics as a vocation, in H.H. Gerth and C.W. Mills (eds) *From Max Weber: Essays in Sociology.* New York: Oxford University Press.

Wuthnow, R. (1995) *Learning to Care: Elementary Kindness in an Age of Indifference.* New York: Oxford University Press.

6 Good death or good life as a goal of palliative care

WIM DEKKERS, LARS SANDMAN AND PAT WEBB

We may all have some idea about the best way to finish our life and we might for different reasons prefer to call this a good death or a good end of life. These ideas about what might be called characteristics of a good death or good life may be very different from person to person and from culture to culture. Indeed many would argue that this should be so. Yet we might still ask whether there are good reasons to articulate these individually and culturally dependent characteristics. This will to some extent depend on what standpoint we adopt concerning more fundamental philosophical problems regarding life and death. In this chapter we do not argue that any characteristic is better or worse at the end of life; we merely illustrate and indicate what kinds of questions need to be asked in relation to such characteristics if indeed we try to find good reasons for them. We will also outline the kinds of questions that need to be dealt with if we want to use these characteristics as a goal of palliative care.

As we began to see in Chapter 3, the problem of a good death or a good life as a goal of palliative care can be analysed from different perspectives: conceptual, evaluative, practical. In this chapter, we focus primarily on conceptual and evaluative issues. We briefly address the issue of how to implement ideas about a good death and a good life in the practice of palliative care. We acknowledge that there is no strict boundary between these different perspectives. This is not crucial however to the thesis of the chapter, since no special conclusions are drawn from these distinctions. Before moving into the discussion we present three patient stories that will be used to illustrate the complexity of the issues at hand: the cases of 'Charles', 'Moira' and 'Bernie'.[1]

Casuistry

Charles

Charles, a 58-year-old barrister working at the London Inns of Court, had received treatment for prostate cancer. At the time of diagnosis, investigations revealed local spread of the disease but there was then no evidence of systemic spread. Following initial treatment, he remained well for one year when the picture had changed radically. The cancer had spread to several bones and, in particular, his spine. He was referred to the palliative care team at the local hospice for pain relief, assessment of mobility and intermittent problems with a high blood calcium from the breakdown of bone, which caused a range of chemical disturbances.

Charles was a very private man. He had never married and had no regular partner. He did not keep in touch with his family but he enjoyed the company of a few professional colleagues. He lived alone and had the help of a non-residential housekeeper. Charles appeared to enjoy a solitary life and had several interests which absorbed him almost as much as the law that he practised – which was his passion and his life. He was fascinated by each new case and admitted to being a workaholic. Nothing would be so distressing to him as to be unable to work.

He accepted his diagnosis and its implications. There was now no treatment or cure and in discussion with his doctors and nurses, the agreed aim of care was to reduce unpleasant symptoms to the minimum so that he could continue to do all of the things he enjoyed. Life was to him 'a great mystery and an opportunity to explore himself and his world'. He had a belief in God but no practising religion and he admitted to wanting to capture as much time as possible in his remaining life in order to complete his ambitions – including work. He did not see any point in thinking about death. It would happen when it did but meanwhile he wanted the best quality of life possible.

His philosophy of life upset many of the staff caring for him. They seemed to want him to talk about the business of dying, presuming that he was denying his condition. This was not at all the case. He was able to have a room of his own so that he could more easily do his work. His papers and computer dominated the room. Despite this and his independence, staff were distressed that he would not take what they thought to be an adequate dose of analgesia for his pain. He refused a larger dose on the basis that it might render him less alert to complete his work. His own remedy was to drink malt whisky with the morphine. He was clearly well used to taking alcohol, as there was never any suggestion that he was out of control, drowsy or inebriated. The drinking worried the staff as well and there were suggestions that the alcohol should be taken away from him and administered at their discretion. This custodial behaviour was not appreciated at all. He became very upset and angry that, as a competent adult, he was not allowed to work out his own way of handling things. The suggestion was dropped.

He had an acute episode of back pain and some suggestion of numbness in his leg for the next few days. Clinical examination revealed that his lumbar spine was crumbling and doctors feared spinal cord compression if the vertebrae were not stabilized with radiotherapy. When this was presented to him, he was not frightened of the treatment but was planning a one-month trip to Peru and did not want to forfeit this. The discussion then moved to the dangers of not treating the spine. He fully accepted and understood the reasoning but preferred to take a chance. He became labelled as uncooperative and difficult. He made a choice and stood by it. His explanation was clear. He did not want to risk the possibility of never seeing Peru. If treatment did not work out, he might be immobile and unable to travel.

During one rare discussion with a younger female consultant, he admitted to his love of life but accepted that it was not his to give or take away. Illness happened as it happened and there was some mystery to it. However, he had much that he wanted to achieve and enjoy and 'medical things' were there to facilitate this. He never accepted the role of 'patient'; he was a dis-eased human being with plans and ways must be found to overcome the effects of the illness in order to achieve his goals. He claimed and it appeared that he had no fear of death – it would come when it came and that was the end of it. He wanted no details and had no questions about the process or the event of death even though it was raised with him by staff on several occasions.

Charles went to Peru and continued to work until the day before his death. On the morning of his death he behaved in the way that he had done all the other days in the hospice except that he asked for one particularly valued colleague to come and visit him with a book that he needed. During the visit, he became drowsy. He died one hour later.

Moira

Moira, a 62-year-old woman with widely disseminated breast cancer, was in the last few weeks of life in a hospital palliative care unit and she had been asking many questions about the process of dying and the event itself. She had become preoccupied if not obsessed with dying; she was very frightened. Her two adult daughters visited her regularly but they were unable to talk to her about her fears. She had always been the dominant member of the family caring for everyone else and this new, dependent role was very hard for her to handle.

The prospect of being cared for with support at home was addressed and practically was a real possibility. However, she was so fearful of death, that being away from a medical institution 'where they know how to deal with it all' was just not acceptable to her.

A variety of staff members tried to help Moira by engaging her in conversation and trying to elicit her concerns, but she just became so anxious focusing on it all that it seemed to make things worse rather than better. She had no religious belief although she believed in some kind of judgment. She perceived her cancer as a punishment for earlier behaviour in her life and on one occasion requested to speak to the hospital chaplain, who was well used to handling similar questions to those she was facing. However, she remained frozen by fear, not enjoying any of the last days of her life. Five days before she died, she became so anxious that she would use every available method to stay awake, rather than risk dying in her sleep. Anxiolytics were offered to her but she believed that these would make her drowsy and she wanted to stay awake at all costs.

She told staff that she knew that death was now imminent but that they must keep her awake 'so that it would not creep up on her and catch her unawares'. Her anxiety became extreme and at a family meeting with her daughters and with the doctors and nurses, she decided that a small amount of an anxiolytic drug would be acceptable to her, providing she could stay awake. The effect of the drug was so soothing after 24 hours that she gradually came to see that her avoiding behaviour could not continue indefinitely. She asked for prayer with the chaplain 'in the vain attempt that my Maker may forgive me my sins and give me some peace'. Although her fear did not go away completely, she was more relaxed than she had been for some weeks. She slipped into unconsciousness and died two hours later. Her daughters were distraught and exhausted. They believed that she had many unresolved issues in her life and that she did not die at peace. Her daughters' distress developed into unresolved grief and both needed the help of long-term therapy to help them through their bereavement process. The story goes on.

Bernie

Bernie, a man of 59 years, began to notice neurological problems only a year ago. He started to drop his teacup and realized that he could no longer feel it in his hand; he could no longer hold a pen to write. The symptoms became progressively and rapidly worse. His diagnosis of motor-neurone disease was a terrible shock to him and his wife Martha. They were a lively couple with grown-up children and the first grandchild had just arrived. Their combined interests ranged from hill walking to jazz and from playing the flute to watercolour painting. Bernie was in the last year of work as a teacher in higher education and he and his wife had been looking forward to enjoying time together in retirement. They were now not going to have much time.

The couple spent time talking about their predicament and began to make plans for Bernie's death, which was clearly now going to be in months rather than years. They decided to do as much together as possible and to continue to pursue most of their interests by adapting equipment and seeking help from disability experts. They also talked together and with their pastor about the process and the event of death. It was clear that both had a firm belief in God and, despite the fact that this illness was so unexpected and unwelcome, they were able to retain their faith and see it grow. Bernie was quite clear that despite the very dependent nature of his illness, he wanted to retain as much independence and dignity as possible. His wife understood this – it was how he had always lived.

When death was just a few days away, Martha was with Bernie constantly in the nursing home. His respiratory muscles were now affected and, even though he was helped somewhat by an artificial ventilator, it was difficult for him not to feel anxiety when drawing breath was so laboured. Nevertheless, Martha and Bernie worked together at producing as many distracting tactics as possible, including reminiscence therapy – remembering all of the good times and friends that had been their pleasure to know. This somehow encouraged Martha that she would still be in touch with these people after Bernie's death and it helped Bernie because he wanted to feel that Martha would not be so desperately lonely in bereavement that she could not continue to enjoy her life.

Bernie died with a smile on his face. His last communication to Martha was that while he had not planned to die so early, the event, though physically uncomfortable and distressing, was not so awful. He had prepared himself with the help of the person he loved most beside him all the way. He was relieved not to have the struggle any more. All his affairs were in order.

On reflection, Martha considered that Bernie had died as he had lived and that somehow he had always considered time on earth as part of a continuum. His body was needed on earth but now he did not need it any more; this episode was over but, while desperately sad at her loss she was content that for him a new episode had begun.

Conceptual issues

When talking in terms of a good death as opposed to a good life, we are looking for some kind of good-making characteristics of something, that is death, a concept that here seems to include also some period of life. So the first question to ask is of course what this something is or in other words, what death is in this context.

Life and death

At least as it is used in the palliative care literature, it seems obvious that 'death' refers to one or more of three different and consecutive situations. These three are 'the process of dying', 'the event of death' and 'the state of death', where the event of death is the passing over from the process of dying to the state of death. In relation to these three consecutive situations, problems of distinctness and vagueness need to be dealt with. When does the process of dying start and when does the event of death occur? Or in other words, when does the person pass from the process of dying to the state of death?

In relation to this, 'a good death' might refer to the whole complex of these three situations or to any single one of them and will hence have to take these complications into account. We can claim that symptom-management is characteristic of a good death in which 'death' refers to the process of dying and, thus, to life. Or we can claim that respectful treatment of the corpse is characteristic of a good death in which 'death' refers to the state of death. Or we can claim that passing away in one's sleep is characteristic of a good death in which 'death' refers to the event of death.

Another important question is whether a specific view of what death is might affect the characteristics of a good death. That is, if we take a religious view on what the state of death implies or if we take a secular view, these views will affect the alleged features of that state and will plausibly also affect what is characteristic of a good death in all of its three different meanings. For example, if we take a religious view on the state of death and believe there will be a kind of (personal) existence after physical death, we might consider it good to prepare for this future existence (a good-making characteristic of the period of dying). It might then also be important what is done to our corpse after we are dead (a good-making characteristic of the state of death). And if we prefer to talk in terms of a good life (after physical death) we could for example say that from a religious view a good life is a life in which we prepare for future life.

In the case of Bernie we saw how his belief in some future existence seemed to affect his dying process and the event of death, and affect them in a positive way. His wife took comfort in believing that he had continued to exist somewhere else after his physical death. Moira, on the other hand, had an idea about judgment after death that plausibly added to her misery and fear in death.

If one believes that persons continue to exist in some more radical form than just as a physical body after death, what characterizes a good state of death will arguably be different from the characterization in cases of the absence of such belief. If we could in some way affect the features of this continued existence before we die, this would plausibly affect the characteristics of a good process of dying or a good life. An example would be that a characteristic of good death is to evaluate one's former life and repent from the bad things done in order to stand a chance at Judgment Day.

Another question, the answer to which might affect the possibility of formulating general characteristics of a good death or a good life concerns what the features of dying and death are like. If the features of death are general – in other words, if most people die in much the same way, and have much the same problems when dying – it might be easier and we might have better reasons to formulate such characteristics for what a good death is. On the other hand, the features of death might be highly dependent on who is dying and in what circumstances. In other words, maybe people almost always die differently from each other, and have different problems. Then it will be more difficult to know and formulate what the good-making characteristics for such deaths are.

The connotations of a good death as contrasted to a good life

A reason for using 'a good death' rather than 'a good life' as a goal of palliative care could be to emphasize that the features of the last period of life are different from the rest of life and hence that the good-making characteristics in relation to that period are different from the good-making characteristics of the rest of life. This could be expressed in terms of emphasizing the *discontinuity* between the different periods of life. One might want to stress that there is a more or less sharp discontinuity between the last period of life (including the event of death) and other periods of life, due to things like an irreversible decay of the human body and mind, an obvious lack of time, a narrowing consciousness and awareness. However, another reason to focus on 'a good death' instead of 'a good life' is precisely the *continuity* of life and death. According to Heidegger (1962), for example, death is inextricably linked with human existence that is essentially characterized as 'being-toward-death'. In the same vein Kübler-Ross (1975) described the last stages of a human being's life (the dying process) as 'life's fulfilment'. Both authors seem to emphasize that human beings are in a sense in the process of dying from the very beginning of life and that life means preparing oneself for death. In the case of Bernie it seemed like he wanted to focus on death and deliberately to prepare for it at the end of his life, at the same time as continuing some aspects of his former life. And the comment from his wife about Bernie having died as he had lived seems to indicate a view of life and death as part of the same continuum, hence voicing an idea that we might focus on death as well as on life without accepting a discontinuity between them.

As was indicated above, in using the notion of a good death we want to emphasize that there are specific good-making characteristics of death, either due to the features of both death and dying or because there are specific characteristics that have death as their subject matter. The difference is that in the first case we have general characteristics such as autonomy and close relationships that must be adapted to the changes related to death (such as declining powers, lack of time left), while in the second case the characteristics are specifically related to death and cannot be generalized to the rest of life (that is, acceptance of death, awareness of death, summarizing of life). In order to emphasize the latter, one uses the notion of a good death. However, in using the notion of a good life one wants to emphasize that the good-making characteristics of this last period are similar to the good-making characteristics of the rest of life.

Besides these fundamental philosophical ideas there are also more practical reasons to focus on a good life or a good death. For example, in using a good death instead of a good life as a goal of care we might express something along the following lines. When you enter into this form of care the focus will be on the fact that you are supposed to die within a short period of time. Life is now practically over and instead of holding on to what has been it is time to look forward to death, deal with it and make the best of it. In emphasizing a good death one might be interpreted as saying something about death on behalf of life. And the other way around, in emphasizing a good life we might be interpreted as saying something about life on behalf of death. For example, a possible interpretation is that we thereby want to deny or de-emphasize the fact that we are soon to die. Another interpretation is the one voiced by Charles in the above case study, though one might be inclined to interpret his living his last days as a denial of his approaching death. Charles wanted to continue with life as he knew and appreciated it and saw no reason whatsoever to focus on death or adapt to the fact that he was dying. For him death seemed only to be what stops the stream of life, nothing more and nothing less.

Good death (or life) for whom?

When talking about a good death or a good life we need to ask 'Good for whom?' The characteristics of a good death (or life) might not be all about the person dying but might also be pertinent to other persons in the vicinity of (or at a distance from) this dying person. When looking for good-making characteristics of death we should include also what is good for the family, friends and the personnel (to limit ourselves to those in the vicinity of the dying person). The reason for explicitly noting this, besides wanting to analyse the goal of good death, is of course that what is characteristic of a good death for the person dying might come in conflict with what is characteristic of a good death for the family or for the personnel.

In the case of Bernie, his wife Martha was deeply involved in trying to arrange a good death for him and as it seems she considered his death good. This in turn seems to have made it good for her too. Moira also illustrated that death, whether good or bad, often affects more than the dying person. In her case her daughters were highly distraught by the way Moira died; and whether Moira finally got a good death or not in the end, it does not appear to have been good for her daughters.

Evaluative issues

As indicated in the introduction, what one means by 'characteristics' of a good death or a good life will to some extent depend on what standpoint one adopts regarding fundamental philosophical problems concerning life and death. Many different assumptions can be made about the characteristics of a good death or a good life, for example, whether these are objective or subjective, substantial or procedural, universal or relativistic. These issues might seem too philosophical to be interesting or important in relation to the goal of palliative care, but it is obvious that the position we take on these issues will influence our claims concerning what is a good death or life.

If we take an objective view on these characteristics we will view these as valid independently of what people think about them, for example, that it is better for us to make a life review whether we like it or want it or not. On the other hand if we take a subjective view, the best way to die will be the way the person likes or wants to die. If we take a substantial view on these characteristics there is an answer to the question about the best way to die independently of the deliberation of the persons concerned. If, on the other hand, we take a procedural view, this answer will come as a result of a procedure, for example, a discourse ethical procedure in which the personnel enter into a dialogue with the dying patient and their significant others. If we take a universal view on these characteristics we will claim that they are valid for all people under all circumstances or at least for all people given certain circumstances. If, on the other hand, we take a relativistic or particularistic view on them we will claim that this is dependent on the context.

It is obvious, when looking at different individuals, cultures and religions, that we find different characteristics of a good death and a good life, but is that due to some of them being wrong or is it how it should be? In the next two sections we examine and analyse two alleged characteristics of a good death. The above comments should therefore be kept in mind as they lead to different interpretations.

Two characteristics of a good death examined

In the literature we find the following characteristics when it comes to the question of what makes a death a good death: death with dignity; being autonomous and having control; acceptance of death; a peaceful death; a natural death; no unnecessary pain or suffering; openness or being aware of one's own dying; independence from others; accepting the timing of one's death; dying in the neighbourhood of significant others; dying in one's sleep; a sudden death; dying at home; and one's death having a positive effect on the family (Momeyer 1988: 65–85; Bradbury 1993; McNamara et al. 1994, 1995; Low and Payne 1996; Payne et al. 1996; Emanuel and Emanuel 1998; Mak and Clinton 1999).

One can distinguish between abstract notions such as dignity, autonomy, acceptance, peacefulness and naturalness on the one hand, and concrete characteristics of a good death such as dying in one's sleep or dying at home, on the other hand. If we start by comparing a peaceful death and to die in one's sleep, it seems they are on different levels of abstraction. To die in one's sleep is a very concrete characteristic because it is descriptively rather clear what it implies, even if it does not in itself have any evaluative content. A peaceful death would seem to be a good example of what is called a *thick concept* with not only a clear evaluative content but also a, supposedly, less clear descriptive content. This more open descriptive content allows us to use the characteristic of a peaceful death in more different ways than are possible with the characteristic of dying in one's sleep. What we suggest here is that different characteristics of good death can be ranked in a hierarchy of abstraction: the higher in the hierarchy, the more descriptively open is the characteristic. On the top of the hierarchy we have *good death*, close to the top we have characteristics like a *dignified death* or a *peaceful death*, and at the bottom we have concrete characteristics as the one mentioned above and, for example, *dying at home*. Here it might also be said that the closer to the top a characteristic is found, the easier it is to use it without definite descriptive content, and hence to use it synonymously with good death. In line with this there is also room for a wider variety of interpretations when using characteristics near the top of the hierarchy and thus for misunderstanding and possibly ideological use (see below). On the other hand, the more concrete characteristics have the disadvantage of leaving less room for interpretation and pluralism.

A peaceful death

The reason why we focus on peacefulness is that it belongs to one of the more abstract characteristics of a good death. Moreover, the idea of a peaceful death is as old as humankind. It has been reintroduced by Callahan (1993, 1997) and has been underlined by several authors as an ideal to strive for (Meier et al. 1997).

The term *peace* has many different meanings. 'Peace' means (1) a state of freedom from war or violence, (2) a treaty ending a war, (3) a (state of) calm or quiet, and (4) a (state of) harmony and friendship (*Oxford Advanced Learner's Dictionary*). From these distinctions we can learn two things. First, meanings (1) and (2) represent a negative description (or defi-nition) of peace. Peace is defined by what it is not: war, violence. The meanings (3) and (4) stand for a positive description (definition) of peace in which it is tried to describe the characteristics of peace in a positive man-ner. Then, peace is considered a state of affairs (for example, a harmonic order accepted by all or an order of commonly accepted justice) that gives no reason to strive for violent changes. Second, the term peace is applied to many different things. Well known is the war–peace dichotomy discussed in western political philosophy and in which peace and war are generally considered to take place within and between communities and states (Nardin 1998). However, when one speaks about a peaceful death in palliative care, 'peace' refers rather to individuals or small communities like families and friends than to bigger communities such as states. These individual connota-tions of peace also have a rich historical tradition.

Also the expression 'a peaceful death' has many different meanings rang-ing from the highly abstract and idealistic to more concrete and practical connotations. It can, for example, simply mean that there is quietness and not a lot of fuss around a dying person or that someone slowly passes away without a death struggle. Referring to the notion of the (late medieval) 'tame death' as has been described by Ariès (1974), Callahan defined a peaceful death as 'a dying that is accepted without overpowering fear and a death that has lost its power to terrorize' (Callahan 1993: 53). Callahan also defined a peaceful death as

> a death that is accepted and not unduly feared, a death that is not marked by excessive pain and suffering, and a death that takes place, so far as possible, in the presence of other people who are there to offer comfort, support, and love.
>
> (Callahan 1997: 1036)

Thus, as the phrase 'being at peace with oneself' seems to imply that one must accept oneself (as one is), a peaceful death is primarily a death that is accepted by the dying person. It is difficult to understand that someone dies a peaceful death (in a strong, idealistic sense of the term) while not accept-ing their own death. This can be said only if someone who has not accepted their death dies in their sleep or smoothly passes away. Then a 'peaceful death' has a less poignant, weaker meaning.

In view of Callahan's description of a good death, a first question is what 'acceptance' actually means. In this context one should at least distinguish between acceptance on a cognitive, emotional or evaluative level. If we look at our cases it would seem that each of the three patients accepted death in a different manner. All seem to have accepted death on a cognitive level, believing that they were in fact going to die. However, on an emotional level they differed from each other. Bernie apparently has accepted death in not fighting against it but rather adapting his life to, in a sense, welcome it.

Moira on the other hand wants to fight death out of an overpowering fear and she cannot emotionally rest assured in front of it. Charles, even if cognitively accepting death, finds a middle ground. He does not embrace death or adapt his life in front of death but he does not fight or defy death either. He rather seems to ignore death.

Further, Callahan probably realized that the above descriptions of the ideal of a peaceful death are on the one hand rather 'thick', but on the other hand meagre and open to debate. This is why he probably added some further characteristics of a peaceful death (Callahan 1993: 54; 1997: 1040). First, a peaceful death should include that the dying person understands that control over fate will pass from their hands. 'Fate' obviously refers here to the event of death and not to the process of dying. Someone might be in control of their life until the precise moment of death, and it might be that the experience of being in control gives someone peace. Charles seems to be a brilliant example of this. But the event of death necessarily means the end of a human being's control over life. Then 'death takes it over'. Thus, Callahan's presupposition here is that peacefulness has something to do with the experience of peace which is supposedly supported by the awareness (and acceptance) of a loss of control. Second, a peaceful death should also be a death marked by consciousness and a self-awareness that one is going to die and by a sense that one is ending one's days awake and alert and not as a body that has long ago lost its mind and self-awareness. The question is whether this is necessarily so. Can someone not die a peaceful death while being somewhat sedated or not fully conscious? Here, again, Callahan's presupposition is that it is more peaceful to be aware of (and accept) the approaching end of one's life, a presupposition which may not be generally accepted. Moira was terrified of death creeping up on her when she was conscious, but for her this was not something that gave her peace. It was rather the opposite, that this anxious wanting to stay conscious kept her from getting peace. Finally, a peaceful death should be a public death in the sense that death is supported by family and loving friends. The cases of Bernie and Martha illustrate this. However, it implies that the surrounding persons do not aggravate the dying person or make them upset. Even if it is not mentioned in the case description of Moira, we might suspect such a problem following the daughters' comments after their mother died. And if not, Moira's death did upset her daughters. A further question in this context is whether dying alone cannot be termed 'peaceful' in any sense.

A formal, but according to Callahan (1993: 196), evident characteristic of a peaceful death is the way it blends personal, medical, and social strands. Concerning the social aspects Callahan defines a peaceful death in a public context as

> a death that, on the one hand, did not require a disproportionate share of resources for fighting illness and death, a practice that leads to

economic violence, threatening other societal goods such as education and housing; and, on the other, rejected euthanasia and assisted suicide as still other forms of violence, though medical and social rather than economic.

(Callahan 1993: 218)

What strikes us in this formulation is the negative description of a peaceful death. A peaceful death is incompatible with a number of unwanted states of affairs. Moreover, this description of a peaceful death seems to imply that not a lot is done with patients at the end of their life and that they are left in peace.

The notion of a 'peaceful death' as used by Callahan is a description of an ideal way of dying rather than a clear and unambiguous (analytical) definition of a peaceful death. Furthermore, though it has its roots in the practice of medicine, it is primarily a regulative idea. It is clearly normative, but it is not prescriptive in the sense of being a blueprint for palliative care. Finally, its focus is not (only) on one particular characteristic of a good death as dignity, autonomy or acceptance, but on a broad context including medical, societal and personal aspects.

With descriptions like these not much is said about the practical implications for palliative care. The question is how to accomplish this ideal of a peaceful death in practice? It is relevant that 'peaceful death' is not an unambiguous term and that the meaning of this term must be interpreted in the context of a particular practice. For example, the death of Charles has been peaceful in an ordinary sense of the concept even if not really in line with the above criteria of acceptance, control, being public. Thus, if one accepts a peaceful death (as a characteristic of a good death) as a goal of palliative care, one must be prepared to be confronted with a number of practical problems, differences in interpretation and interpersonal conflicts. Due to a lack of resources, for example, people might have to die in rooms with more than one bed, where a lot of activity is going on in relation to other patients. Symptoms can cause much trouble or the dying patient might have psychological or emotional problems, so that it is difficult to achieve peace in one or another sense. Sometimes pain is not relievable other than by terminal sedation that does not seem to be in line with Callahan's ideal of a death marked by consciousness and self-awareness that one is going to die.

Die in one's sleep

The alleged characteristic of a good death as dying in one's sleep is not as descriptively unclear or vague or open as the more abstract characteristic discussed above. What it says is something along the following lines. It is better for a person if the event of death takes place when this person has a lowered degree of consciousness. An important question will then be to what degree it should be lowered. Perhaps this notion can be interpreted as implying that the less conscious the person is when the event of death takes place, the better. It is possible to provide a number of reasons why this would be good for the person in question. There will be no psychological distress or fear as it might be in the conscious waiting for death. Depending on the context, there might be an aspect of surprise, which might be considered good: I live my life the way I want it or in a good way and it is just cut short of death, without any former loss of anything that is good in life. However, this is generally not relevant in relation to patients within palliative care because they know that they are incurably ill and that death possibly is not so far away. On the other hand, one may claim that if I am not conscious just before I die I cannot say a last goodbye to my close ones or make a last evaluation of my life, all of which are considered important characteristics of a good death. I may also claim that I want to face death with open eyes, that I want to be conscious at this important event of my life. As we have seen earlier, Moira was terrified of not facing death fully awake, even if her fear receded somewhat and she actually did die in her sleep.

These reasons can plausibly be further supported by other reasons and perhaps by even more fundamental reasons. The reasons we allow into this account will also depend on what stand we take on the fundamental philosophical questions mentioned earlier. If we take a subjective view on what is good, to die in one's sleep will be good to the extent someone prefers it or wants it. If we take an objective view it might be good or bad independent of what people prefer or want. If we take a procedural view on what is good, to die in one's sleep will be good to the extent that is the outcome of the dialogue between the patient, the family, the friends and the personnel.

Dying in one's sleep may be regarded as an ideal way of dying that sometimes happens, but often does not. One can be lucky or not. Another question is whether we should actively strive for letting patients die in their sleep. Given that we accept that it is indeed good to die in one's sleep, we are still left with the more practical issue of what that implies in terms of care or what palliative care professionals should and could do. It seems there are two different ways to achieve this characteristic. One is to give terminal sedation to patients so whenever they die they will die in their sleep. The other is to give them a lethal drug when they happen to be asleep. A possible problem here is that we can accept the characteristic of good death without accepting the means to achieve it. That is, it does not necessarily follow that what is characteristic of a good death should automatically be achieved with whatever means possible. We might have restrictions due to the values and norms of the personnel, due to the care-worker being a professional, due to what is morally acceptable, or what is legal.

Evaluative conflicts and problems

A problem indicated by the above discussion is that reasons or arguments provided in relation to alleged characteristics of a good death (or good life for that matter) will be inconclusive. There are counter-arguments to any argument we try to provide and even if we believe in the possibility of rational argument in value issues this in turn will be based on the acceptance of more basic values. In the end we might be left with insoluble value differences of a fundamental kind. If this is true, we might be less prone to make definite statements about characteristics of a good death and maybe we also should be less prone to make such statements, at least not without carefully stating our reasons for adhering to that set of characteristics instead of another set.

Therefore, even if it is the case that a peaceful death or to die in one's sleep are indeed characteristics of a good death, we cannot prove it (since all we can do in philosophy is to provide better or worse reasons for and against something) and hence there is always some insecurity to whatever such claim we are prone to make. And when looking at different claims about what is a good death or a good life we find a plurality of different ideas, many of which are conflicting as our cases illustrate. Some ideas are based on different religions, ideologies or cultural traditions and find their *raison d'être* only if accepting the underpinnings of that religion or tradition. And depending on how we answer the above fundamental philosophical questions about objectivism, subjectivism, relativism and universalism, we will arrive at different ideas of how to deal with this pluralism.

More substantial claims about a good death or a good life may also come in conflict with other values in palliative care. Such a value that is found in palliative care, at least in some countries, is the value of autonomy. Autonomous decision-making and control are often considered a precondition for a death with dignity, but are also mentioned as characteristics of a good death without reference to the dignity-doctrine. In some interpretations autonomy includes the right to choose what is not in one's best interest or what is not good for someone. However, whether there arises a conflict or not will depend on what we claim autonomy to be and what scope and role it is given within a person's care. For example, if autonomy is not restricted so that the person is fully free to choose what is in their best interest or what is rational, and if autonomy is given priority over all other norms and values, any characteristic of a good death will be overturned by the person to the extent it is not in line with their own preferences. The more autonomy is restricted in different ways, the greater might be the role for these characteristics of good death and life. But to the extent autonomy is given any role within palliative care there might be a conflict with these characteristics of a good death or a good life. Charles illustrates this well in not adapting to the accepted characteristics for a good death that were found at the place where he was treated. He exercised his autonomy and chose to live life to the very end according to his own opinion about how it should be lived. And this obviously caused a conflict with the established opinion of the staff about how someone dying should live their lives.

This is also pertinent in relation to another problem mentioned above, namely the possible ideological use of characteristics of a good death (or a good life). The preoccupation with death and dying in the practice and theory of hospice and palliative care has led to what might be called the 'Good Death Model' (McNamara et al. 1994) or the 'ideology of the good death' (Clark and Seymour 1999: 79). Hospice and palliative care have become synonymous with 'good death'. What is meant by this 'ideology of the good death'?

Any goal in the context of palliative care is based on a number of value assumptions as well as on scientific facts and experiences about what is possible or realistic to do in relation to patients. If these goals are the focus of care without explicating the underlying value assumptions in order to get the patient to accept them then they are put to what may be called 'ideological use'. By ideological use we mean here the attempt to get people to accept certain ideas about death and dying, particularly *good* death and dying, without allowing or giving these people opportunity to examine critically these ideas and to take a deliberated stand in relation to them. The problem with this is that it does not seem to be in line with the strong emphasis on patient autonomy and informed consent we find in the western care context.

If a good death is used as a goal of care, implying a number of characteristics, and if these characteristics are presented as indisputable or objective, or at least as characteristics for which there are good reasons, then someone not wanting to die accordingly, is choosing a bad death. So it would take a lot of courage for the patient to question these characteristics. Instead of justifying these characteristics with reasons and arguments, it is possible to support them with references to the authoritative education and experience of the caregiver or the established tradition of the institution. To some extent the higher up in the above presented hierarchy, the more easily will the characteristic of good death or life be put to ideological use, since it will then have a rather clear positive value that might be difficult to question and at the same time a less clear descriptive content. While, on the other hand, a characteristic like to die in one's sleep would seem easier to question and hence less easy as a means to manipulate people, it is not free from the risk of ideological use. The case of Charles demonstrates that healthcare professionals to some extent used their opinions about a good death in an ideological sense and, as we saw, tried to get Charles to adapt to it. Even if it was not always explicit, their distress and aggravation with his decisions may have been shown implicitly in the way they treated him. Charles, being an influential member of society, a barrister, managed to get his way, but obviously we are not all barristers used to arguing our case.

Now, it has to be pointed out that a value conflict does not necessarily involve a moral conflict per se. Moral conflicts can be avoided or 'solved' in different ways. First, we might agree to differ and one way to avoid the types of moral conflicts indicated here is to have an explicitly *pluralistic* goal of palliative care when it comes to ideas about good death and life. Other ways of solving this type of conflict without having to give up the ideas about a good death or life is to put restrictions on what we are allowed to do in relation to patients given these ideas: for example, that we are allowed to enter into a dialogue with the patient about issues concerning a good death, but that we are not allowed to try to influence the patient or manipulate the patient. Here it is also important to point out that if we take a subjective view on good death we leave it to the patient to decide what a good death is and then this type of conflict does not seem to arise. And if we take a procedural view, a good death is what comes out of a certain procedure, for example a dialogue between patient and carer. This seems to minimize the above problem even if not eradicating it, since there is still inequality of power in such a dialogue.

However, even given a pluralistic goal of care we might still end up with moral conflicts due to different ideas about a good death. For example, to some people it is essential that they are allowed to end their life in a quiet and peaceful environment and to others (perhaps due to cultural traditions) it may be important to have family, relatives, and friends gathered around and loudly expressing their grief over the oncoming loss of this person. Obviously this constitutes a possible moral conflict if these two persons are cared for at the same institution, for example, in making it impossible for them both to achieve a good death according to their views at the same time. To enable these two people to die at home would be one possible solution to this and other problems of conflicting value. Still, this is not possible in relation to every patient. Hence, another idea is to have different institutions for people from different cultural traditions. On the other hand, this might be problematic from the perspective of social integration. So, a third way to solve this type of conflict is to put restrictions on what we can do in order to get a good death (that it should not interfere too much with other people or be harmful to other people) in a way similar to the restrictions we put on all social activities.

Conclusion

In this chapter a number of philosophical-ethical questions and problems concerning the notions of good life and death, especially in relation to palliative care, have been examined. We have illustrated the complexity of these notions in contrast with the ease and routine with which they are sometimes used within palliative care. We have neither advocated a particular conception of a good death or a good life as a goal of palliative care, nor have we argued that any characteristic of a good death or a good life is better or worse at the end of life, nor have we wanted to present one of the three cases, mentioned above, as an ideal way of living and dying. On the contrary, we have simply emphasized the vagueness and ambiguity of many concepts that are currently used in the debate on the goals of palliative care (see also Chapter 3).

This philosophical stance may be disappointing for care providers in palliative care. However, we hope that our analysis will inspire them to (re)start thinking about how these notions are used and should be used. As we said in the introduction, we all have some idea about the best way to die ranging from some preliminary thoughts on this matter to more elaborated philosophical views in which attention is also paid to underlying norms and values. Callahan's notion of a 'peaceful death' is one example of such an elaborated description of an ideal way of dying. Callahan's notion is a regulative idea rather than a clear and unambiguous definition of a good death. It is clearly normative, but not prescriptive in the sense of being a clear blueprint for palliative care.

Again, patients at the end of life and caregivers in palliative care all have implicit or explicit ideas about a good way of dying. An adequate palliative care is unthinkable without some shared view on all these different (intuitive) ideas. Thus, thinking about what a good life or death could be is a task not only for philosophers and ethicists, but also for patients at the end of their life, for caregivers in palliative care, and for every human being. This is not to say that it will be possible to define, once and for all, or even for a particular context of palliative care what are the characteristics of a good death. Though we have emphasized in this chapter the necessity of a clear analysis of relevant concepts and notions based on reasons and arguments, we realize that this analysis must start (and end) with our intuitive ideas on death and dying. We also realize that a clear philosophical analysis never can replace being inspired by (intuitive) ideals of living and dying.

In this respect, there are two different but related questions that need to be answered. First, what is within the power of the caregivers to do, and second what is their responsibility, that is, what should they do? What one *should* do, is obviously dependent on that one *can* do, but it is not necessarily so that one should do something just because one can do it. Take the problem touched upon by Randall and Downie (1996) when they claim that the patient has implicitly approved of physical care by seeking the help of a hospital or other healthcare institution, but has not necessarily approved of anything beyond this, for example, emotional care, or in this case, of help to die a good death or in living a good life. We must be careful about finding that out first before we can do anything along those lines. The case of Charles seems to be an example of this.

Another practical problem that concerns the implementation of the idea of a good death and a good life is what may be called the 'messiness' of death. At the end of life we sometimes have painful and distressing symptoms that will preclude us from having a good death or a good life, or our consciousness can be affected in a way that prevents it, or other losses of functions might be present. Moira is an example of how the distress caused by oncoming death can make it very difficult to do anything else but try to cope with the distress. It was not until her distress was treated that she could try to achieve some of the alleged characteristics of a good death, even if her daughters did not find it sufficient. A way to accommodate to this 'messiness' is to talk about a *comparatively* good death or life, that is, to adapt one's characteristics to the messiness of death.

We hope this chapter (with all its questions) might inspire some much needed discussion on the issues of good death and good life within palliative care.

Note

1 The following case studies are derived from cases in a south London independent hospice, a Belgian hospice and a London-based hospital palliative care unit.

References

Ariès, P. (1974) *Western Attitudes toward Death: From the Middle Ages to the Present*. Baltimore, MD: Johns Hopkins University Press.

Bradbury, M. (1993) Contemporary representations of 'good' and 'bad' death, in D. Dickenson and M. Johnson (eds) *Death, Dying and Bereavement*. London: Sage.

Callahan, D. (1993) *The Troubled Dream of Life: Living with Mortality*. New York: Simon and Schuster.

Callahan, D. (1997) The value of achieving a peaceful death, in C.J. Cassell et al. (eds) *Geriatric Medicine*, 3rd edn. New York: Springer.

Clark, D. and Seymour, J. (1999) *Reflections on Palliative Care*. Buckingham: Open University Press.

Emanuel, E.J. and Emanuel, L.L. (1998) The promise of a good death, *The Lancet*, 351: SII21–SII29.

Heidegger, M. (1962) *Being and Time*, translated by J. Macquarrie and E. Robinson. New York: Harper and Row.

Kübler-Ross, E. (1975) *Death: The Final Stage of Growth*. Englewood Cliffs, NJ: Prentice-Hall.

Low, J.T.S. and Payne, S. (1996) The good and bad death perceptions of health professionals working in palliative care, *European Journal of Cancer Care*, 5: 237–41.

McNamara, B., Waddell, C. and Colvin, M. (1994) The institutionalization of the good death, *Social Science and Medicine*, 39(11): 1501–8.

McNamara, B., Waddell, C. and Colvin, M. (1995) Threats to the good death: the cultural context of stress and coping among hospice nurses, *Sociology of Health and Illness*, 17(2): 222–44.

Mak, J.M.H. and Clinton, M. (1999) Promoting a good death: an agenda for outcomes research – a review of the literature, *Nursing Ethics*, 6(2): 97–106.

Meier, D.E., Morrison, R.S. and Cassel, C.K. (1997) Improving palliative care, *Annals of Internal Medicine*, 127(3): 225–30.

Momeyer, R.W. (1988) *Confronting Death*. Bloomington, IN: Indiana University Press.

Nardin, T. (1998) Philosophy of war and peace, in E. Craig (ed.) *Routledge Encyclopedia of Philosophy*, Vol. 9. London and New York: Routledge.

Payne, S., Hillier, R., Langley-Evans, A. and Roberts, T. (1996) Impact of witnessing death on hospice patients, *Social Science and Medicine*, 43(12): 1785–94.

Randall, F. and Downie, R.S. (1996) *Palliative Care Ethics: A Good Companion*. Oxford: Oxford University Press.

7 Palliative care: a relational approach

PAUL SCHOTSMANS

As early as the 1950s, Cicely Saunders recognized the beginnings of the gross divergence of medical care for the curable and for the dying at a time when the 'ability to diagnose, intervene, and technologically support patients was growing exponentially' (Saunders 1993: 1). Thanks to her insights and contributions hospice and palliative care of the dying began to develop as a fully inter-human event, with a particular kind of conceptualization:

> In the palliative phase there is a shift in emphasis from quantity of life to quality of life . . . this shift has an important consequence: a requirement to listen to the patient's views . . . Here, care is as concerned with the whole person as with the pathology of the disease.
>
> (Jeffrey 2000: 22)

From the viewpoint of the ethicist, this interest in the relational structure of palliative care is very similar to some twentieth-century developments in philosophical anthropology and ethical theory. For within the phenomenological and existential traditions, several philosophers have developed fundamental theories concerning the basic relational structure of human existence. Influential philosophers, like Gabriël Marcel, Emmanuel Levinas, Martin Buber and Paul Ricoeur, exemplify this evolution in philosophical and ethical reflection.

Surprisingly enough, these philosophers and their relational approach are relatively unknown to the majority of fieldworkers in palliative care, although many tendencies of the theoretical approach in palliative care can be linked directly to their philosophical insights. Greater awareness of these philosophical foundations therefore has considerable potential to enhance the ethical culture of palliative care. From another perspective, it is important to recognize that the mainstream within European anthropology, philosophy and ethics represents a very different tradition to that of the principle of autonomy which has tended to dominate Anglo-American bioethics in recent times. Anglo-American bioethics creates the impression that there is very little space for the relational encounter between the patient, the caregiver and other human beings surrounding them. This is also clear in the Anglo-American ethical debate concerning the end of life, where the relational approach, unfortunately, is almost totally absent.

To understand fully the relational structure of palliative care, it is necessary to stress the multidimensional character of the human person. As Martien Pijnenburg (1998: 246) observes: 'There is too much one-dimensional focus on the human person as an autonomous entity making autonomous choices. Autonomy is an ideal but not an absolute value'. Harry Kuitert, the protestant Dutch theologian who is in favour of the legalization of euthanasia, also makes clear that 'the autonomy of the patient is not, has never been, and cannot be the sole reason for performing euthanasia' (Kuitert and van Leeuwen 1998: 224). The theologian Theo Beemer has commented on this disproportionate interest in the principle of autonomy, by referring to the withdrawal from a common search for the meaning of life. He calls it a movement of retreat because, as experience is teaching us, the difficult common search for insight into what is truly human and good is often broken off prematurely because everyone starts insisting on his or her rights. The question 'who may decide?' thus short circuits the discussion what is 'the good and human to decide?' The question then becomes one of competency, debating who has the right to decide, rather than being a discussion that is concerned with the fundamental aspects of the matter (Beemer 1981, 1984).

It is also evident that some supporters of palliative care take a critical view of the one-sided application of the principle of respect for the autonomy of the patient:

> If an ethical framework is to be of practical use to patients and staff, respect for autonomy needs to be combined with a caring approach. Such a model has the advantage of acknowledging that feelings, compassion, integrity and virtue play a vital part in the holistic approach to care.
>
> (Jeffrey 2000: 35)

Ben Zylicz captures this admirably: 'we can help to carry the suffering with the patient. This is a concept introduced by hospice long ago. Palliative care is to help walk along with the patient for this last part of life' (Zylicz 1998: 197).

This issue is more important than simply a matter of ethical analysis: the exclusive affirmation of the autonomy principle can prevent us from seeing the wonder of being human in its multidimensionality. To grasp the whole of this mystery, we must consider as well the openness of each human being toward fellow human beings. As early as 1923, Martin Buber, the Jewish philosopher, wrote his pioneering work on being human, *Ich und Du*.[1] With this most valuable contribution, a new insight broke through: one can never be a human being on one's own. As humans, we essentially stand in an open relationship, involved with the reality in which we live, with other humans to whom we owe our existence and who continue to surround us, and ultimately – for those who believe – with God. If humans wish to be fully themselves, they stand in need of encounter with others and of being encountered by others. This is a fundamental insight that can also guide us in our approach to the dying person and in the understanding of the relational structure of palliative care (Schotsmans 1992).

Even more crucial to this description of the caring relationship is the work of Emmanuel Levinas, who was born in 1906 in Lithuania and died in Paris in 1995.[2] His contribution has been explained thus:

> *Autrui* is arguably the key term in all of Levinas's work and, in line with common French usage, it is Levinas's word for the human other, the other person. The claim here is that the relation with the other goes beyond comprehension, and that it does not affect us in terms of a theme or a concept. If the other person were reducible to the concept I have of him or her, then that would make the relation to the other a relation of knowledge or an epistemological feature. For Levinas, this relation to the other irreducible to comprehension, what he calls the 'original relation', takes place in the concrete situation of speech. Although Levinas's choice of terminology suggests otherwise, the face-to-face relation with the other is not a relation of perception or vision, but is always linguistic. The face is not something I see, but something I speak to. Furthermore, in speaking or calling or listening to the other, I am not reflecting upon them, but I am actively and existentially engaged in a non-subsumptive relation, where I focus on the particular individual in front of me . . . this leads to a significant insight . . . it is the relation which is ethical, not an ethics that is instantiated in relations.
>
> (Critchley and Bernasconi 2001: 15–16)

These fundamental insights on relational anthropology will now be clarified. They present us with a foundational ethical framework for an adequate integration of palliative care in an ethical project. An illustrative case may guide us in discovering the richness of the anthropological clarification of Levinas.

A case history

The following case description illustrates the strongly relational and ethical structure of the caring relationship surrounding the dying patient. The case was presented to the author by a physician who works in a palliative care unit that had recently celebrated its tenth anniversary.

Mr A (and Mr B)

Mr A is more than 80 years old. He has lived for some 50 years with his friend, Mr B. About six years ago, he developed an otorhinolaryngeal cancer which was treated with surgery and radiotherapy. As a consequence of this treatment, he now has a dry mouth and a facial asymmetry. For three months he has had serious problems with swallowing. Sometimes he vomits and pushes food out by his nose. His general practitioner has decided to send him to an academic hospital. Several diagnostic examinations are applied to find the cause of his problems. Unfortunately, these do not clarify the specific aetiology. The medical team discovers a mycosis (mould) and spasms of the inferior oesofagus. After treatment of the infection, they propose to the patient the insertion of a gastric tube in order to feed him. His problems are without any doubt secondary effects (late but irreversible) of the cancer therapy. Mr A returns home with the doctors' reassurance that there is no other cause for the problems he is having. Nevertheless, he remains feeling sad and believes that he is going to die. Some days later, he arrives in the emergency unit of St John's Hospital in Brussels. He still feels sad and wants to know why. He is hospitalized in a medical unit (Internal Medicine). New diagnostic tests are applied. These reveal anaemia, a minor renal insufficiency but most important of all, the presence of multiple hepatic metastases. The change to his general condition is now proceeding rapidly and the emaciation has become a state of cachexis.

His facial paralysis is definite, also the paralysis of a vocal cord makes it difficult for him to make himself understood. The late secondary effects seem to develop further and together with the presence of his hepatic metastases, they explain his pathology. During his stay, Mr A develops pneumonia due to bad swallowing, which is duly treated.

During the month of his stay in the Internal Medicine Unit, the patient makes regular requests for assisted suicide and eventually also euthanasia. He receives anxiolytic doses. He is transferred then to the palliative care unit in the same hospital. His situation is critical. The patient is in a terminal condition.

During his admission to the palliative care unit, the team finds a sad, even depressed patient, but is he really depressed? He cries a lot and speaks continuously about his wish to die. He requests also – with the same intensity – that he needs someone at his bedside. He tells the nurses that he feels abandoned and that he is cold, despite the fact that the nurses give him several blankets to warm him up. He maintains that he feels cold inside himself.

During the clinical examination, a light bronchitis is diagnosed, but his tender liver does not cause pain. Mr A often repeats his request to see his friend, who comes every evening for a visit but cannot stay long for reasons he describes as private. Continuously, Mr A requests 'something' which will allow him to die quickly without any suffering. He also tries regularly to come out of his bed and to go to the window in what may be a suicidal intention.

The symptoms of his bronchitis become more and more serious. He must therefore be regularly aspirated. He has frequent diarrhoea, probably due to the artificial feeding, and also due to the digestive interventions in the past. The symptomatic treatment of Internal Medicine is of course continued.

The physician starts wondering whether the artificial feeding must be continued, well knowing that Mr A's physical condition is degrading and that he remains cachectic, while continuously asking to die. She discusses this with the team. After some days of evaluation and discussion within the team, after attentive listening to the patient and his friend, the team proposes to diminish progressively the amount of feeding, while continuing hydration. With a lot of humour Mr A observes that he prefers to receive 'champagne' instead of water.

A very light sedation will be applied with this therapeutic limitation (désescalade), in order to help him forget his suffering. The patient quickly reaches a peaceful acceptance under the explicit condition that the physician should stay very close to him, which she does. This decision is communicated to the whole team, as also is his request that the nurses should be present at his bedside. Volunteers take over regularly from the nurses and stay with him. His friend and his relatives are contacted and informed, as also his general practitioner. Several contacts with his general practitioner have helped the palliative care team to better understand Mr A and his background.

Nevertheless, a meeting between his friend and the physician is planned: the nursing team observes that both share a secret. During this conversation his friend decides to reveal an intimate part of his life. Indeed, they share a secret. With great kindness his friend describes the lifestyle of Mr A: he was always very 'coquet', 'raffiné', proud of his appearance. He invested a lot of energy in his 'good looks'. Since the vomiting has started, he could not stay at the table and he felt he gave a bad impression and was ashamed about his self-image. He felt he had lost every seductive attraction.

The physician became aware that both men needed a moment of reconciliation: they wished to be reconciled with each other, but were not able to do so. But from that moment on, his friend was more available and paid more visits to the unit.

Meanwhile, the disease is progressing, the patient gets weaker and he is somnolent. But he has stopped repeating his wish to die. This is a surprise for the team, as is the fact that he is not dying, despite the fact that his treatment is limited and he is lightly sedated. Is there not a contradiction between his requests for euthanasia and his desire?

His friend has finally decoded this mystery: Mr A indeed wants to die, but is anxious to encounter his mother about whom he has until now never spoken. Yet his mother has played an important role in his life, through her authority, her lack of recognition of the worth of her son, and her denial of his homosexuality. The palliative care team asks his friend to intervene, to communicate about this anxiety in a long conversation with his partner.

The team did not ask him what were the words he said and what helped Mr A to let his life go and to die peacefully. The initiative was very difficult for everyone involved, certainly not comfortable, indeed courageous, but also confidential. But it created the opportunity for Mr A to pass away in the peace he requested.

This narrative is full of inter-subjective and dialogical challenges and comprises much more than the story of the dying patient alone. It is clear that the relationship between the professional caregivers and the patient, between the patient and his friend, between the patient and his mother, are all crucial elements in understanding the existential crisis of Mr A. It is evident that the quality of life of this patient is linked to the quality of the relationships with those significant others who are surrounding him and taking care of him. Cicely Saunders described this experience very accurately:

> A short time of true attention can often reach such bitterness and quieten angers and fears. Answers are not really expected and long sessions are not always needed. Old structures and values emerge almost unbidden to make sense again, and sometimes new discoveries develop from the interchange with a committed person.
>
> (Saunders 1993: 11)

Care for the dying as an inter-human process

Very often, the world of the dying person is wrongly assessed through the eyes of the bystanders and the life context of the dying person is frequently misunderstood. The narrative story of Mr A and Mr B is illustrative of the difficult process of encounter and understanding. A number of elements make clear how frequently and how easily people speak about the dying, but how little the voice and the reality of the dying person is heard and represented. Too often, the wrong criteria are used to judge the commitment of those who sit by the deathbed for hours, those who can bring human nearness alive with a small gesture. For the dying person, all of this has a totally different dimension than what may simply be observed.

The exchange between the one seeming to be in need of assistance and the one who is offering care is strongly influenced by the life history of the dying patient and by the ethical claims on the caregivers. The most difficult kinds of questions are obviously those which touch the companion as a human being (for example, the friend, the physician and the nurses around Mr A). Those who have the courage to go into these challenges do not escape a confrontation with the meaning of their own lives. Where the dying person may become a question to themselves, this happens simultaneously to the accompanying person as well. Being with a dying person, therefore, really means actually participating in the process of dying: the companion comes to deal with their own death, the fate that every human being has to face. Human accompaniment of the dying person is not possible therefore unless the relationship between the dying person and the companions is taken with utmost seriousness. This is the revolutionary insight of palliative care, when fully established as relational care.

Responding to the ethical claim of the dying person

Within modern healthcare, until recently, the physician and other caregivers attended to a patient on the basis of their own specialization: they knew, and some still consider they know, what is best for the patient on the basis of their insight into what is good for the patient's health. In other words, the responsibility of the caregiver was formulated in the first person: 'I (as doctor, nurse . . . member of the family) take the responsibility for such and such a decision, for this unique person or for this concrete action'. The patient entrusted themselves fully to this strange world full of expertise without, however, considering themselves to be a partner in the process. In other words, the patient remained passive in what was decided and done for them.

Since 1970, bioethics has reacted to this overwhelming paternalism with the 'principlist' approach. The authors of the *Principles of Biomedical Ethics*, a standard textbook for Anglo-American bioethics, developed four prima facie principles: beneficence, non-maleficence, autonomy and justice. In their own words:

> We defend what has sometimes been called the *four-principles* approach to biomedical ethics, and also called, somewhat disparagingly, *principlism* . . . That four clusters of moral 'principles' (in another framework they might be developed as 'rights', 'virtues', or 'values') are central to biomedical ethics is a conclusion we have reached by the search for considered judgments and coherence, not a position that receives an argued defense . . . The four clusters of principles are (1) respect for

autonomy (a norm of respecting the decisionmaking capacities of autonomous persons), (2) nonmaleficence (a norm of avoiding the causa-
tion of harm), (3) beneficence (a group of norms for providing benefits
and balancing benefits against risks and costs), and (4) justice (a group
of norms for distributing benefits, risks, and costs fairly). Nonmaleficence and beneficence have played a central historical role in medical
ethics, whereas respect for autonomy and justice were neglected in
traditional medical ethics but have come into prominence because of
recent developments.

(Beauchamp and Childress 1994: 37–8)

Unfortunately, 'principlists' have been unable to give expression to the caring
relationship and have stressed more the process of decision-making than
the process of care. Even more, the principle of autonomy has been used as
an ethical instrument to change medical paternalism into a paternalism
emanating from the patient.

It can however be argued that this self-determination by the patient is not
an adequate answer to medical paternalism. Stressing the importance of the
principle of autonomy as radically as do the 'principlists' is more an expression of a one-sided anthropological insight in human existence than a good
pathway for the patient–caregiver relationship. This change can also be described in medical experience. Therefore, the concept of responsibility needs
to be reconsidered in the light of a full relational anthropology. This has led
to another understanding of responsibility: no longer 'I am responsible', but
'I have been made responsible by the patient', that is with all of my expertise I lend myself to the promotion of the well-being of the patient. In this
way the patient has become a real and full partner in the process of care.

This new understanding of responsibility is indeed influenced by the relational anthropology of Martin Buber and Emmanuel Levinas (Levinas [1961]
1969, [1974] 1981, [1963] 1990; Burggraeve 1981, 1985; Critchley and
Bernasconi 1991). The ethical relationship is interpreted as a relationship in
which the other offers themself to me in their being other. Thus they no
longer subject themself to a meaning relative to my attitude to them. That
most proper to the countenance of the other is that it appeals to me, hence
there is a real ethical claim of the patient on the caregiver. The core ethical
question is then: to what extent do I permit myself to be appealed to by the
patient who has entrusted themself to my care? Through this appeal the
patient directs themself radically towards me as the caregiver. I can perhaps
run away from my responsibility, but I can never pretend it does not exist.

When the patient beholds me

One of the most essential conditions for the development of this dialogical
encounter is undoubtedly that the caregiver experiences a sense of being

made responsible for the patient. This means that one attempts to respond to the appeal or the ethical claim that comes from the patient: that one turns to them with a willingness to meet them, to devote attention to them and to care for them. An expert reply – and expertise itself – remain a prerequisite. But the relative value of this expertise must be situated correctly: fundamentally one is dealing with an inter-human event, involving both the attendant and the dying person. This relationship, furthermore, is entirely ethical in nature: the other confronts me and encounters me as a radical arrest of my egocentric desires, but they can do this only from a situation of extreme vulnerability. This reality of extreme vulnerability is quite familiar for everyone who is involved in the development of adequate palliative care. Thus, it should be clear how intense the concept of ethical appeal can become. In any case, healthcare is placed in a new perspective: it is no longer the intention of the caregivers or the maintenance of the institution that is of primary importance, but rather the well-being of each patient and the promotion of dignity.

As became quite clear in the narrative of Mr A, the dying Mr A challenged strongly the ethical responsibility of his friend, his doctor and the caregivers surrounding him. The complex but dialogical and interrelated process of care nevertheless made it possible to realize for Mr A a death with dignity. All were challenged by his extreme vulnerability and all were made responsible for a humane dying process. For others, looking Mr A in the face at the same time broke open the possibility of the acceptance of their own life and their own death.

The way we describe this relational structure of palliative care is a simplistic translation of the relational approach of Levinas. We can now clarify more philosophically what we understand by this ethical claim, coming from the Face of the Other. In doing this, it is helpful to follow the clarification of Levinas and his translator Burggraeve (1977, 1985).[3]

The face's epiphany

To show the Face's radical otherness, we must indeed briefly clarify what Levinas understands by the pre-eminent otherness of the 'Other'. Now, to describe the Other, he begins with the classic western definition of 'metaphysics', *ta meta ta physica*, that is what lies behind the *fusis*, the nature of humanity and the world; what surpasses the sensual, the material, the earthly or worldly toward the 'supra-natural', the invisible, the spiritual, immaterial or divine. Therefore, metaphysics in its general and formal guise appears in the history of thought as a movement which proceeds from a familiar world toward a foreign country, from a *chez-soi*, which we inhabit to an unknown *hors-de-soi*. It is thus directed toward the 'elsewhere', the 'other than', the 'beyond', the 'other'.

According to Levinas, not every 'otherness' is of a radically metaphysical character. The metaphysical Other is different in an eminent sense: it is not relatively but absolutely other. The realities which I meet in my world, such as the bread I eat, the country or house where I live, the object I am holding, originally do not possess a certain otherness. Yet from my neediness I integrate them into my existence and reduce them to myself or an extension of myself as food, shelter or an instrument. In this way they lose their 'foreignness' and they shed their otherness, or better: they possess only a relative otherness.

However, the metaphysical Other knows how to maintain its otherness before every reducing covetousness. This otherness, of course, can persevere only when it does not come from elsewhere, that is when it is not based on mere contradiction or an opposition to the other than itself. Only the Other that obtains its otherness intrinsically and constitutively from itself can maintain itself. This implies that metaphysical otherness cannot be a 'border idea'. It cannot arise from the nostalgia of an unfulfilled and failed being that from its needy disaster situation designs a 'better existence in another world' without having any touchstone in reality. Only a real otherness (compare the *autrui*) can be radical.

The Other appears before the narcissistically totalizing I as a given fact that the I cannot reduce to its own totality. The I that self-confidently draws the world to itself is, as it were, startled by the Other's appearance.

The Face's nakedness is further concretized through its glance and word. The eyes are the pre-eminent facial zone from which appears the Other's unmediated presence. The manner in which a being breaks through the form in which it appears is concretely the being's glance. This breakthrough does not precede the glance, to break through one's form is precisely to look: the eyes are absolutely naked. The glance manifests from itself the hard substantial core which makes the Other different. In his glance the Other shows his totally independent manner of being which comes from within. In this context, Levinas speaks of an 'absolute', 'pure' and 'heteronomous' experience: in the Face's glance I experience a totally absolute fact that I cannot avoid. The Other looks me straight in the eyes: via the glance we stand 'eye-to-eye' with one another (*face à face*) in a totally immediate manner. In this way I experience the Other as the pre-eminent fact that 'traumatizes' and 'surprises' me (*traumatisme de l'étonnement*).

However, most characteristic of the Face is that it speaks, or better, that it addresses me. The Other comes from itself toward me and addresses me. On so doing, it comes into direct contact with me. Therefore, within inter-human relationships the vocative linguistic form is more fundamental than the indicative or thematising. Now, in this addressing, the Face is pre-eminently 'self-expression'. The content of the Other's self-expression is nothing other than the essential quality of its existence, namely its absolute otherness. It is not what the Face says that is here essential, but the fact that it speaks, the fact of its expression, of its appearance.

A closer look at this 'self-revelation' shows that it has an ethical character: the face is the fact that a being touches us not in the indicative but in the imperative. The Other's radical otherness implies this ethical-imperative structure. The Face's metaphysical strangeness must be described as an *étrangeté-misère*. We see this from the Face's very essence. As radical otherness it possesses not only an absolute irreducibility and hard resistance, but also an extreme vulnerability. The strangeness which is freedom is at the same time strangeness-as-misery. The Face's nakedness proceeds to the nakedness of its body, which suffers cold and is ashamed of its nakedness. Existence *kath'auto* is a misery in this world.

It is just this 'depth of misery' or 'humility' in which the Other lives, that makes the Face's command ethical. As strangeness or otherness the Face indeed demands my recognition and hospitality. But as helpless poverty, it can neither from physical nor from moral superiority compel me to give it. The Other is not only my superior, but also my subordinate. Therefore, they can only ask me to come to their aid in their misery. Because of the Face's powerlessness the Other turns their absolute demand to the begging 'please'. In his own evocative, nearly poetic style, Levinas speaks here of the Face's timidity that 'does not dare to dare'. It is a 'solicitation' that is not sufficiently hard and brutal to be a request or an 'application for' hospitality. It is a 'beggar's plea', almost inaudibly mumbled with bowed head. Or to use another image, the Face looks to me pleadingly with a timid, half-lowered glance.

Only through this begging does the demand become ethical. A demand is ethical only when it is directed toward and calls upon a freedom, that is when there is a summons or appeal which cannot physically – or in any other way – manipulate or force this freedom. On the other side, the begging is ethical only when it includes an absolute and unavoidable *ought*, otherwise it remains an uncommitted question, to which one may or may not respond according to one's wish or will. In short, the Face is ethical because it is simultaneously demand and begging, or rather because it may beg only to the extent that it also demands and may demand only to the extent that it also begs.

If we translate this emphatic (continually self-deepening and 'over-exerting') analysis of 'accusation' into ethical terms, then we must posit that in the Face I discover that my freedom is an egocentric imperialism, which overwhelms and murders. I realize that the spontaneity and the vital drive towards self-development from which, up to that moment, I proceeded without even a glance to the right or left, is not nearly as innocent as I thought in my self-sufficient autonomy. The activity of the conscience in me is therefore my ascertaining the 'bodies' beside me and my revulsion at my existence as a murderer. This discovery brings forth in me a feeling of being ashamed of myself.

From this we see that the responsibility for the Other, which flows forth from the Face's appeal, essentially begins as an absolute 'heteronomy': I am no longer the law, rather, the Other is. I am no longer the 'measure of all things', but rather the one being 'measured'. Without being asked I become responsible because of the Other's appearance. To stand in the Other's place is at the same time to be answerable for the Other, or put more strongly: a 'responsibility' for the Other's responsibility. Levinas concretizes this radicality by positing that my responsibility extends up to and includes the obligation to render account concerning the Other's freedom, which directly implies that I continually have to go one step further, that I have one additional degree of responsibility.

Levinas also likes to express the same idea with a quotation from Dostoevsky's *The Brothers Karamazov*: 'each of us is guilty before all, for all, and I more than all others'. In his typical expansive manner he speaks of the whirlpool or spiral of responsibility:

> the Other's suffering, my compassing with his suffering, his suffering as a result of my compassion, my pain as a result of this suffering etc . . . stop with me. In all this repetition I am the one who has to make one movement more.
>
> (Levinas [1974] 1981: 186)

This spiral implies that I am also responsible for the Other's failures and faults. I stand accused of the evil they perform; I am an 'accessory' to their faults, nevertheless, without being personally guilty of them. In the Face's radical claim, I cannot wash my hands in innocence as if what the Other does is no concern of mine. I cannot retreat to my ivory tower and be satisfied with my quiet conscience with regard to what I have done, because the evil in the world touches me and gives me no peace. For Levinas, the one who closes himself up in his subjective responsibility on the basis of his freedom and the thereto related 'ability to be called to account' is the image of the *Pharisee*.

The relational approach and palliative care

As described by Levinas, the Face's metaphysical strangeness must be described as an *étrangeté-misère*. The narrative of Mr A and Mr B may help us to clarify more clearly the relational structure of palliative care. The extreme vulnerability of Mr A is undeniable: his facial paralysis is marked, likewise the paralysis of a vocal cord makes it difficult for him to make himself understood. He cries a lot and speaks continuously about his wish to die. It is difficult to imagine greater vulnerability and dependency.

But at the same time, his demand is strong: he needs someone at his bed-side. This is an imperative demand, although Mr A is totally dependent on the willingness of his caregivers to accept his request. A little bit later he requests the physician to stay very close to him. His vulnerability is also exemplified in the short visits of his friend: 'both share a secret'. The caregivers and the physician became aware that both Mr A and Mr B need a moment of reconciliation. They promote this through the relational encounter between the two men and the subsequent possibility of a peaceful dying process.

Finally, there is the anxiety about the encounter with his mother, who has never accepted his homosexuality. Again, the caregivers and Mr B pro-mote the communication about this anxiety and this initiative creates the opportunity for Mr A to pass away in the peace he has requested.

The physician recognizes that all words (like anxiety and despair, but also like hope, trust and even transcendence) are relative. Promotion of the relations between Mr A and his friend, his doctor, his nurses and volunteers and finally, his mother becomes something eminently ethical in character.

The narrative of Mr A (in the words of his physician) may help us to understand that the human accompaniment of the dying is not possible unless the relationship between the dying person and the caregivers is taken with utmost seriousness. The work required will take a great deal of effort on the part of all involved. This indicates clearly that the relational structure of palliative care is a crucial aspect in the promotion of a dignified death. Dying is indeed human only when it is lived through as an inter-human process. Even when the dying patient is unconscious or cannot express themself, the relational structure of the dying process remains strongly present in the caring responsibility of those being made responsible by the dying patient.

Conclusion

Cicely Saunders has described the palliative care experience in these words of a patient: 'I thought it so strange. Nobody wants to look at me. And then doctor, I came here and you listened to me. I felt you understood. It seems the pain went with me speaking to you!' (Saunders 1993: 11). We must continue to clarify palliative care as a form of relational care. This chapter is intended to function as an invitation to take relational philosophy in general and Levinas in particular as a significant guide in developing an ethical foundation to the experience of palliative care as a relational challenge.

Notes

1 The first words of a human being are not words on their own, but coupled words. The first word is the coupleword I–thou, the other word is the coupleword I–it. (Buber 1923: 9).

2 E. Levinas (1906–95) was born an orthodox Russian Jew in Kaunas, Lithuania. In 1923 he emigrated to France, of which he was made a citizen on 6 April 1931. There he became simultaneously philosophically active and engaged in the life of the so-called 'third' of French Jewry (esp. as director from 1946 to 1975 of the 'Ecole Normale Israélite Orientale' in Paris). See Burggraeve (1985; see also Burggraeve 1981). The most important works of Levinas are *Totalité et infini* (1961), *Autrement qu'être ou au-delà de l'essence* (1974) and *Difficile liberté* (1963).

3 Roger Burggraeve is professor of fundamental moral theology at the Catholic University of Leuven in Belgium. He has also published a bibliography of studies both by and on Levinas (see Burggraeve 1977).

References

Beauchamp, T.L. and Childress, J.F. (1994) *Principles of Biomedical Ethics*, 4th edn. New York: Oxford University Press.

Beemer, T. (1981) Een voorstel tot kernontwapening, *Tijdschrift voor Theologie*, 21: 245–64.

Beemer, T. (1984) Je leven: in de waagschaal of op de weegschaal?, *Tijdschrift voor Theologie*, 24: 36–55.

Buber, M. (1923) *Ich und Du*. Leipzig: Insel-Verlag.

Burggraeve, R. (1977) Emmanuel Levinas: une bibliographie, *Salesianum*, 39: 634–92.

Burggraeve, R. (1981) The ethical basis for a human society according to Emmanuel Levinas, *Ephemerides Theologicae Lovanienses*, 57: 5–57.

Burggraeve, R. (1985) *From Self-development to Solidarity: An Ethical Reading of Human Desire in its Socio-political Relevance According to Emmanuel Levinas*. Leuven: Peeters.

Critchley, S. and Bernasconi, R. (eds) (1991) *Re-reading Levinas*. Bloomington, IN: Indiana University Press.

Critchley, S. and Bernasconi, R. (eds) (2001) *The Cambridge Companion to Levinas*. Cambridge: Cambridge University Press.

Jeffrey, D. (2000) Care versus cure, in P. Webb (ed.) *Ethical Issues in Palliative Care: Reflections and Considerations*. Manchester: Hochland and Hochland.

Kuitert, H. and van Leeuwen, E. (1998) A religious argument in favor of euthanasia and assisted suicide, in D.C. Thomasma, T. Kimbrough-Kushner, G.K. Kimsma and C. Ciesielski-Carlucci (eds) *Asking to Die: Inside the Dutch Debate about Euthanasia*. Dordrecht: Kluwer.

Levinas, E. ([1961] 1969) *Totality and Infinity*, trans. A. Lingis. Pittsburgh, PA: Duquesne University Press; *Totalité et infini*. The Hague: Martinus Nijhoff.

Levinas, E. ([1974] 1981) *Autrement qu'être ou au-delà de l'essence* (*Otherwise than Being or Beyond Essence*), trans. A. Lingis. The Hague: Martinus Nijhoff.

Levinas, E. ([1963] 1990) *Difficult Freedom*, trans. S. Hand. London: Athlone; *Difficile liberté: essais sur le Judaïsme*. Paris: A. Michel.

Pijnenburg, M.A.M. (1998) Catholic healthcare and the Dutch national character, in D.C. Thomasma, T. Kimbrough-Kushner, G.K. Kimsma and C. Ciesielski-Carlucci (eds) *Asking to Die: Inside the Dutch Debate about Euthanasia*. Dordrecht: Kluwer.

Saunders, C. (1993) Introduction – history and challenge, in C. Saunders and N. Sykes (eds) *The Management of Terminal Malignant Disease*, 3rd edn. London: Edward Arnold.

Schotsmans, P. (1992) *En de mens schiep de mens: Medische revolutie en ethiek*, 3rd edn. Kapellen: Pelckmans.

Zylicz, Z. (1998) Palliative care: Dutch hospice and euthanasia, in D.C. Thomasma, T. Kimbrough-Kushner, G.K. Kimsma and C. Ciesielski-Carlucci (eds) *Asking to Die: Inside the Dutch Debate about Euthanasia*. Dordrecht: Kluwer.

PART III

Ethics and palliative care practice

Introduction to Part III

The final part of this book turns to some of the most central (and in some cases more familiar) bioethical issues which relate to palliative care. Again, in several cases the authors develop their arguments in contradistinction to the concerns of 'principlist' bioethics, but they also build on this work, seeking out its relevance in the palliative care context.

Simon Woods contributes a chapter which explores the argument concerning respect for autonomy and begins by examining the evolution of its place within healthcare ethics and the extent to which autonomy is something distinctive of persons. He examines the notion that central to respect for persons is the idea of respect for their capacity for self-determination. But of course a person's self-determined choices may make demands on others, or society in general, raising an argument for limiting personal autonomy. Here Woods brings in the concept of axiology – a vision of the good life which is greater than the particulars in which people take pleasure. It is in this context that palliative care can be seen to possess a distinct set of values and it is here that a number of moral principles of palliative care become important. Woods discusses the 'good' death and family-centred care in particular. He also examines the stance of palliative care *vis-à-vis* euthanasia and finds here a contradiction between the palliative care opposition to euthanasia and its claim to respect autonomy.

In Chapter 9 an ethicist and a physician combine their efforts to address the important question of sedation at the end of life. Bert Broeckaert and Juan Manuel Núñez Olarte offer considerable conceptual clarity to this foggy area, where much discussion and some research evidence is now appearing in the literature. These authors eschew the usage of 'terminal sedation' in favour of the term 'palliative sedation' and they offer their own definition. In particular they establish clear water between the practices of euthanasia and sedation in the final phases of life. Their key to this is the concept of proportionality: interventions, drugs and dosages must be proportional to the relief of symptoms and a match achieved between symptoms present and the degree of sedation required. Their helpful discussion of this issue is good evidence of the gains which can result when ethicists and clinicians combine their efforts in the search for solutions to complex problems.

Chapter 10, on euthanasia and physician-assisted suicide, is also written by medical doctors and an ethicist. As elsewhere in the book, Bert Gordijn, Ben Crul and Zbigniew Zylicz make good use of case studies, one in which euthanasia takes place and the other in which it does not. This chapter does several important things: it exposes some serious flaws in the arguments of beneficence and respect for autonomy used as supports for euthanasia; it also questions some assumptions within the principle of double effect; finally, although it exposes weaknesses in the 'slippery slope' argument, it does find a certain veracity within it. The chapter ends by briefly suggesting that palliative care may serve a useful purpose in helping to reassess some of our cherished cultural values of control and independence.

In Chapter 11, Franz-Josef Illhardt and Henk ten Have explore the theme of research ethics in palliative care. Concentrating in particular on research conducted within the biomedical paradigm, they also examine the ethical issues which should govern the conduct of research in palliative care. In particular, they argue that terminally ill patients should be regarded as autonomous and capable of giving consent to participation in studies. However, the risks of participation must also be balanced with the benefits, and here the role of research ethics review committees is important.

Chapter 12, by Henk ten Have and Rien Janssens, raises a less discussed topic within the ethics of palliative care: the issue of futility. Although futility has been much discussed by writers concerned with the limits of both life-prolonging and curative healthcare interventions, there is a sense in which, until very recently, it has been ignored as an issue for palliative care, which might generally be thought to begin when 'futile' interventions have been largely abandoned. Needless to say, this is an oversimplification. In particular it raises the question of whether care itself can ever become futile. From the deontological perspective, the answer to this would be no; but utilitarians might take a different view.

By the end of Part III of the book a broad picture of the ethics of palliative care in the European context has been offered: from historical and sociological analyses of conceptual and institutional development; through a consideration of underlying moral principles; to the analysis of some crucial ethical issues confronting contemporary practice. Finally, the editors offer a concluding chapter, drawing out key issues for further analysis and highlighting the benefits of a wide-ranging approach to both empirical and theoretical issues in bioethics as they relate to palliative care.

Respect for autonomy
and palliative care

■ SIMON WOODS

One of the central concerns of ethics is to establish what sort of entity has moral value and this in turn involves a consideration of both the sorts of *thing* to which we owe moral duties and the nature of those duties. In healthcare ethics we think almost exclusively in terms of humans as the focus of moral significance. Yet the question of what makes a human of moral worth remains a debated question, whether it is being *human* per se or whether it is the possession of particular *properties* which some humans may have and some may not. In ethics there has been a move towards the view that merely being human is not sufficient to establish the moral status of a thing. In one sense being human is too inclusive, since cells, corpses and cancers can all be *human* yet clearly they are not of the same moral status as a human person. In another sense being human is too exclusive, a form of *speciesism*, seemingly ruling out the possibility of morally valuable entities of a non-human kind. There is some consensus that it is in virtue of certain properties that humans gain their moral status and the concept of autonomy, the capacity to think and choose for oneself, has become a dominant contender as a necessary condition of moral value (Harris 1985; Beauchamp and Childress 2001). Autonomy has emerged as a modern criterion of moral worth providing the grounds to distinguish between being merely *alive* and being *meaningfully* alive. The importance of this capacity for autonomy has led to the recognition that a principle of respect for autonomy ought to have a central role in demonstrating respect for persons. It is therefore not surprising that such a principle should have gained a prominent place within contemporary (particularly Anglo-Saxon) healthcare ethics given that respect for autonomy underpins several of the important foundations to ethical practice such as consent, confidentiality and effective communication. If respect for autonomy is both relevant and important to healthcare practice it is ever more so to the delivery of palliative care. But what exactly does respect for autonomy imply?

In this chapter some of the implications of this principle for palliative care will be explored. First, the meaning and evolution of autonomy will be discussed. The debate concerning autonomy in the context of palliative care will take into account the evolving nature of palliative care and consider the extent to which the principle of respect for autonomy is compatible, or in conflict with, the core values of palliative care. The aim of discussing issues such as euthanasia, terminal sedation and family-centred care is to indicate the work that needs to be done in order to fully integrate the principle of respect for autonomy into palliative care, and at the same time defend the other important values which palliative care advances.

Autonomy and healthcare ethics

There is no single historical source for the meaning of autonomy. Its ancient origin lies in Greek political theory which refers to the *autos* (self) and *nomos* (governing) nature of the citizens who made their own laws. In the modern era autonomy has been associated with the ethics of Immanuel Kant who argued that autonomy and the mutual respect for others' autonomy are a prerequisite of moral action. Farsides (1998), in her discussion of autonomy in palliative care, captures the Kantian influence on the concept of autonomy when she says that 'the most valuable form of autonomy entails voluntarily choosing to do that which is right' (Farsides 1998: 148).

Other influences on the contemporary meaning of autonomy include the evolving concept of the 'self' and individuality. The now commonplace notion of the autonomous self has evolved out of a backdrop of rebellion against traditional sources of authority such as the church and state. The contemporary concept of the 'self' or 'person' is bound up with a politics of non-interference into the personal life of the individual and this is strongly reflected in the legislatures of many nations across the globe. In the context of healthcare, autonomy or the principle of respect for autonomy, has been championed by ethicists of many different theoretical persuasions as a central if not *the* most important ethical principle. Although there may be differences in the priority and scope accorded this principle, there is general agreement that autonomy has challenged and now seems set to replace the ethic of paternalism.

However, it is one thing to accept that autonomy is of *general* importance in healthcare but quite another to suggest that autonomy is of pre-eminent importance. The idea that we ought to respect a person's autonomous choices may be seen to conflict with the other important moral goals of healthcare, namely to do actual good for people with regard to their healthcare needs.

There are several important questions that must be addressed in order to establish the place of autonomy within the ethics of healthcare. Are all individuals equally autonomous? Are the different decisions made by one individual equally autonomous? To what extent are we obliged to respect autonomous assertions? Individuals live within a network of meaningful relationships such as family and friends, individuals are also part of a community, all of which suggests that the degree to which an individual's wishes are respected may be curtailed out of consideration for the interests of others or for the common good.

While it may be possible to determine the goals of healthcare in terms of the good that healthcare aims to promote, it requires a different set of considerations to justify how such goals may be legitimately met. It would seem to follow, at least, that no person should be compelled to comply with a healthcare regime even for their own good, saving for the most exceptional circumstances.

Autonomy as a valued capacity has particular prominence in the liberal political framework (Kymlicka 1990). Liberals value autonomy because of a scepticism about the possibility of identifying any *single* conception of the good life for a person. Liberals would therefore always challenge any interference by another individual or external authority in the life of a person, thereby defending the right of the individual to choose for themselves (Dworkin 1993; Savulescu 1997). This said, autonomy is by no means clearly conceived either by liberals or by others. There is first the problem of definition and second the problem of deciding what exactly is entailed by the claim that autonomy ought to be respected. The second question is impossible to address without addressing the question of definition first.

There are at least three key, but by no means exhaustive, aspects of autonomy, which contribute to its contemporary meaning. These are autonomy as a defining feature of persons, autonomy as an aspect of axiology and autonomy as an ethical principle, the principle of respect for autonomy. I shall say something about each aspect in turn while also raising questions of their relevance to palliative care.

Autonomy as a definining feature of persons

John Locke defines 'person' as 'a thinking intelligent Being, that has reason and reflection, and can consider it self as it self, the same thinking thing in different times and places' (Locke 1976: 162). This definition has proved influential on modern thinking, placing the essence of the person in intellectual rather than spiritual or even uniquely *human* characteristics (Woods 2000). Locke's account does however provide a basis for attributing a *moral* value to persons since it is by exercising such capacities that persons reveal their power to choose for themselves, to direct and control their own lives, to value themselves, arguably to value anything at all (Harris 1985).

The exercise, indeed the mere possession, of such capacities has become synonymous with autonomy. The capacity to value is linked to those capacities that are distinctive of persons outlined in Locke's account, the capacity for reason and reflection. Locke's account has been widely influential, hence in Kant's ethics an individual is a moral agent only in so far as the individual has the capacity to think and reflect.

The formal account of personhood therefore seems essentially bound up with a *moral* account of the person. It is the exercise of autonomy that many contemporary ethicists regard as *the* defining characteristic of a morally valuable entity, namely a 'person' (Harris 1985; Dworkin 1988). It is often argued that as a criterion of moral worth autonomy ought to command the highest respect although it remains an ongoing debate just *how* important autonomy is. For convenience I shall refer to this account of autonomy as the Lockean view.

The Lockean view raises further questions concerning what it implies in terms of general moral outlook. The emphasis upon an intellectual criterion of personhood can seem deeply counter-intuitive. According to the Lockean view a human corpse is *human* but no longer a *person*; does this mean that the dead have no moral significance? The *infant* is both human and alive but again on this account not yet a *person*. Similarly, there are adult humans who are alive but would be judged to be no longer persons because they lack the relevant characteristics, the *irreversibly* comatose for example, but even amongst fully conscious individuals there are great variations in their capacities.

If the Lockean view is correct then we are left either to abandon moral considerations with regard to 'non-persons' or to argue for some other ground of moral significance. I would suggest, without here offering an argument, that the former view is repugnant. The latter option constitutes the very business of healthcare ethics and a fortiori for palliative care ethics, where the focus of care from diagnosis through to death is often directed towards the individual with an altered and diminishing capacity for autonomy.

It seems uncontroversial to claim that the practice of healthcare aims at promoting a form of human good, the health, welfare or well-being of patients. It is on the grounds that it is *right* to promote such goods that the moral justifications for the practice of healthcare rests. However, moral debate raises questions that challenge the legitimacy of this claim. For those who place a high premium on autonomy, welfare considerations have no or only minor significance in determining what is good for a person, hence Harris's claim:

> So autonomy, as the ability and the freedom to make the choices that shape our lives, is quite crucial in giving to each life its own special and peculiar value . . . So that where concern for welfare and respect for

wishes are incompatible one with another, concern for welfare must give way to respect for autonomy.

(Harris 1995: 11)

For Harris the welfare of a person, even their very life are legitimate trade-offs in order that a person's autonomy be respected. In a similar vein Dworkin (1986) argues that the value of autonomy is independent of considerations of an agent's welfare since 'autonomy encourages and protects the capacity competent people have to direct their own lives at least generally in accordance with a scheme of value each has recognized and chosen for himself or herself' (Dworkin 1986: 9). Respect for autonomy is therefore crucial to the moral respect for persons and suggests autonomy should be given high regard in the context of healthcare where many decisions will influence the length and quality of a person's life.

However, one of the difficulties we face when trying to put such a principle into practice is that of determining the extent of a person's capacity. People differ in their capacities and even the same individual may alter from moment to moment when under the influence of drugs, pain or extreme emotion. What does respect for autonomy require when an individual has a diminished capacity? Does a person's earlier autonomous self have authority over their later less or non-autonomous self? If we believe that autonomy is important then this suggests that we make serious attempts to identify the means of judging a person's capacity and perhaps set the criteria at a fairly modest level so as to be as inclusive as possible. It also suggests that advance directives be regarded as authoritative even though these instructions may conflict with an individual's current interests.

Any thorough account of a principle of respect for autonomy must consider whether autonomy brings with it *positive rights* or whether it is more concerned with protecting liberty, freedom from interference for example. To what extent does an individual have a right to expect their autonomous decisions to be respected, does a person have the right not only to refuse treatment but also to make positive requests for treatment and care? It is at this point that we turn to consider a further aspect of autonomy, that of axiology.

Autonomy as an aspect of axiology

Axiology is the theory of the good usually taken to mean a theory of the good life without reference to ethics so that when one asks what sort of life is the good life for a person this is usually considered to be a question about self-interest (Parfit 1991). Axiological theories have traditionally attempted to give an account of the good life in terms of a single criterion. Plausible candidates can be roughly grouped under the headings of *subjective* theories and *objective* theories (Parfit 1991; Bowling 1995).

Subjective theories usually try to account for the goodness of a life in either hedonistic terms, that is in terms of the quality of a person's experiences, or in terms of the satisfaction a person feels when their life is going well according to their wishes and preferences. The problem with subjective theories alone is that they may be *necessary* components of a good life but they are far from sufficient to guarantee a good life. The idea that the good life is a life entirely devoted to the pursuit of pleasurable experiences is unconvincing. Pleasurable experiences are, tautologically, *good*, and we no doubt seek such experiences as the end of some of our endeavours. Indeed pleasurable experiences may be essential to a good life but a life that consisted of nothing but the pursuit of pleasurable experiences would be lacking as an account of the good life, in Dworkin's words such a life would not be 'pure but preposterous' (Dworkin 1993: 201). In life we do distinguish between different kinds of pleasure and between pleasure and other more valued ends. The marathon runner will forgo the pleasure of languishing in a warm bed in order to get the training miles in preparation for the race they hope to win. A patient may choose to take a lower dose of analgesia knowing that their pain may be worse but in order to be more alert at visiting time.

Similarly there are limitations on the extent to which the goodness of one's life is truly reflected in the level of satisfaction one experiences. The claim that the goodness of a life is judged by the feeling of satisfaction that we enjoy when our preferences and wishes are fulfilled may be challenged on two fronts. First, with regard to the importance of the *feeling* of satisfaction, and second, with regard to the preferences themselves. Take for example the view that the success of my life is entirely contingent upon the fulfilment of my ambition to climb the highest mountain, Mount Everest. After years of planning and training I eventually struggle up the summit slopes in storm conditions and upon reaching a natural peak I raise my ice axe in triumph, believing my ambition fulfilled. However, what if I was deceived by the storm and mistook a false summit well below the actual summit for the real thing? Imagine further that I never discover my mistake and live out my years satisfied, happy in the belief that my life's ambition to climb Mount Everest has been fulfilled. Clearly it would not be true of me that my life was the success I believed since my life would have failed in this one defining interest. So it is possible to judge the goodness of a life independently of the judgement of the person whose life it is.

Similarly with regard to preferences it would seem reasonable to accept a person's choices and requests as a veridical account of their preferences. But it is odd to claim that what is good for a person is good simply because they *choose* it and are content with their lot. It is clear that the goodness of the life of a person can be judged poor, even if many of their wishes and preferences are satisfied, because their set of preferences is so meagre as to be satisfied by the meanest of existence. Take for example a person referred for palliative care who, having a paralysing fear of death and a lack of insight into the possibilities of symptom control, steadfastly refuses any intervention or care. What this person chooses on the basis of their fear and lack of knowledge will restrict the quality of life they may enjoy even with a terminal illness. It is possible therefore to judge the goodness, at least of some aspects, of a life from a more objective perspective. This said, one must be cautious not to interpret this as an argument justifying the *imposition* of palliative care upon this person. At most it is an argument that it may be right to attempt to allay their fears and persuade them that palliative care has something to offer them, to do more would not be kindness but tyranny.

When considering subjective theories of axiology it is clearly possible to contrast 'experiential interests' with more abiding interests, with ends that even the individual whose life it is, would, all things considered, regard as necessary for a good life. The possibility of judging the goodness of a life independently of the 'felt' qualities of a life suggests there is room for an objective theory of axiology.

First, what do we mean by 'objective'. One sense of 'objective' is to claim that there are certain *necessary* components of a good life of a non-experiential kind or at least of a kind that are not dependent upon the *experiences* of a subject for their evaluation. These are often expressed in very general terms and may be concrete or abstract in nature, health, nourishment, liberty and so on – what Rawls (1971) for example refers to as 'primary goods'. A second sense of 'objective' refers to the possibility of adopting a perspective from which it is possible to judge the goodness of a life so that one could determine whether a component of a life was really good or not. In principle such judgements could be made equally well by the person whose life it is or by a third party. For example drug addicts may recognize that for all the pleasure and satisfaction they gain from their addiction, their life would really be better without their addiction. But it must be recognized that between different people there will be differences of opinion about the relative value and importance of different lifestyles that will not be resolved by appeal to objective qualities in the first sense of objective. People do have different views and beliefs, different ideas about what constitutes a good life when seen as a whole without at the same time rejecting the possibility that such beliefs and plans could be revised. Broadly speaking this view supports the liberal view that there is no absolute authority with regard to what is good hence the priority given to the individual in judging their own good life. As Jeremy Waldron suggests, it is an axiom of liberalism 'that there is something like *pursuing a conception of the good life* that all people, even those with the most diverse commitments, can be said to be engaged in' (Waldron 1987: 145).

The liberal view does not amount to a denial of the objective but argues instead that any objective conception of the good must of necessity be a 'lean' one since any substantive theory of the 'good' life will always be underdetermined by individual conceptions of the good (Rawls 1971). The political implication of this view is that governments should adopt a position of neutrality between different possible conceptions of the good life allowing the greatest possible freedom for individuals to pursue their own conception of it. What holds for governments holds for any institution that makes up society, including relationships between health professional and patient and hence individuals should be allowed to determine the meaning and values of their own life. The upshot of our discussion is that any adequate axiology will attempt to combine both subjective and objective components. No way of life can be endorsed as *the* good life since any objective account of the good will of necessity be very general and lacking in the felt quality that contributes to the goodness of a life. A person may be compelled to adopt a wholesome and healthy lifestyle but it cannot make their life better if they do not also regard such a lifestyle as worthwhile.

Axiology must inevitably involve ethics since it is not enough to consider in what way a life may be judged a good life without considering the sort of life it is permissible to pursue, otherwise axiology becomes nothing more than a report of what people in fact take pleasure in. Unless we are totally sceptical with regard to moral values, some ways of living ought to be condemned as immoral and a person's right to pursue such a life restricted. Generally the liberal view regards a person's own good as insufficient grounds for interference in that person's life. However, the degree to which this principle is adhered to in practice varies greatly even between the most liberal of societies. Many societies accept that some interference, even of a quite draconian kind is justified where an important public interest is at stake, although most restrict interference to cases concerned with the interests of *others* and not the interests of the individual concerned.

The liberal position has had a dominant place in our discussion of axiology because the importance ascribed to autonomy in contemporary ethics relies on such an axiology as a rationale. However, it is still possible to recognize autonomy as important within a more general ethic of respect for persons without accepting the individual person as *the* authoritative source of value. I, like many critics of the liberal position, am disturbed by the rather negative vision of humanity that is implied by liberalism at its extreme. This vision sees humanity as a colony of isolated individuals engaged in competitive negotiations with other equally independent individuals, attempting to agree on the set of compromises that will secure the best sort of life for themselves.

However, not all liberals are wedded to such an extreme view. Indeed some candidly admit that an individual's view of what is good for them may be improved by being challenged by someone with a quite different view (Savulescu 1997). This said there is still disagreement over the relative priority of autonomy both within and between cultures. Some commentators have argued that where autonomy is given a high priority (North America and Northern Europe) there is greater emphasis placed upon the individual over the family or wider community, although this is by no means homogenous. There are other critics who simply reject the priority given to the 'liberal' individual out of hand, such critics argue that individual choices are themselves only possible against a background of shared values (Taylor 1990). So where does palliative care sit with regard to the importance of autonomy? Before addressing this question I will say something about the principle of respect for autonomy.

Autonomy as an ethical principle: the principle of respect for autonomy

Respect for persons is partially understood as respect for *the* person that each person is, the unique ways in which they define themselves through their own choices, actions and beliefs. Respect for persons in general is premised upon this distinctive capacity. So central to respect for persons is respect for their capacity for self-determination, their autonomy. One way in which respect for persons is demonstrated is by equal concern for people's interests, and given the diversity of interests a person may have, this can be achieved only by letting each person choose for themselves the life they wish to pursue.

In the context of palliative care much of what has been said can be accommodated without difficulty. It seems uncontroversial to accept at face value what people say they take pleasure in. It is almost an axiom of palliative care to accept as authoritative what people say about their pains and comfort. Ethics requires that we have good reasons for interfering in another's life and that such interference, in the context of healthcare for example, is limited to advising, informing and challenging, intervening, if at all, only in the most extreme circumstances.

Whether we agree or not with the claim that autonomy is a necessary condition of being a person there is no denying that the capacity to reflect upon different possible goals and choose some over others *is* important in distinguishing one person from another. Making choices and deciding one's goals is what makes an individual unique and if there is value in being an individual then there is good reason to respect such choices and the liberty to exercise them. But what is troubling with the principle of respect for autonomy is that someone's choices may, and often do, make demands of either other individuals or of society. This problem has been variously dealt with by arguing for necessary *limiting* conditions to autonomy such that an individual may exercise their autonomy only to an extent compatible with the same degree of autonomy for others.

The essence of the ethical principle of respect for autonomy therefore is that in order to show respect for a person we ought to respect their capacity for, and liberty to make, their own choices. This said there is the further task of determining the weight attached to autonomy relative to other important values. Such values as the shared goals of social living, the mutual goals and interests shared by a loving couple or a family, the shared goals of a community and the other interests an individual may have. These and other common values may provide good reasons for constraining what an individual may claim for themselves in the name of their autonomy. No individual lives in a vacuum and therefore it seems indefensible to argue that morality demands respect for unbridled autonomy since much of what one chooses for oneself will impinge on others who have an equal claim to their own life and choices. The problem of defining the balance between liberty and justified interference remains a perennial moral problem. Jack's demand to indulge simultaneously in his passion for fast cars and fine wines will conflict with Gill's desire to transport her family along the roads with some guarantee of safety. This seems reason enough for limiting Jack's liberty to indulging in only one of his passions at a time but not reason enough to demand that Jack replace his wine cellar with mineral water because mineral water would be so much better for him, just as in healthcare it is no longer acceptable to coerce a patient in their best interests. The wide consensus on this point is reflected in the concept of consent, that a competent person's permission is required before they may be treated or even touched.

Acknowledging that there are good reasons for limiting a person's autonomy in terms of what they may demand of, or impose on, others is not to say that such limiting clauses are *absolute*. There are circumstances where morality demands that we sacrifice something of our own autonomy in order to respect the specific wishes of another or indeed the important interests of others. Jury service, military conscription and donating blood are all examples where we may be morally required to sacrifice our own autonomy for others.

Palliative care: ethics and axiology

This account of theories of the good is by no means a complete one. There is another important category of what can be called 'transcendental' theories, which adopt a vision of the good life that transcends the particulars in which people take pleasure or satisfaction. The moral implication of such a view is that there is a positive duty to promote a *particular* vision of the good life even though this vision may not be recognized or shared by the individuals concerned. Versions of this form of axiology are evident in both Plato and Aristotle and in religious or politically inspired axiologies. To a limited extent healthcare may be regarded as falling within this category. Healthcare aims to promote a particular good, 'health' that many people, as witnessed through their lifestyle choices, seem not to value or even recognize. The very aim of health promotion for example is to influence and ultimately change people's behaviour even in the face of their expressed desire to behave in a contrary manner. The *raison d'être* of healthcare is that there *is* a version of the good that ought to be promoted. But while in most cases there is no question that this might justify enforcing compliance it does not necessarily mean that individuals should be left simply to choose for themselves. Across the spectrum of healthcare, sophisticated measures are employed to persuade and influence individuals in their choices because a *healthier* life is believed to be a *better* life. An important dilemma within the ethics of healthcare therefore turns on the question of how far it is legitimate to pursue this welfare agenda and at what cost to the individual's autonomy?

An interesting point raised by the possibility of a 'transcendental' theory is that such a theory could challenge scepticism with regard to the good life since it could provide the grounds for challenging the claims of individuals to know with authority what is good for them. There is of course an obvious danger of paternalism with such a claim. However, *if* such a position were tenable it could be seen not as a ground for rejecting autonomy completely, but rather for rethinking the priority of autonomy *vis-à-vis* other important values. Something like this more attenuated account may be an appropriate model for ethical healthcare.

However, there is no consensus as to which version of autonomy should underpin healthcare ethics. At one extreme is Veatch's (1995) view that the only judge of what constitutes 'good' healthcare is the patient. At the other extreme are views like those of Tobias (1997) who argues that since the public has charged doctors to seek the cure for cancer this permits conducting trials even without informed consent, regarded by most as a necessary condition to respect autonomy in research. In the middle are views such as those of Savulescu (1997) who, while defending the individual's right to non-interference, believes it possible to improve one's view of the good through rational discourse. Indeed Savulescu goes so far as to say it is the doctor's duty to engage the patient in such discourse. These differences not only reflect different opinions within healthcare but also are sometimes belied by important cultural differences in attitudes toward autonomy and the status of the individual within society (Clouser and Gert 1999).

We turn now to consider the place of palliative care within this spectrum. One view of palliative care is to see no significant difference between it and any other health discipline. On this narrow view, palliative care is just palliative *medicine* and as such accepts autonomy as part of the secular liberal spectrum that is arguably the foundation of contemporary medical ethics. This is of course a controversial account, and one that continues to be debated within the field. It is perhaps nearer the truth to claim that while it may not be entirely accurate to say that palliative *care* is synonymous with palliative *medicine* this state of affairs is becoming increasingly nearer the truth as palliative care evolves as a health speciality (see Chapter 3).

An alternative view sees the history of palliative care as standing outside that of healthcare, and drawing explicitly upon a moral foundation of 'theological' axiology rather than a secular liberal one. On this view palliative care can be seen as having a transcendental axiology of its own, a vision of the good life which includes a particular view of the good death. Evidence for this can be seen in the religious, and specifically Christian, foundation of modern hospices that formed the first phase in the evolution of contemporary palliative care (Clark 1993, 1998). More space than this chapter allows is needed for the detailed discussion this topic requires. The view presented here is a *feasible* account in the knowledge that other interpretations are possible. For example, it is arguable that the history of palliative care is much younger and quite distinct from that of the hospice movement as evidenced by the coining of the term 'palliative care' to describe a more 'acute' hospital-based model (Mount 1997). However, given Mount's own experience within the hospice movement, and the core principles held in common between hospice and palliative care it is as feasible to see hospice and palliative care as a continuation of a single tradition rather than separate ones.

Several commentators have identified medicalization and secularization as sources of tension, even crisis, within contemporary palliative care (Biswas 1993; Field 1994; Bradshaw 1996). The very fact that such transitions are identified as sources of tension suggests that there is a background of more or less homogenous values against which to judge such changes. At the very least such critical commentary suggests a non-secular or religious component to palliative care, and that palliative care has its origins in a system of *care* and not a medical speciality.

It is therefore plausible that the values of the modern palliative care movement have their roots within a 'Christian' axiology, which has continued to influence some of the key values within contemporary palliative care. Values such as the sanctity of life, the importance of death as an 'event' in life, and the family-centred model of care. It seems almost inevitable that the price of becoming a modern health speciality is secularization and with it an inexorable secularization of palliative care ethics requiring secular rather than theological justification for its core values. We can see evidence of this in the *Pallium* European survey described in Chapter 4. This is not to say that justification is not possible but rather that to date those values remain largely unexamined axioms of palliative care.

One issue on which there is near universal agreement within palliative care is the acceptance of death but the denial of a right to die. Viewed in the context of the history of palliative care and its underpinning Christian axiology this stance has the tenor of an objection to voluntary euthanasia that is theological rather than philosophical in nature. Admittedly it would be going too far to generalize the claim that the whole of modern palliative care shares the same specifically Christian prescription against voluntary euthanasia, clearly objections to euthanasia may have a secular basis, a point acknowledged by the palliative care community (Association of Palliative Medicine 1993). My point is rather that given the Christian influence on palliative care, it is reasonable to suppose that the origins of this position are under the same influence. The significance of this point is that although autonomy is recognized within palliative care as an important component of respect for persons, the scope of autonomy is constrained by an overarching axiology, which takes a broadly Christian view of the good life. It is against such a background, I suggest, that the anti-euthanasia stance of palliative care is taken. But if the evangelism of palliative care as a health speciality requires it to be secularized one must question how defensible such a stance is. The imposition of a Christian axiology appears overly prescriptive and is open to challenge on the same grounds that medical paternalism has been challenged.

The alternative is for palliative care to turn to secular bioethics to support its stance against euthanasia and in favour of 'good death', and this is beginning to happen. Bioethics offers a number of approaches. One approach argues that the principle of respect for autonomy requires a distinction between autonomy as a *liberty* claim and autonomy as a *rights* claim and thereby argues that respect for autonomy is best understood as a liberty claim carrying no obligation to fulfil positive requests. The second, but as yet underdeveloped approach, turns to axiology and the claim that a good life requires a good death (see Chapter 6 for a further discussion). To pursue this approach requires an account of the good death, and an argument that a good death is achievable for all. These lines of argument conform to two possible general strategies, one bold and the other more modest in purpose. The bolder aim is that a core purpose of palliative care is the *prevention* of euthanasia, the more modest purpose sees palliative care merely as an *alternative* to euthanasia. My general point is that so far, if one can speak of the palliative care 'community' then this community has not clarified which of these strategies it is committed to, though Chapter 3 suggests that, within palliative care, the former view has been the more dominant. An important implication of the more modest strategy is the possibility of palliative care existing alongside 'euthanasia services'. Space does not permit a longer treatment of these issues, so a number of specific points about the difficulties that pro-autonomy but anti-euthanasia arguments face will be briefly discussed.

There have been attempts to maintain the anti-euthanasia stance of palliative care within a broadly autonomy respecting framework and without the necessity for a theologically based sanctity of life argument (Farsides 1998; Gordijn and Janssens 2000). The pro-autonomy, anti-euthanasia position has been defended in the following way. When a person requests euthanasia then sincerely listening to the request and facilitating discussion around the issue is all that respect for autonomy requires. The 'sincerely listening' approach works as an account of respect for autonomy only if the point of the request was really aimed at the catharsis achieved by having one's concerns taken seriously and being given the opportunity to talk about them. However, if the real point of the request is actually to *receive* euthanasia then it seems overly ambitious and unnecessary to claim that by sincerely listening to the person's request autonomy has been respected.

Where the response to an autonomous request falls so far short of fulfilling the substance of the request it clearly begs the question about what it means to have one's autonomy respected. A further argument is required as to why a general principle of respect for autonomy does not require the fulfilment of such autonomous requests. While there are such arguments to be made they should not be mis-described as part of what it means to respect autonomy since they are precisely reasons for *constraining* autonomy, and denying an autonomous request. It goes without saying that nothing in the principle of respect for autonomy requires compliance with every request a person makes. However, good reasons are required for denying such requests particularly where what is requested carries greater moral weight than the imposition imposed upon the person requested.

So what would constitute good reasons? In considering this question the legal status of euthanasia will be ignored, since although it may provide an important pragmatic reason for denying the request, the law does not necessarily provide a moral reason for doing so. A moral reason frequently cited concerns the autonomy of others. As discussed earlier, a condition of the principle of respect for autonomy requires a reciprocal and equal respect for the autonomy of others. Clearly a good reason to deny one person's wish is where their request impinges unfairly upon the autonomy of another. But while respect for the autonomy of others is an important constraint on the autonomy of every individual it is by no means an *absolute* constraint. There are many circumstances, which furnish good reasons for requiring that one endure some risk of harm and sacrifice a degree of one's autonomy for the sake of others. However, to argue that the denial of euthanasia is justified because it represents an unjustifiable encroachment on the autonomy of others, requires reasons why this constraint on what others may request of you is sacrosanct. A compelling reason for this claim might be the objection of the person who is requested to perform the task. But given that not everyone shares this conviction a further argument is required to establish a valid and compelling general objection. It is my suggestion that by offering a view of the 'good death' palliative care offers an alternative to euthanasia based upon an axiological claim about the nature of the good life. A way in which this point is often made (for example in Chapter 7) is via a case history in which, for example a terminally ill person requests euthanasia because their life now lacks meaning but they subsequently discover that, with good palliative care, their last days are in fact meaningful. The conclusion from such accounts is that 'euthanasia poses the risk that an opportunity for growth will be lost and that life will be devalued' (Association of Palliative Medicine 1993: 4).

Perhaps a fitting compromise between the prohibition against euthanasia and respect for autonomy can be found in the use of terminal sedation where a dying person is rendered insensible to their suffering through heavy sedation until they die (Tännsjö 2000). The question of terminal sedation is discussed in detail in Chapter 9; however, terminal sedation is itself autonomy denying if the dying person's request was to be killed rather than to be rendered insensible but alive. Furthermore the use of terminal sedation may itself be seen as contrary to the goals of palliative care again denying a person the opportunity for meaningful life and growth at the end of their life. Gordijn and Janssens (2000) develop some arguments against euthanasia that, if valid, apply also to terminal sedation. One of their arguments is made within an autonomy framework, that a decision for euthanasia made at a time of pain and suffering could not be autonomous in any full sense (Gordijn and Janssens 2000: 44). However, this claim is too strong since not only does it rule out requests for euthanasia and terminal sedation, but also it rules out any other requests made under the same circumstances. The requirement that a person's decision can be judged autonomous only when it is seen as being free from duress or other influence is too stringent a criterion for autonomy. This is not to say that people's capacity for making autonomous decisions is never affected by their health or other circumstances. Rather it is an argument to take pains to establish the degree of impairment to a person's capacity for autonomous decision-making, which may differ with respect to the complexity of the decision. It is therefore reasonable to suppose that some terminally ill people will lack autonomy and some will not. However, questions about *an* individual's capacity are quite separate from the question of whether a request for terminal sedation or euthanasia ought to be respected on the grounds of the principle of respect for autonomy. If autonomy is relevant to the practice of palliative care, and at least some terminally ill people are autonomous, then a further argument is needed to justify the limits imposed upon certain wishes.

One possibility is to argue for the modest thesis, that palliative care is an alternative to euthanasia, and to do so upon axiological grounds. A plausible account might argue that palliative care aims to promote the total good of the patient which means promoting the patient's *objective* interests. Where there is uncertainty as to what these are then this speaks in favour of respect for a person's wishes. But respect for autonomy not only is an important moral claim, but also implies an epistemological claim, namely that an autonomous person has authoritative knowledge not only of their best interests, but also of their wishes. If however there is reason to judge that what a person wishes for is not really in their best interests, as *they* would define them, then this may justify overriding someone's wishes in favour of the interests they really value. For example, a terminally ill person who believes that their best interests lie in a painless death, and on this basis requests euthanasia as a *means* of meeting that end, may be judged to be mistaken. Although the request may be a sincere wish voluntarily expressed, pain relief by *death* may *not* be in the best interests of someone who sees their best interests as *dying* painlessly, and there are means of achieving this end still unexplored. Clearly the question of whether symptom relief measures have been exhausted in this case is an objective one. But even this case does not provide a reason for refusing euthanasia to someone who, even with the best possible palliation, continues to request euthanasia. This approach has still less to offer where the request is made on different grounds, for example a person who wishes to control the moment of their death. Here the principle of respect for autonomy speaks in favour of granting their request.

Arguments against voluntary euthanasia are implicitly also arguments against the priority of autonomy. For these to be sustained it must be established not only that palliative care can achieve the goal of a peaceful and symptom free death but also that this is what we *ought* to aspire to. But since there are competing views about what constitutes a good ending, a further argument is required to move from the factual possibility of achieving a 'good' death to the moral imperative that this is what we ought to aim for to the exclusion of all other forms of ending. If the stance the palliative care community takes against euthanasia is, as suggested above, premised upon a Christian axiology, then it seems feasible to defend only the more modest claim that palliative care offers an alternative way of dying. Of course the issue of euthanasia is not an issue for palliative care alone, it is an issue for the whole of healthcare and for every society. A general moratorium against euthanasia is not one that can be sustained by the mere fact that good palliative care is possible. The compelling cases in favour of palliative care can be matched with an equal number of compelling cases in favour of euthanasia. Citing the fact that someone may enjoy a better ending than they think possible attempts to weigh welfare considerations against those of autonomy. However, welfare considerations diminish in moral weight as they cease to contribute to autonomy. Where imposing interventions designed to increase welfare serve only to frustrate a person's attempts to direct and control their own life, including their ending, then we have a compelling reason not to impose such interventions.

Autonomy and family-centred care

As we see at several points in this volume, the World Health Organization's definition of palliative care states: 'the goal of palliative care is the achievement of the best quality of life for patients and their families' (WHO 1990: 11). In the United Kingdom, the National Council for Hospices and Specialist Palliative Care Services (NCHSPCS) defines palliative care as 'the active total care of patients and their families' (NCHSPCS 1995: 5). The family focus of care is emphasized in the definitions of palliative care of other European countries, many of which are also derived from the WHO definition indicating a degree of consensus regarding the purpose of palliative care (but see Chapter 3). The fact that palliative care philosophy is *family* centred raises further issues with regard to the importance of autonomy within palliative care. This represents further evidence that palliative care relies upon an axiology that, while not denying *any* importance to autonomy sees good reason to limit the priority of autonomy where there is a competing good, such as family interests. Family care within palliative care is one area where the autonomy-centric view seems inadequate to the task of dealing with the range of ethical issues raised (Hardwig 1990; Nelson 1992).

Since the family unit is so central within palliative care this seems ground enough for seeking an alternative to individual autonomy. The fact that a patient's family not only may receive care but at the same time may be providers of care complicates further the usual professional–client relationship, blurring the conventional ethical boundaries between carer and cared-for.

Autonomy plays an important role in contemporary healthcare ethics, used as it is to justify common ethical norms such as consent and even confidentiality. These norms are challenged in contexts where the family argues a right to both confidential information and to participate in decision-making (Woods et al. 2000). Transcending such moral norms in the face of respect for autonomy requires justification. Advancing the priority of family interests over that of individual autonomy seems most convincing when the claim is limited to a restricted context such as that of palliative care. However, this position is itself vulnerable.

The claim that the family should be regarded as the unit of moral authority in the palliative care context has a number of specific problems (Kissane and Bloch 2002). First, what actually is a family? There are different ways in which 'family' can be construed, for example: as a genetic entity although married couples are often not genetically related; as a legally defined entity although this also seems lacking since a person may be married yet have a more significant partner or friend. Even a broader more inclusive definition of family is still faced with the problem of how to weigh the relevance of the conflicting views of different family members. What has to be determined is the relevance of the views of the family to decision-making in palliative care. Is the family view a mere adjunct to medical decision-making or is the family to be regarded as authoritative? If so is it *their* view of the patient's best interests that matters or their view of what the patient would judge their interests to be had they been able to do so? Is the family view elicited only to provide an opportunity for them to ventilate their own feelings about the situation?

Problems with the family-centred view arise because the general claim about the place of the family in palliative care does not sufficiently distinguish between two issues. There is good reason to take the family, however construed, as a legitimate focus of concern within palliative care. However, this can be regarded as a separate issue from the more important ethical question of determining who should be involved when making important decisions for another? Clearly it is the same problem whether this question is posed within palliative care or elsewhere.

The role of the family or significant other in deciding for the patient has to be established either because the patient has so empowered them or because they have been invited to contribute to a debate aimed at improving the patient's own decisions through rational discourse. For example, a person's decision to die at home may impose a heavy burden on family members who will be relied upon to provide the additional support and care in order to respect such a decision. In such circumstances the decision is no longer an issue of the individual's autonomous wishes. Where the patient is no longer autonomous, then the family's view must be weighed as one among others when attempting to determine what is best for the patient.

Conclusion

There is no question that autonomy is both relevant and important within contemporary healthcare ethics and therefore to palliative care also. But autonomy is a complex concept relevant to political theory, theories of the self, and to ethics, and therefore requires more than a chapter-length analysis. In this chapter the contemporary meaning of autonomy has been explored, considering a number of its more important aspects, their relationship to one another and their relevance to palliative care. Each aspect of autonomy discussed is important because it reveals something of the evolution of the concept and its pervasive presence in modern thought. Even those who question the priority accorded to the concept cannot but recognize its place in ethical debate.

There are no grounds for regarding palliative care ethics as distinct from healthcare ethics in general and so the account of the liberalization of healthcare ethics and the role of autonomy in rejecting paternalism as the modus operandi of healthcare practice is again a relevant one. Ethical debate within palliative care has now begun to adopt the language of bioethics, itself significantly autonomy-centric. Some critics would see this as yet another symptom of the medicalization and secularization of palliative care but in order to sustain this criticism the argument for a palliative care alternative needs to be made.

It has also been argued that the most robust form of liberal autonomy is vulnerable to a number of criticisms, for example in terms of what is actually entailed by respect for autonomy. Liberal theories of autonomy are perhaps most vulnerable to criticism in the context of axiology, where, to a limited extent at least, some objective theories of the good gain ground against liberal scepticism. It is in the context of axiology that palliative care could be regarded as possessing a distinctive set of values and it is against such a background that a number of important moral principles of palliative care gain their credence. Two such principles, the good death, and the family-centred goal of palliative care, have been considered here. In the context of euthanasia the secularization of palliative care, substantially removed as it now is from its Christian hospice roots, requires those who reject voluntary euthanasia to employ autonomy-based arguments to defend palliative care's antithesis towards taking life. However, the argument that palliative care aims to prevent all euthanasia yet respects autonomy is much tougher to defend than the more modest claim that palliative care is an alternative to euthanasia.

A brief analysis of the family orientation of palliative care reveals that the moral implications of such a principle stand in need of more rigorous analysis and justification. A robust commitment to family care is quite rightly regarded as a challenge to some of the conventions of contemporary ethics. However, what is lacking are the detailed arguments which provide the consistent alternatives to established, predominantly autonomy-based, practices. The future challenge for palliative care is to decide whether a distinctive axiology underpinning its most important values is feasible and hence to go about defending it or to accept that palliative care is one option, which a discerning and autonomous patient may choose among others.

References

Association of Palliative Medicine (1993) *Submission from the Ethics Group of the Association of Palliative Medicine of Great Britain and Ireland to the Select Committee of the House of Lords on Medical Ethics.* 1F/PJH/3/Lords.

Beauchamp, T.L. and Childress, J.F. (2001) *Principles of Biomedical Ethics*, 5th edn. New York: Oxford University Press.

Biswas, B. (1993) Medicalization: a nurse's view, in D. Clark (ed.) *The Future for Palliative Care*. Buckingham: Open University Press.

Bowling, A. (1995) *Measuring Disease: A Review of Disease-specific Quality of Life Measurement Scales*. Buckingham: Open University Press.

Bradshaw, A. (1996) The hospice: the secularization spiritual dimension of an ideal, *Social Science and Medicine*, 43: 409–19.

Clark, D. (1993) Wither the hospices?, in D. Clark (ed.) *The Future for Palliative Care*. Buckingham: Open University Press.

Clark, D. (1998) Originating a movement: Cicely Saunders and the development of St Christopher's Hospice, 1957–67, *Mortality*, 3(1): 43–63.

Clouser, K.D. and Gert, B. (1999) A critique of principlism, *Journal of Medicine and Philosophy*, 15(2): 219–36.

Dworkin, R. (1986) Autonomy and the demented self, *Milbank Quarterly*, 64(suppl. 2): 4–16.

Dworkin, G. (1988) *The Theory and Practice of Autonomy*. Cambridge: Cambridge University Press.

Dworkin, R. (1993) *Life's Dominion: An Argument about Abortion, Euthanasia and Individual Freedom*. New York: Alfred A Knopf.

Farsides, C.C.S. (1998) Autonomy and its implications for palliative care: a Northern European perspective, *Palliative Medicine*, 12: 147–51.

Field, D. (1994) Palliative medicine and the medicalization of death, *European Journal of Cancer Care*, 3: 58–62.

Gordijn, B. and Janssens, R. (2000) The prevention of euthanasia through palliative care: new developments in the Netherlands, *Patient Education and Counselling*, 41: 35–46.

Hardwig, J. (1990) What about the family?, *Hastings Center Report*, 10(2): 5–10.

Harris, J. (1985) *The Value of Life*. London: Routledge and Kegan Paul.

Harris, J. (1995) Euthanasia and the value of life, in J. Keown (ed.) *Euthanasia Examined: Ethical, Clinical and Legal Perspectives*. Cambridge: Cambridge University Press.

Kissane, D. and Bloch, S. (2002) *Family Focused Grief Therapy*. Buckingham: Open University Press.

Kymlicka, W. (1990) *Contemporary Political Philosophy: An Introduction*. Oxford: Clarendon.

Locke, J. (1976) *An Essay Concerning Human Understanding*. London: Dent.

Mount, B. (1997) The Royal Victoria Hospital Palliative Care Service: a Canadian experience, in C. Saunders and R. Kastenbaum (eds) *Hospice Care on the International Scene*. New York: Springer.

National Council for Hospices and Specialist Palliative Care Services (1995) *Specialist Palliative Care: A Statement of Definitions*, occasional paper 8. London: NCHSPCS.

Nelson, J.L. (1992) Taking families seriously, *Hastings Center Report*, 22(4): 6–12.

Parfit, D. (1991) *Reasons and Persons*. Oxford: Clarendon.

Rawls, J. (1971) *A Theory of Justice*. Oxford: Oxford University Press.

Savulescu, J. (1997) Liberal rationalism and medical decision making, *Bioethics*, 11(2): 115–29.

Tännsjö, T. (2000) Terminal sedation – a possible compromise in the euthanasia debate?, *Bulletin of Medical Ethics*, November: 13–22.

Taylor, C. (1990) *Sources of the Self*. Cambridge: Cambridge University Press.

Tobias, J.S. (1997) BMJ's present policy (sometimes approving research in which patients have not given fully informed consent) is wholly correct, *British Medical Journal*, 314: 1111–14.

Veatch, R.M. (1995) Abandoning informed consent, *Hastings Center Report*, 25(2): 5–12.

Waldron, J. (1987) The theoretical foundations of liberalism, *Philosophical Quarterly*, 37(147): 127–50.

Woods, S. (2000) Persons and personal identity, *Nursing Philosophy*, 1(2): 169–72.

Woods, S., Beaver, K. and Luker, K. (2000) User's views of palliative care services: ethical implications, *Nursing Ethics*, 7(4): 314–26.

World Health Organization (1990) *Cancer Pain Relief and Palliative Care*. Geneva: WHO.

9 Sedation in palliative care: facts and concepts

BERT BROECKAERT AND JUAN MANUEL NÚÑEZ OLARTE

The need to sedate terminally ill patients for the management of uncontrolled symptoms has been a contentious issue in the palliative care literature since a seminal report in 1990. In this report Ventafridda and colleagues stated that more than 50 per cent of terminal cancer patients die with physical symptoms (the most important being dyspnoea, pain, delirium and vomiting) that are controllable only by sedation. Only by increasing the dosages of opioids and/or psychotropic drugs until sleep was induced, could symptom control be achieved in these patients (Ventafridda et al. 1990). Though recent clinical studies on sedation show a frequency that is significantly lower (Porta Sales et al. 1999a; Fainsinger et al. 2000b; Porta Sales 2001), the use of sedation still seems necessary with so-called refractory symptoms (those which cannot otherwise be controlled) in a significant number of terminally ill patients.

Some authors have equated the concept of sedation to that of 'slow euthanasia' (Billings and Block 1996), while others have stressed the need for clinical evidence and reliable definitions in this discussion (Mount 1996). Though recent research has provided important information on the clinical facts regarding this therapeutic procedure, there are still serious differences of opinion regarding the ethics surrounding the practice (Quill and Byock 2000; Sulmasy et al. 2000). The purpose of this chapter is to clarify what sedation in palliative care is all about, opting for an interdisciplinary approach that combines a philosophical-ethical analysis with a careful review of the available clinical data. The first section of the chapter deals with terms and definitions. The second section discusses the reasons for sedation, the frequency of this practice and the medication used to induce sedation. The importance of both a good term and definition and a sound knowledge of the clinical facts is shown in the final section, which deals with the relationship between sedation and euthanasia.

From terminal to palliative sedation

The best known but also the most controversial term used to denote sedation in palliative care is *terminal sedation*. This term was introduced by
Enck (1991) in a review article that was published in the *American Journal
of Hospice and Palliative Care*. Since then, terminal sedation has been a
widely used term, though the term is remarkably absent in several important studies on this topic (Cherny and Portenoy 1994; Stone et al. 1997;
Fainsinger et al. 2000a,b) and plays only a marginal role in most other
international clinical studies. This is not a coincidence. One of the conclusions of a study by Chater et al. (1998), which examined the response of
61 selected palliative care experts to a proposed definition for terminal
sedation, was precisely that the term 'terminal sedation' should be abandoned and be replaced with another. Several other authors object explicitly
to the use of the term (Carver and Foley 2000; Krakauer 2000; Portenoy
2000; Sulmasy et al. 2000).

In our opinion there are three good reasons for not using the term 'terminal
sedation'. First, there is the negativity associated with the word terminal.
Precisely in order to avoid this misleading suggestion of negativism and
passivity we talk rather about palliative than about terminal care (Doyle et
al. 1998). Though heavy sedation is indeed a palliative treatment of last
resort (Quill et al. 2000), it is still an active and positive treatment addressing refractory symptoms and thus relieving suffering. Therefore a more
positive term is called for.

Second, there is the problem that the term 'terminal sedation' does not
give a clear idea of what sedation is all about, of the reason or intention
behind this intervention. Whether a patient is sedated with the intention of
shortening life or just to relieve a refractory symptom, there is nothing in
the term terminal sedation that suggests that this term is not appropriate in
both cases, however different these cases are from an ethical point of view.
In this way the confusion between sedation and euthanasia (the intentional
shortening of life) is nourished. Accordingly, this sedation is put in a bad
light, which could bring caregivers, patients suffering from refractory symptoms and their families to oppose or refuse sedation. The effect of this
vagueness and confusion could also be that physicians, who still call what
they are doing terminal sedation, do actually cross the border between
sedation and euthanasia.

Our last and most important argument against the use of the term 'terminal
sedation' is the fact that, rather than being just vague and unspecified, this
term actually suggests that terminal sedation is about terminating the life of
the patient. Seen from this perspective, the confusion between sedation and
euthanasia, resulting from the use of this term, becomes even more likely.

It is not surprising therefore that other terms have been suggested, such
as *controlled sedation*, a term that was briefly mentioned in Cherny and

Portenoy's (1994) influential article on sedation. Since the advice on sedation of the Medical Ethics Committee of the Faculty of Medicine of the Catholic University of Leuven was published in 1998, this has become the standard term in Flanders (Vermylen and Schotsmans 2000). Several problems exist with this term. First, whereas we can clearly understand the meaning and the meaningfulness of the terms 'physician-controlled sedation' and 'patient-controlled sedation' (as used in anaesthesiology), we find it quite meaningless and pleonastic (superfluous) to talk about controlled sedation. If one is convinced that the addition of the word 'controlled' is meaningful and necessary, one should also start to talk about controlled pain-relief and controlled chemotherapy. Second, the use of the adjective 'controlled' could give the impression that the physician is totally in control, and is always capable of restoring the consciousness of the patient whenever this seems necessary or is asked for. This is, however, certainly not the case. The Spanish definition of 'terminal sedation' even limits the use of this term to those cases in which there is a presumably *irreversible* reduction of consciousness (Porta Sales et al. 1999b, our italics). Third, just as with the term 'terminal sedation', the term 'controlled sedation' also does not tell us what sedation is all about, or for what reason it is given. Finally, the term 'controlled sedation' does not make clear that we are talking here about sedation of patients who are terminally ill.

Two other terms that have been introduced recently are *sedation for intractable distress in the dying* (Chater et al. 1998; Krakauer et al. 2000) and *sedation in the imminently dying patient*, a term coined by Carver and Foley (2000; Wein 2000). The problem with these terms is that they have become sentences, and are therefore not very handy and unlikely to become widely embraced. Nor does the term 'sedation in the imminently dying' tell us why sedation is performed, or with what purpose. In this way confusion between sedation and euthanasia becomes unavoidable. Moreover, in palliative care sedation, even full and irreversible sedation, is *not* limited to those patients who are imminently dying, that is those who are dying within hours or one or two days. For example, the period of sedation in a multicentre international study by Fainsinger et al. (2000b) was in all participating centres between 1 and 6 days. In a South African study (Fainsinger et al. 1998) it was between 4 hours and 12 days. In a Leuven study (Menten 2000) it was between 1 and 18 days. Moreover, using the words 'imminently dying' could be or become something of a self-fulfilling prophecy. Indeed it is easy to sedate a patient in such a way that they are bound to die in a few days' time, thus retrospectively 'proving' that the patient was indeed imminently dying. Adopting the term 'sedation in the imminently dying' does not prevent unwarranted use of sedation; the contrary might even be true.

As none of the terms we have discussed so far seems convincing, we suggest the adoption of the term *palliative sedation* (Broeckaert 2000b). As with palliative care itself, this term has a positive connotation and suggests an active effort to relieve suffering. Moreover, this term makes it perfectly clear in what context and to whom sedation is being given: we are talking about the sedation of palliative patients, the sedation of patients in palliative care. Even more importantly and unlike the other terms that have been proposed, the term 'palliative sedation' clearly suggests the purpose of sedation in palliative care: sedation is about palliation, it is about symptom relief. So, because it is in no way suggesting that sedation is about terminating the life of a patient, the term 'palliative sedation' actually prevents the confusion of sedation with euthanasia. Sedating a patient in order to shorten their life is clearly not to perform palliative sedation, but to do something fundamentally different.

Palliative sedation defined

Having a term is not enough, we also need a good definition of palliative sedation. As palliative sedation is about symptom control, it would be a good idea to start our discussion with a definition of pain and symptom control. What is typical of pain and symptom control is not just the subjective intention behind what is done, but also and even more importantly, the adequacy or the proportionality of what is done. Therefore, we would define pain and symptom control as 'the intentional administration of analgesics and/or other drugs in dosages and combinations required to adequately relieve pain and/or other symptoms' (Broeckaert 2000a: 100).

Focusing on this adequacy or proportionality, namely a clear match between the drugs given and the drugs needed, is absolutely essential in differentiating pain control from euthanasia. That all this is not about splitting hairs, can easily be seen from the Dutch and Flemish data on end-of-life decisions. Knowing that pain relief, even when heavy medication is given in extreme doses, is remarkably safe (Bercovitch et al. 1999), it is puzzling to read that both in the Netherlands and in Flanders in no less than 18.5 per cent of all deaths nationwide, physicians have shortened the life of the patient while alleviating pain and symptoms with opioids (van der Maas et al. 1996; Deliens et al. 2000). If one takes a closer look at these figures, one learns that in 3 per cent (4100 cases in 1995 in the Netherlands) or even 5 per cent (2966 cases in Flanders in 1998) of all deaths, this pain relief with life-shortening effect was 'also intended to terminate life'. One may assume that in these cases, physicians may not mind giving an inadequate dose, or rather that they often deliberately – in order to terminate the life of the patient – give a higher dose than is needed to relieve the pain. Here the importance of a good definition of pain and symptom control immediately becomes clear, for a doctor who willingly and knowingly overdoses, intending to terminate life, thus not respecting this notion of adequacy or proportionality, is not providing pain relief at all, but, without a shadow of doubt, is carrying out (in)voluntary euthanasia.

A clear definition of palliative sedation is extremely important too, for it helps again to avoid confusion with euthanasia. In line with our definition of pain and symptom control, we define palliative sedation as 'the intentional administration of sedative drugs in dosages and combinations required to reduce the consciousness of a terminal patient as much as necessary to adequately relieve one or more refractory symptoms' (Broeckaert 2000b: 58).

This new definition has been developed in order to overcome the limitations of previous ones and it incorporates the following elements. First, there is the often neglected but nevertheless crucial notion of adequacy or proportionality. Sedation is certainly not just a matter of subjective intention. If a subjective intention to relieve a refractory symptom does not translate itself into an adequate and proportional intervention – 'giving as much as needed' – this stated intention is not the real intention; or it is, we would say, real but perverted by other competing intentions. Whoever knowingly and willingly gives more than is needed to relieve the refractory symptom is not doing sedation anymore, but performing euthanasia when this overdosing shortens the life of the patient. On the other hand, whoever clearly gives more than is needed, albeit understanding very well what is being done when overdosing shortens the life of the patient, is guilty of medical malpractice. In neither case are we dealing with (adequate) palliative sedation.

Second, whether sedation is continuous or intermittent, reversed or not, mild or deep ('total'), all these types of sedation are included in our definition. We think it is important *not* to restrict our definition of sedation just to deep, continuous, unreversed or even irreversible sedation, as for example in the Spanish definition of 'terminal sedation':

> the deliberate administration of drugs in order to induce a sufficiently profound and presumably irreversible reduction of consciousness in a patient close to death, with the intention of alleviating refractory physical and/or psychological suffering and with the explicit, implicit or delegate consent of the patient.
>
> (Porta Sales et al. 1999b: 110)

If one does this, one runs the risk of losing track of the crucial notion of adequacy or proportionality. Sedation is *not* about bringing deep and continuous sleep, but about reducing the consciousness of a patient as much and as long as necessary. Individual titration is therefore absolutely essential. Any definition that suggests otherwise is misleading and dangerous.

A third element of our definition is the prerequisite of a limited expected survival of the patient. The key conditions that define a patient as terminally ill in the course of a disease are:

- progressive, incurable, advanced disease
- lack of a reasonable possibility of response to active specific treatment
- multiple problems or symptoms that tend to be intense, multifactoral and subject to change
- high emotional impact in patient, family and team related, explicitly or not, to the proximity of death
- expected survival of less than six months

(Sanz Ortíz et al. 1993)

Cancer, AIDS, motor-neurone disease, specific organ failure (renal, cardiac, hepatic) fulfil the previous criteria up to a certain degree in the final stages of the illness (Sanz Ortíz et al. 1993). Terminal sedation is usually considered in the setting of patients with a very limited life expectancy – either days or weeks. In Spain, due to its cultural peculiarities, the phases of *agonía* and *preagonía* (see p. 172) approximately match with this limited prognosis of days or weeks, and are therefore regarded as an acceptable time frame in which to consider terminal sedation (Núñez Olarte and Gracia Guillén 2001). An adequate combination of clinical experience and laboratory data (Rich 1999) and/or validated prognostication tools (Maltoni et al. 1999) are essential in determining whether a patient fits these categories.

Fourth, what about the withholding of hydration and nutrition? We think the only right answer here is to say that this is a totally different discussion. Such withholding is *not* in our definition and should certainly not be standard practice (Morita et al. 1999; Wein 2000). If sedation is combined with the withdrawing of hydration and nutrition, what is done is not just sedation (inducing sleep), but sedation *and* the withdrawing of hydration and nutrition. Withdrawing hydration and nutrition is *not* an intrinsic part of sedation or the treatment of refractory symptoms. Moreover, it is clearly misleading to state that one is 'only' sedating, inducing sleep or reducing the consciousness of the patient, when at the same time these seemingly innocent words cover up the fact that knowingly and willingly (artificial hydration is a distinct possibility) vital fluids are withdrawn, thus making short-term death inevitable.

Are we suggesting here that one always has to start artificial nutrition and hydration as one starts palliative sedation? Not at all. It would rightly be considered pointless, futile and not in line with palliative care philosophy to begin (once sedation is started) artificial hydration, still less artificial nutrition, in patients who had not been eating and drinking and were not artificially hydrated during the days before sedative drugs were administered. We are not discussing and certainly not advocating the artificial lengthening of the life of sedated patients. What we do advocate here is honesty and openness when the life of sedated patients is artificially *shortened*.

The issue of nutrition and hydration in the terminal phase is a contentious one and has prompted expert consensus groups of the European

Association for Palliative Care on Nutrition (Bozzeti et al. 1996), and systematic reviews of the literature on hydration (Viola et al. 1997). Withholding nutrition is generally not a problem in the setting of terminal disease, and withholding hydration is certainly *indicated* in the setting of Spanish *agonía*, 'the last 48 hours of life'. We also know from research that the perception of thirst as a symptom diminishes with the decrease of cognition (Burge 1993). Therefore the ethical problem is located basically in the setting of terminal patients with weeks to live (Spanish *preagonía*) who are receiving sedation. In these patients careful clinical judgement has to guide decisions about providing artificial hydration. In the initial phases of the sedation process, when the sedation is still not sufficiently deep to avoid the patient from perceiving thirst, probably artificial hydration should be provided. On the other hand when *agonía* ('the last 48 hours') arrives it should be removed.

A fifth and last element of our definition has to do with the fact that the notion of refractory symptoms is not specified in it, thus acknowledging the possibility of sedating for both physical and psychological suffering. What these refractory symptoms might be is discussed in the next section.

Refractory symptoms

Any given symptom can be considered *refractory* to treatment when it cannot be adequately controlled in spite of every tolerable effort to provide relief within an acceptable time period without compromising consciousness. It is extremely important not to misinterpret these refractory symptoms as *difficult* symptoms. It is quite possible to find symptoms that seem impossible to alleviate without the help of sedation. However, when referred to more specialized programmes, these same patients are usually managed successfully without the need to reduce consciousness. This situation has already been demonstrated with the development of advanced cancer pain protocols in Spain (Núñez Olarte et al. 1997). Likewise the arrival of palliative care in France has meant the dismissal of the frequently abused 'lytic cocktail' (Meunier-Cartal et al. 1995).

A recent Canadian report has shown that 50 per cent of patients receiving palliative sedation at the beginning of the study were sedated in response to symptoms that were not refractory. In this study the implementation of 'clinical practice guidelines' on palliative sedation dramatically reversed the tendency to oversedate (Braun et al. 2000).

The most frequent reasons for inducing sedation are delirium, dyspnoea and pain and these are shown in Table 9.1. There might, of course, be more than one reason in any given patient to start sedation.

The issue of psychological distress or suffering as a reason for palliative sedation is a recent arrival in the literature. Significantly the studies that

Table 9.1   Reasons/indications for sedation (percentage of total patients sedated)

Symptoms	(Porta Sales 2001)	(Porta Sales et al. 1999a)	(Fainsinger et al. 2000b)
Delirium	39.00	10.70	72.70
Dyspnoea	38.00	23.20	9.00
Pain	22.00	23.20	4.50
Haemorrhage	8.50	8.90	9.00
Nausea/vomiting	6.00	6.20	0.00
Fatigue	20.00	1.70	
Psychological	21.00	54.46	40.90

Table 9.2   Frequency of palliative sedation (percentage of total of patients cared for)

(Porta Sales 2001)	(*Porta Sales et al. 1999a)	(Fainsinger et al. 2000b)
25.00	23.05	22.00

accept this indication have all been performed outside the North American Anglo-Saxon cultural environment: four studies in Spain (Porta Sales et al. 1999a; Fainsinger et al. 2000b; Pascual and Gisbert 2000; Viguria Arrieta et al. 2000), one study in Italy (Peruselli et al. 1999), one study in Japan (Morita et al. 1999) and one study in the United Kingdom (Stone et al. 1997). Cultural factors indeed have an impact on decisions about and the social acceptability of sedation due to psychological suffering (Fainsinger et al. 2000b; Núñez Olarte and Gracia Guillén 2001). A recent comparative study has shown that Spanish terminally ill patients and their families ascribe less relevance to the preservation of cognition and diagnosis disclosure, than do their counterparts in Canada (Núñez Olarte et al. 2000).

The proportion in any given setting of patients who need palliative sedation does not vary a great deal, but there are differences in the studies depending on the methodology (prospective versus retrospective) and the definition of sedation used (Porta Sales 2001). No important differences have been found in the frequency of sedation between early studies which considered only physical symptoms as a reason for sedation, and later ones in which both physical and psychological factors were taken into consideration (Porta Sales 2001). Table 9.2 gives an overview of reported frequencies of the need for palliative sedation.

Nevertheless, although percentages are relevant, it is important to emphasize that variability of criteria for sedation, depending on the centre, allow for substantial differences in the decision to sedate (Stone et al. 1997; Chater et al. 1998; Peruselli et al. 1999).

In summary, palliative sedation (as we prefer to call it) is a useful therapeutic procedure, needed in approximately one out of every four or five patients in a palliative care setting.

Drugs used

Several sources give us sufficient patient numbers to analyse the issue of which drugs are used in palliative sedation. A recent review of the literature (Porta Sales 2001) encompasses 13 studies published since 1990 (Ventafridda et al. 1990; Fainsinger et al. 1991; McIver et al. 1994; Turner et al. 1996; Morita et al. 1996; Stone et al. 1997; Ojeda et al. 1997; Fainsinger 1998; Fainsinger et al. 1998; Porta Sales et al. 1999b; Morita et al. 1999; Peruselli et al. 1999; Viguria et al. 2000). Two recent prospective studies also exist (Porta Sales et al. 1999a; Fainsinger et al. 2000b). Together, these contribute several hundreds of patients, together with information about the drugs used. Table 9.3 summarizes the relevant data.

These drugs might be classified by their sedation-inducing capacity:

- tranquillizers: haloperidol, chlorpromazine, methotrimeprazine
- sedatives: midazolam, diazepam, chlometiazole
- anaesthetics: propofol, phenobarbitone

(MacLeod 1997)

It is important to remember that there is a clinical 'ceiling effect' with benzodiazepines (midazolam, diazepam). On reaching a certain dose maximum inhibition through the GABAergic system is achieved, and further increases are futile (e.g. 160–200 mg/day of midazolam). Furthermore there is always the risk involved of paradoxical agitation with benzodiazepines. Therefore sedative neuroleptics (methotrimeprazine, chlorpromazine) are always a reasonable alternative.

Table 9.3 Medications used in palliative sedation

Medication frequency % / mean dose mg/day	(Porta Sales 2001)	(Porta Sales et al. 1999a)	(Fainsinger et al. 2000b)
Midazolam	65%/25	79.5%/38.4	82%/61
Haloperidol	31%/7	25.0%/14.6	0%/0
Diazepam		4.5%/20	5%
Methotrimeprazine		5.4%/197.9	5%
Chlorpromazine		0.9%/30	
Chlometiazole		1.8%/2.000	
Phenobarbitone		0.9%/1.200	14%/900

The use of anaesthetics, especially barbiturates, has been considered ethically unacceptable by some authors in the management of reversible terminal delirium if administered without life-supporting systems (MacLeod 1997). On the other hand the same author, and standard reference textbooks in palliative medicine (Twycross and Lichter 1998), readily accept the fact that a small percentage of patients requiring palliative sedation will require anaesthetics after failing on benzodiazepines and sedative neuroleptics. Nevertheless as shown in Table 9.3 the most widely used drugs are midazolam and haloperidol.

Slow euthanasia?

That terminal or palliative sedation raises serious ethical questions and causes a great deal of controversy is apparent from well-known discussions in the *Journal of Medical Ethics* (Craig 1994; Wilkes 1994; Ashby and Stoffell 1995; Dunlop et al. 1995) and the *Journal of Palliative Care* (Billings and Block 1996; Dickens 1996; Brody 1996; Mount 1996; Portenoy 1996) and also from the legal case *Vacco* et al. *v. Quill* et al., ultimately decided by the United States Supreme Court (26 June 1997, no. 95–1885). One could also look at the euthanasia debate in Belgium where one finds similar discussions. Though several people involved in palliative care, during the hearings in the Belgian senate (February–May 2000), defended sedation as a possible alternative to euthanasia, some senators regarded this as nothing but euthanasia in disguise; slow euthanasia, but euthanasia nonetheless.

How should we view these allegations? Is palliative sedation a form of euthanasia? We take the view that it is not. If the sedation that is given is indeed adequate or proportional, then it is symptom control which is carried out, not euthanasia. At least three things, not present in this instance, can be said to be typical of euthanasia (see also Chapter 10). First, the subjective intention of the physician must be the death of the patient. Second, the medication and the dosages that are given must reflect this aim. Third, the result of this act must be, per definition, the death of the patient. Now if one looks at sedation, at least if one starts from our definition, one gets a totally different picture. First, the subjective intention of the physician is different: the physician does not wish to kill the patient but simply to control the refractory symptom(s). If the patient dies sooner as a result of sedation, this shortening of life is and should be seen as an unintended side-effect, nothing else. There is more, however, for the difference between sedation and euthanasia should not only be looked for, as is often done, at this subjective, intentional level. Hence our second point. When sedating, there is and there should be a clear match between the dosages given and the dosages needed for symptom control, not a match between the dosages

Table 9.4   Mean survival of patients after starting sedation

(Porta Sales 2001)	(Porta Sales et al. 1999a)	(Fainsinger et al. 2000b)
2.4 days	3.2 days	2.4 days

given and the dosages needed to end the life of the patient. Third, what about the result of palliative sedation when compared to that of euthanasia? Our answer here is that, unlike euthanasia, sedation has not *per definition* a life-shortening effect. The question then remains whether in reality giving adequate symptom relief through sedation has a life-shortening effect or not. This is of course an empirical question not settled by choosing certain terms and definitions, but if we look at the available empirical studies, the clear suggestion is that this is generally *not* the case. The mean survival of patients after sedation can be read from Table 9.4.

Would these patients have lived longer if they had not been sedated? According to the available studies there are no significant differences in survival between patients receiving palliative sedation and those patients in the same palliative care setting not receiving this procedure (Ventafridda et al. 1990; Stone et al. 1997; Thorns and Sykes 1999; Waller et al. 1999; Morita et al. 2001). Due to the insurmountable ethical difficulties involved (one simply cannot deny sedation to a patient who clearly needs it) prospective controlled studies that would produce harder data are rendered impossible.

Conclusion

Unlike the other terms used hitherto to denote sedation, the term *palliative sedation*, introduced in this chapter, makes it perfectly clear in what context, to whom and, most importantly, why this form of sedation is given. Therefore using this term is an important way of preventing confusion between sedation and euthanasia. Equally important in this context is of course a good *definition* of *palliative sedation*. Crucial to the definition proposed in this chapter is that it concentrates not only on the subjective intention of the physician, but also and even more importantly, on the adequacy or proportionality of what is objectively done. There should be a clear match between the drugs given and the drugs and degree of sedation needed to relieve the refractory symptom. From the conceptual and factual clarification offered in this chapter it becomes clear that palliative sedation, as reflected in our definition, is *not* a form of euthanasia, but a useful and indispensable therapeutic approach in a significant number of terminal patients.

For the philosopher and the ethicist discussing sedation in palliative care it is of crucial importance to start from medical reality. Ethical studies that do not respect this reality and are ignorant of the relevant clinical studies on sedation that have been published run the risk of completely missing the point and having nothing to offer to the actors in the field. On the other hand, both ethical and clinical studies can work with poor and misleading concepts and definitions. Without the kind of clarification we have tried to offer in this chapter, requiring a close cooperation between ethicists and clinicians, then ethical discussions of the delicate subject of sedation in palliative care all too easily become confused and are of little use. What is true for palliative care patients – that they benefit from an interdisciplinary approach – seems also true for palliative care ethics.

References

Ashby, M. and Stoffell, B. (1995) Artificial hydration and alimentation at the end of life: a reply to Craig, *Journal of Medical Ethics*, 21: 135–40.

Bercovitch, M., Waller, A. and Adunsky, A. (1999) High dose morphine use in the hospice setting: a database survey of patient characteristics and effect on life expectancy, *Cancer*, 86(5): 871–7.

Billings, J.A. and Block, S.D. (1996) Slow euthanasia, *Journal of Palliative Care*, 12(4): 21–30.

Bozzeti, F., Amadori, D., Bruera, E. et al. (1996) Guidelines on artificial nutrition versus hydration in terminal cancer patients, *Nutrition*, 12: 163–7.

Braun, T., Hagen, N., Wasylenko, E., Labrie, M. and Wolch, G. (2000) Sedation for intractable symptoms in palliative care: do CPGs improve care? Abstract, 13th International Congress on Care of the Terminally Ill, September 2000, Montreal (Canada), *Journal of Palliative Care*, 16(3): 88.

Brody, H. (1996) Commentary on Billings and Block's 'Slow Euthanasia', *Journal of Palliative Care*, 12(4): 38–41.

Broeckaert, B. (2000a) Medically mediated death: from pain control to euthanasia, 13th World Congress on Medical Law, August 2000, Helsinki, *Book of Proceedings*, 1: 100.

Broeckaert, B. (2000b) Palliative sedation defined or why and when terminal sedation is not euthanasia. Abstract, 1st Congress RDPC, December 2000, Berlin (Germany), *Journal of Pain and Symptom Management*, 20(6): S58.

Burge, F.I. (1993) Dehydration symptoms of palliative care cancer patients, *Journal of Pain and Symptom Management*, 8(7): 454–64.

Carver, A.C. and Foley, K.M. (2000) The Wein article reviewed, *Oncology*, 14(4): 597–8.

Chater, S., Viola, R., Paterson, J. and Jarvis, V. (1998) Sedation for intractable distress in the dying – a survey of experts, *Palliative Medicine*, 12: 255–69.

Cherny, N.I. and Portenoy, R.K. (1994) Sedation in the management of refractory symptoms: guidelines for evaluation and treatment, *Journal of Palliative Care*, 10(2): 31–8.

Craig, G.M. (1994) On withholding nutrition and hydration in the terminally ill: has palliative medicine gone too far?, *Journal of Medical Ethics*, 20: 139–43.

Deliens, L., Mortier, F., Bilsen, J. et al. (2000) End-of-life decisions in medical practice in Flanders, Belgium: a nationwide survey, *The Lancet*, 356: 1806–11.

Dickens, B.M. (1996) Commentary on 'Slow Euthanasia', *Journal of Palliative Care*, 12(4): 42–3.

Doyle, D., Hanks, G.W.C. and MacDonald, N. (eds) (1998) *Oxford Textbook of Palliative Medicine*, 2nd edn. Oxford: Oxford University Press.

Dunlop, R.J., Ellershaw, J.E., Baines, M.J., Sykes, N. and Saunders, C.M. (1995) On withholding nutrition and hydration in the terminally ill: has palliative medicine gone too far? A reply, *Journal of Medical Ethics*, 21: 141–3.

Enck, R.E. (1991) Drug-induced terminal sedation for symptom control, *American Journal of Hospice and Palliative Care*, 8(5): 3–5.

Fainsinger, R.L. (1998) Use of sedation by a hospital palliative care support team, *Journal of Palliative Care*, 14(1): 51–4.

Fainsinger, R., MacEachern, T., Hanson, J., Miller, M.J. and Bruera, E. (1991) Symptom control during the last week of life on a Palliative Care Unit, *Journal of Palliative Care*, 7(1): 5–11.

Fainsinger, R.L., Landman, W., Hoskings, M. and Bruera, E. (1998) Sedation for uncontrolled symptoms in a South African hospice, *Journal of Pain and Symptom Management*, 16: 145–52.

Fainsinger, R.L., de Moissac, D., Mancini, I. and Oneschuk, D. (2000a) Sedation for delirium and other symptoms in terminally ill patients in Edmonton, *Journal of Palliative Care*, 16(2): 5–10.

Fainsinger, R., Waller, A., Bercovici, M. et al. (2000b) A multicentre international study of sedation for uncontrolled symptoms in terminally ill patients, *Palliative Medicine*, 14: 257–65.

Krakauer, E. (2000) Responding to intractable terminal suffering, *Annals of Internal Medicine*, 133: 560.

Krakauer, E., Penson, R.T., Truog, R.D. et al. (2000) Sedation for intractable distress of a dying patient: acute palliative care and the principle of double effect, *The Oncologist*, 5: 53–62.

McIver, B., Walsh, D. and Nelson, K. (1994) The use of chlorpromazine for symptom control in dying cancer patients, *Journal of Pain and Symptom Management*, 9: 341–5.

MacLeod, A.D. (1997) The management of delirium in hospice practice, *European Journal of Palliative Care*, 4(4): 116–20.

Maltoni, M., Nanni, O., Pirovano, M. et al. (1999) Successful validation of the Palliative Prognostic Score in terminally ill cancer patients, *Journal of Pain and Symptom Management*, 17: 240–7.

Menten, J. (2000) *Gecontrolleerde sedatie: een therapeutische mogelijkheid voor refractaire symptomen bij de terminale palliatieve patient?* Leuven: K.U. Leuven.

Meunier-Cartal, J., Souberbielle, J.C. and Boureau, F. (1995) Morphine and the 'lytic cocktail' for the terminally ill patients in a French general hospital: evidence for an inverse relationship, *Journal of Pain and Symptom Management*, 10: 267–73.

Morita, T., Inoue, S. and Chihara, S. (1996) Sedation for symptom control in Japan: the importance of intermittent use and communication with family members, *Journal of Pain and Symptom Management*, 12: 32–8.

Morita, T., Tsunoda, J., Inoue, S. and Chihara, S. (1999) Do hospice clinicians sedate patients intending to hasten death?, *Journal of Palliative Care*, 15(3): 20–3.

Morita, T., Tsunoda, J., Inoue, S. and Chihara, S. (2001) Effects of high dose opioids and sedatives on survival of terminally ill cancer patients, *Journal of Pain and Symptom Management*, 21: 282–9.

Mount, B. (1996) Morphine drips, terminal sedation, and slow euthanasia: definitions and facts, not anecdotes, *Journal of Palliative Care*, 12(4): 31–7.

Núñez Olarte, J.M. and Gracia Guillén, D. (2001) Cultural issues and ethical dilemmas in palliative and end-of-life care in Spain, *Cancer Control*, 8(1): 46–54.

Núñez Olarte, J.M., Conti Jiménez, M., López, C. and Luque Medel, J.M. (1997) Protocolos de manejo del dolor refractario canceroso de la UCP del Hospital Gregorio Marañón de Madrid, *Medicina Paliativa*, 4(2): 81–92.

Núñez Olarte, J.M., Fainsinger, R.L. and deMoissac, D. (2000) Influencia de factores culturales en la estrategia de tratamiento. Ponencia, III Congreso SECPAL, May 2000, Valencia, *Medicina Paliativa*, 7(2): 76–7.

Ojeda Martín, M., Navarro Marrero, M.A. and Gómez Sancho, M. (1997) Sedación y enfermo oncológico terminal, *Medicina Paliativa*, 4(3): 101–7.

Pascual, A. and Gisbert, A. (2000) Sedación en una Unidad de Cuidados Paliativos. Comunicación oral, III Congreso SECPAL, May 2000, Valencia, *Medicina Paliativa*, 7(suppl.1): 16.

Peruselli, C., DiGiulio, P., Toscani, F. et al. (1999) Home palliative care for terminal cancer patients: a survey on the final week of life, *Palliative Medicine*, 13: 233–41.

Porta Sales, J. (2001) Sedation and terminal care, *European Journal of Palliative Care*, 8(3): 97–100.

Porta Sales, J., Yllá-Catalá Boré, E., Estíbalez Gil, A. et al. (1999a) Estudio multicéntrico catalano-balear sobre la sedación terminal en Cuidados Paliativos, *Medicina Paliativa*, 6(4): 153–8.

Porta Sales, J., Guinovart, C., Yllá-Catalá, E. et al. (1999b) Definición y opiniones acerca de la sedación terminal: estudio multicéntrico catalano-balear, *Medicina Paliativa*, 6(3): 108–15.

Portenoy, R.K. (1996) Morphine infusions at the end of life: the pitfalls in reasoning from anecdote, *Journal of Palliative Care*, 12(4): 44–6.

Portenoy, R.K. (2000) The Wein article reviewed, *Oncology*, 14(4): 592, 601.

Quill, T.E. and Byock, I.R. (2000) Responding to intractable suffering: the role of terminal sedation and voluntary refusal of food and fluids, *Annals of Internal Medicine*, 132: 408–14.

Quill, T.E., Coombs Lee, B. and Nunn, S. (2000) Palliative treatments of last resort: choosing the least harmful alternative, *Annals of Internal Medicine*, 132: 488–93.

Rich, A. (1999) How long have I got? Prognostication and palliative care, *European Journal of Palliative Care*, 6(6): 179–82.

Sanz Ortíz, J., Gómez Batiste, X., Gómez Sancho, M. and Núñez Olarte, J.M. (1993) *Cuidados Paliativos: recomendaciones de la Sociedad Española de Cuidados*

Paliativos (SECPAL), Serie Guías y Manuales. Madrid: Ministerio de Sanidad y Consumo.

Stone, P., Phillips, C., Spruyt, O. and Waight, C. (1997) A comparison of the use of sedatives in a hospital support team and in a hospice, *Palliative Medicine*, 11: 140–4.

Sulmasy, D.P., Ury, W.A., Ahronheim, J.C. et al. (2000) Responding to intractable terminal suffering, *Annals of Internal Medicine*, 133: 560–1.

Thorns, A. and Sykes, N. (1999) Opioid use in the last week of life and the implications for end of life decision making. Abstract, 6th Congress EAPC, September 1999, Geneva, Switzerland. *Abstract Book*. Geneva: EAPC Onlus.

Turner, K., Chye, R., Aggarwal, G. et al. (1996) Dignity in dying: a preliminary study of patients in the last three days of life, *Journal of Palliative Care*, 12(2): 7–13.

Twycross, R. and Lichter, I. (1998) The terminal phase, in D. Doyle, G.W.C. Hanks and N. MacDonald (eds) *Oxford Textbook of Palliative Medicine*, 2nd edn. Oxford: Oxford University Press.

Van der Maas, P.J., van der Wal, G. and Haverkate, I. (1996) Euthanasia, physician-assisted suicide, and other medical practices involving the end of life in the Netherlands, *New England Journal of Medicine*, 335: 1699–705.

Ventafridda, V., Ripamonti, C., deConno, F., Tamburini, M. and Cassileth, B.R. (1990) Symptom prevalence and control during cancer patients' last days of life, *Journal of Palliative Care*, 6(3): 7–11.

Vermylen, J. and Schotsmans, P. (2000) *Ethiek in de kliniek. 25 jaar adviezen van de Commissie Medische Ethiek, Faculteit Geneeskunde, K.U. Leuven*. Leuven: Universitaire Perss.

Viguria Arrieta, J.M., Rocafort Gil, J., Eslava Gurrea, E. and Ortega Sobera, M. (2000) Sedación con midazolám: Eficacia de un protocolo de tratamiento en pacientes terminales con síntomas no controlables con otros medios, *Medicina Paliativa*, 7(1): 2–5.

Viola, R.A., Wells, G.E. and Peterson, J. (1997) The effects of fluid satus and fluid therapy on the dying: a systematic review, *Journal of Palliative Care*, 13(4): 41–52.

Waller, A., Bercovitch, M., Fainsinger, R.L. and Adunsky, A. (1999) Symptom control and the need for sedation during the treatment in Tel Hashomer in-patient hospice. Abstract, 6th Congress EAPC, September 1999, Geneva, Switzerland. *Abstract Book*. Geneva: EAPC Onlus.

Wein, S. (2000) Sedation in the imminently dying patient, *Oncology*, 14(4): 582–92.

Wilkes, E. (1994) On withholding nutrition and hydration in the terminally ill: has palliative medicine gone too far? A commentary, *Journal of Medical Ethics*, 20: 144–5.

10 Euthanasia and physician-assisted suicide

BERT GORDIJN, BEN CRUL AND ZBIGNIEW ZYLICZ

Euthanasia is a topic which creates ardent debate and presents serious moral challenges within contemporary medicine. In principle, however, both opponents and advocates agree that requests for euthanasia are frequently symptoms of rather tragic situations. Hence, the prevention of such requests has become a matter of interest. In this regard, palliative care can play a pivotal role (Zylicz and van Dijk 1995; Aulbert et al. 1998; Husebø and Klaschik 1998; Gordijn and Janssens 2000). However, even in hospices and palliative care units euthanasia requests do occur (Seale and Addington-Hall 1995).

In this chapter we intend to analyse some of the ethical issues connected with euthanasia. Following a brief conceptual clarification, we present two cases in which patients develop and bring forward a wish for euthanasia. In the first case, a situation is described in which euthanasia is finally performed. The second case depicts circumstances in which the physician refuses to perform euthanasia, despite a lot of pressure to do so from both the patient and the family. These cases serve as a starting point for further reflections on the ethical dimensions of the different ways in which physicians can cope with requests for euthanasia. First, however, we focus on two of the most important arguments that have been brought forward in favour of euthanasia: beneficence (compassion, relief of suffering) and respect for autonomy. A closer analysis of these arguments as sources of support for euthanasia reveals that they are problematic. In addition, we analyse other ethical considerations such as the argument from the wrongness of unnecessary killing of innocent life, the slippery slope argument and the role of euthanasia within palliative care.

Conceptual clarification

The word 'euthanasia' comes from the Greek and, taken literally, signifies a good (*eu*) (happy and painless) death (*thanatos*). Nowadays, however, the concept of euthanasia signifies different forms of medically induced death. In the palliative care literature there is a good deal of conceptual confusion surrounding euthanasia (Janssens 2001). Let us consider three different distinctions made in the international discussion on the ethical aspects of euthanasia.

First, *passive* and *active* euthanasia are distinguished. Passive euthanasia means letting die by forgoing or withdrawing life-sustaining treatment. Examples of this would include removing life-support equipment (turning off a respirator) or not delivering cardio-pulmonary resuscitation and allowing a person whose heart has stopped to die. Active euthanasia, on the other hand, means causing the death of the patient by giving a certain life-shortening treatment. Mostly, this is done by injecting controlled substances into the patient, thus causing death.

Second, there is the distinction between *direct* and *indirect* euthanasia. The latter means inducing the death of the patient as a foreseen but un-intended side-effect of treatment of pain or other symptoms, rather than bringing about the death of the patient as the intended effect of the treatment.

Finally, *voluntary*, *involuntary* and *non-voluntary* euthanasia are distinguished. This last distinction assumes that euthanasia can either be an object of the will of the patient or not (non-voluntary euthanasia). Moreover, if it is an object of the will, it can be contrary to it (involuntary euthanasia) or conforming with this will (voluntary euthanasia).

In contrast to euthanasia, physician-assisted suicide (PAS) means that a physician supplies information and/or the means of committing suicide to a patient (such as a prescription for a lethal dose of pills), so that they can easily terminate their own life (for an extensive discussion of both euthanasia and physician-assisted suicide, see Uhlmann 1998).

Two cases of a request for euthanasia

As both cases presented here are embedded in a Dutch context, which in certain regards is rather idiosyncratic, a few words of commentary are necessary (for more information on euthanasia and palliative care in the Netherlands see Janssens et al. 1999; Zylicz and Finlay 1999; Gordijn and Visser 2000; ten Have and Janssens 2001). In the Netherlands, the term 'euthanasia' means the intentional termination of the life of a patient at their request by someone other than the patient. This means that the Dutch use of the term 'euthanasia' presupposes that there is a *voluntary* request of the patient, that there is an act of *active* termination of life and that this act is carried out *deliberately*, that is the act is performed with the intention to end the life of the patient (Leenen 1984).

The Dutch policy of pragmatic tolerance towards euthanasia continues to cause concern in other countries. Up to 2001 euthanasia was illegal in the Netherlands. Conforming to article 293 of the Dutch penal code, euthanasia was a penal offence that could be punished by a prison sentence of up to 12 years or a fine of up to Dfl.100,000. Nevertheless, most reported cases of euthanasia were not criminally prosecuted. Many cases in which article 293 of the Dutch penal code was clearly offended against were dismissed after an inquest. Generally, this happened when a physician, when performing euthanasia, had observed certain well-described conditions. In these cases, the public prosecutor would not further prosecute the illegally acting physician (Gordijn 1997, 1998).

This situation has now changed. In the summer of 1999, a new government bill concerning euthanasia and PAS went to Parliament for discussion (Bill on certification of life termination on request and PAS 1999). Through this bill, the government intended to legally embody a ground for exemption from punishment for physicians who conducted euthanasia or PAS and who complied with certain requirements. On 28 November 2000, the Lower House of the Dutch Parliament accepted this new bill; on 10 April 2001, the Upper House did the same. Setting aside discussion on specific details, the main effect of the new law is the transformation of a practice of pragmatic tolerance into a legally codified practice of euthanasia. Hence, the Netherlands is the first country in the world legally to allow euthanasia under specific circumstances.

Euthanasia performed

Mr C was suffering from a severe form of disseminated plasmocytoma, a malignant condition characterized by multiple localizations in the bones. He was 42 years old and married with three daughters and his prognosis was poor. The cancer was treated with chemotherapy and radiotherapy. As the tumour responded only partially, further chemotherapy followed. In addition, a bone marrow transplant was carried out, which was accompanied by many cumbersome side-effects such as mucositis, neuritis and a very painful dermal graft-versus-host reaction with skin toxicity. Finally, treatment proved to be effective and a symptom-free period began. Mr C experienced the therapy as very demanding and on several occasions, he was about to give up. Strong support from his wife and children and indeed a certain pressure from their side had moved him to carry on.

Unfortunately, six months later tumour growth recurred. The pain returned and increased gradually. Because the situation at home had

*become unmanageable and further chemotherapy was considered, Mr C
was admitted to the hospital. He complained of severe pain in the lower
back radiating to the right leg. Pain treatment consisting of morphine
and amitriptylin did not relieve his pain and caused nausea and vomiting.
His Numeric Rating Scale (NRS) for pain amounted to 8 (0 = no pain at
all, 10 = pain at its worst). The pain rapidly expanded to the whole lower
half of his body and a paraparesis became apparent. An MR (magnetic
resonance) scan revealed a massive compression of the spinal cord. Since
pain treatment with regular oral analgesics (morphine and co-analgesics)
failed, a spinal infusion with a combination of morphine and local
anaesthetics was started (van Dongen et al. 1993). Within one week,
Mr C developed a complete paraparesis and he became fully bedridden.
Pain control could be maintained only with additional intravenous
infusions with midazolam and ketamine. Mr C remained conscious and
reported a NRS in rest of 1–2. During daily care manoeuvres the NRS
increased to 5–6. He had to be nursed on a sand-floating mattress bed
and became completely immobile. Further increase of infusion therapy
with analgesics was not possible without compromising his vital functions
(van Dongen et al. 1997).*

*On several occasions soon after admission to the hospital, Mr C
made clear he wished to consider euthanasia. He had no hope of any
improvement of the situation and his suffering was intense. He discussed
the topic regularly with his attending nurses and physicians. His wife said
she respected his wish and six days before his death the patient made a
formal written request for euthanasia.*

*A gradual but continuous increase of the dosage of intravenous
midazolam and ketamine would have resulted in deep sedation and coma,
finally resulting in the patient's death. However, the administration of
these drugs was meant exclusively for the treatment of pain. Therefore,
the dosages remained restricted to those necessary for pain control. The
physicians involved in this case wanted to avoid a grey zone between
control of pain and euthanasia. Hence, for the euthanasia procedure,
a completely separate path was chosen. This approach allows a strict
separation between medical treatment (symptom control) and the active
ending of a patient's life (euthanasia). The fact that Mr C's suffering was
excruciating was obvious to everybody involved in his treatment. Hence,
his wish for termination of suffering was judged to be realistic and fully
comprehensible.*

*According to the rules prevailing in the Netherlands in 2000, a
second independent physician must be consulted, and this was done.
The physician judged the request of the patient consistent and well based.
Euthanasia was planned for Sunday, 2 p.m. Because he had been given
midazolam Mr C was somewhat obtunded but when addressed he was
fully coherent. In the presence of his wife and brother, the doctor*

administered pentothal followed by a muscle relaxant resulting in the immediate death of the patient. The persons present described the procedure as peaceful and dignified. In later encounters, during bereavement, his wife was convinced that her husband had made the right decision. To have supported him in accomplishing his last wish was a great solace to her.

An autopsy revealed an epidural tumour growth extending from the sacrum to the second thoracic vertebra. There were extensive retroperitoneal tumour masses around the great abdominal vessels and lumbo-sacral nervous plexus and multiple bone metastases in skull and vertebrae.

Euthanasia refused

Mrs D was a proud mother of four adult children and many (adult) grandchildren. She was 82 years old and had been widowed ten years ago. Her husband died of bronchial cancer. His death was very difficult for her as she had nursed him at home for several months. She did not want to admit him to the nursing home. At the very last moment, her husband suffocated. Unfortunately, there was no adequate medical help available at the time as the general practitioner was on holiday. After this, Mrs D signed an advance directive, which included discontinuation of futile treatment and even euthanasia in the case of prolonged suffering.

Mrs D had seen her general practitioner four months earlier because of problems with swallowing. She was found to be anaemic and was referred to the specialist, who diagnosed upper oesophageal carcinoma. As a course of radiotherapy was given, Mrs D improved considerably. However, little attention was given to her symptoms of pain, burning and difficult swallowing, which were exacerbated in the weeks after radiotherapy.

One month before admission to the hospice, Mrs D started to complain of pain in her left shoulder and left occipital region. Her left arm became weaker and she was not able to lift a cup of coffee in her left hand. In addition, she started to experience tinitus in her left ear. The specialist found a small (3 cm) tumour located under her left ear, which was probably the secondary of the oesophagus carcinoma diagnosed earlier. Again, radiotherapy was suggested, but she refused because of her unfortunate previous experience. She also informed the specialist that she would now prefer euthanasia rather than a new course of radiotherapy.

Her pain was treated with paracetamol and later with morphine and transdermal fentanyl. However, the pain increased and the therapy was not very successful. Mrs D became restless, was not sleeping well and her mind was sometimes clouded. In addition, she was at times rude to her children. In the evenings, Mrs D's symptoms of restlessness increased. Her general practitioner suggested increasing the dose of fentanyl, which he believed would improve pain control and maybe hasten the impending death. However, the increase of the dose of transdermal fentanyl to 100 μg/hour did not have any effect on the pain, but instead increased her restlessness and anxiety.

Mrs D, supported by three of her children, began requesting euthanasia. The general practitioner, well known to her, considered her wish for euthanasia valid and promised to comply with it. However, her eldest son John opposed this view and began looking around for alternatives. John's wife was also ill, suffering from disseminated breast cancer and her prognosis was poor at that moment. John and his wife were practising Christians, as opposed to John's siblings, who were not.

John suggested admission to the local hospice and Mrs D agreed to this, albeit with some hesitation. At the admission she stated that she would like to live longer, but only if the pain could be adequately controlled. The neuropathic pain syndrome was diagnosed, involving several nerves and branches that originate at the skull basis and cervical spine. Mrs D continued to refuse radiotherapy. Fentanyl was gradually decreased from 100 to 25 μg/hour and gabapentin (Neurontin®) was administered in a dose of 1800 mg a day. Additionally, she was treated with dexamethazone 12 mg a day, but this drug was gradually discontinued and stopped three weeks later.

Mrs D improved considerably and the pain decreased from originally NRS 9 to NRS 1. She started to eat and became fully ambulant again. Her evening and night restlessness and anxiety disappeared. Many relatives, including her children, who were very optimistic about the treatment, visited her. At that time she never mentioned euthanasia again.

Four weeks later, the pain returned. This time, however, swallowing problems accompanied the pain. Gabapentin capsules needed to be opened and the patient was swallowing the drugs mixed with some thick fluids. Hence, she became depressed and her hope faded away. Knowing that the hospice staff did not perform euthanasia on principle, she avoided discussing the topic, even when asked. John avoided bringing up the issue too, but the rest of the family, convinced that their mother should request euthanasia again, persuaded her to do so.

At that time, Mrs D was not able to swallow at all, and her condition deteriorated rapidly. There was a real danger that the (neuropathic) pain would recur because, unfortunately, gabapentin is not available as an injectable drug. For this reason, the hospice physician chose to switch to clonazepam subcutaneous infusion and to titrate this drug rapidly against the pain. He informed Mrs D and her relatives that this drug would probably sedate her and that consequently she would not be able to communicate any more.

Therefore, Mrs D said farewell to all her children and grandchildren, most of whom thought that the new drug would soon kill Mrs D, which they considered to be very similar to euthanasia. The dose of clonazepam was increased rapidly from 2 to 6 mg per 24 hours as Mrs D experienced sharp pains in her left arm. She fell asleep within several hours, but sometimes she screamed when the nurse changed her position in the bed. This was distressing for the relatives and some of them began requesting instantaneous euthanasia, bringing up the advanced directive signed by Mrs D several years earlier. John's brother even stated that he felt cheated by the hospice; he expected clonazepam to end his mother's life quickly. John opposed the request, explaining to his siblings that euthanasia was not necessary and that their mother would die anyway within one or two days. The hospice physician, who felt himself under pressure to intentionally shorten Mrs D's life, supported this view.

As Mrs D was still experiencing pain while changing position in bed, it was agreed that morphine 20 mg/24 hour would be added to clonazepam (subcutaneous infusion) and the fentanyl transdermal patch. This resulted in better control of symptoms and a full coma that lasted for another two days. During this period, the family did not communicate with the hospice physician or with the nurses. However, they stayed day and night in the hospice waiting for Mrs D's death.

From the start of the initial clonazepam infusion, five days had passed and the family was really exhausted by the time Mrs D died. She died peacefully at night. Several hours later, John's brother, aged 53, while still in the hospice, experienced severe chest pain; he was transported by ambulance to a nearby hospital. Fortunately, his condition was not serious and he recovered several days later. However, his wife blamed John for all this. John and his wife were desperate. After their mother's death, they visited the hospice to thank the staff for their good care. They agreed to visit the bereavement counsellor afterwards, though John's siblings did not take up this service.

Ethical dimensions

The cases of Mr C and Mrs D bring up different ethical questions. First, the case of Mr C demonstrates that extensive anti-tumour treatment can be a heavy burden for the patient involved. Sometimes this treatment can postpone death only at the price of increased suffering. Everybody involved in his treatment concurred in holding that Mr C's suffering was agonizing. Accordingly, his wish for termination of suffering was judged to be realistic and fully comprehensible. The excessive suffering of Mr C led to an extreme measure: euthanasia. Since the attending physicians regarded euthanasia as the only way to reduce the suffering, considerations of beneficence led them to perform euthanasia. This case calls for a more elaborate analysis of the role of the principle of beneficence with regard to euthanasia.

Second, in the case of Mrs D the hospice physician did not perform euthanasia, in spite of considerable pressure from the patient's family. Instead, terminal sedation was chosen, thereby not complying with the wish of the patient. Here, it can be asked whether respect for autonomy must always imply doing what the patient wants. In other words, has the physician failed to respect the autonomy of the patient in this case?

The third topic brought up by the two cases is the difference between euthanasia and terminal sedation as a last resort in palliative care, which is also discussed in Chapter 9. Both measures result in death but the intentions of the physicians differ. What is the ethical meaning of intentions in decisions at the end of life?

The fourth issue brought to light by the two cases is what happens if physicians start actively to terminate the lives of their patients. Will this gradually reduce the power of certain inhibitions to kill? Will situations arise that are clearly morally undesirable? Might, for example cost pressures within the healthcare system lead to situations in which suffering patients would be more easily killed non-voluntarily or even against their will? These questions call for a reflection on the slippery slope argument.

Finally, the place of euthanasia within palliative care is discussed. Medicine has certain ends that physicians should try to achieve. Up to now active killing has never been such an end. Has the traditional set of goals of medicine been incomplete up to now? Is euthanasia compatible or incompatible with palliative care? What happens to the ethos of palliative care if euthanasia becomes an option?

We shall now consider these five issues in turn.

Beneficence

In different ethical theories, considerations of beneficence have played an essential role and various views on the defining properties of beneficence have been developed. Frankena (1973), for example, holds that beneficence implies four different obligations:

- One ought not to inflict evil or harm.
- One ought to prevent evil or harm.
- One ought to remove evil or harm.
- One ought to do or promote good.

In contrast, Beauchamp and Childress (1994) distinguish between non-maleficence and beneficence. Accordingly, they distinguish the first above-mentioned obligation that one ought not to inflict evil or harm from the other three duties, categorizing the first as an obligation of non-maleficence.

Arguments relating to beneficence play a central role in debates on euthanasia. The traditional argument from mercy, for example, states that no person should have to endure pointless terminal suffering. If the physician is unable to relieve the patient's suffering in other ways and terminating the life of the patient is the only way to bring the torment to a close, then the physician should be allowed to bring about the death of the patient (van den Berg 1969; Wilkinson 1990; Overberg 1993; Prouse 2000).

This argument is not unproblematic. It presupposes that there are conditions in which relief of the patient's suffering cannot be brought about in ways other than death. This is not unmistakably evident on first sight. Hence, further arguments are needed to sustain this premise. Are there really situations in which relief of suffering cannot be brought about in ways other than by death? Could not even in extreme cases terminal sedation always bring about the same relief of suffering without any direct termination of the life of the patient? Supposing that palliative care specialists have done everything in their power to relieve the distress of a patient and nothing has worked, complete sedation seems still to be an option of coping with the otherwise untreatable agony. Complete sedation implies total obtundation. Accordingly, a completely sedated patient cannot communicate or perceive or suffer. Therefore, terminal sedation can be regarded as a last resort in palliative care when nothing else works (see Chapter 9).

On the other hand there seem to be a few problems connected with terminal sedation as a last resort. First, there are patients who plainly do not want to be terminally sedated. In their view, sedation would imply total dependency and giving up entirely any control over their life, the thought of which causes great distress. Second, how can we really know with absolute certainty that a terminally sedated patient does not suffer any more? For example, in the second case, after having been sedated Mrs D still seemed to experience pain while changing position in bed, for a certain period. Could the pain have still been the same, although the perception was blocked with drugs? We do not seem to have definite criteria to determine whether a terminally sedated person does indeed not suffer any more and more research is needed in this respect.

There is also a second problematic aspect of referring to considerations of beneficence in trying to justify euthanasia. Normally we presume that a genuine relief of suffering consists in reducing the amount of distress or agony after which the subject of suffering will be able to feel relieved. Essential for the phenomenon of feeling relieved of suffering is the capacity to notice the reduced level of torment. In the case of euthanasia, however, the suffering is brought to an end by annihilating the subject of the suffering. Here, the means to achieve the end consist of an irreversible elimination of the subject of all conscious experience. Accordingly, the reduced level of suffering is never really experienced by the suffering subject. This objection, however, could also be brought forward against terminal sedation.

After all, in terminal sedation all conscious experience is also eliminated. However, here the elimination is not as definitive and irreversible as in euthanasia. In principle, the sedation could be reversed if there are good reasons to do so.

Respect for autonomy

The case of Mrs D brought up the question of whether respect for autonomy demands that physicians terminate the life of an autonomous patient if they are being asked to do so. Since the 1960s, the concept of autonomy has dominated the bioethical debate, especially the Anglo-Saxon discussion (see Chapter 8). This supremacy of the principle of autonomy has had important ramifications for debates on euthanasia. In these discussions, respect for autonomy has become one of the most important arguments in favour of euthanasia. It is stated that respect for autonomy is the foundation of the right to determine the course of one's own life. Analogously, the same principle calls for the right to determine the way we die. Therefore, if a terminally ill person seeks assistance in dying from a physician, the physician ought to comply, provided the request is made autonomously (see for discussion Boisvert 1988; Roscam Abbing 1988; Birnbacher 2000; Prouse 2000). However, it can be seriously questioned whether the autonomy of patients is truly respected in performing euthanasia as a solution to extreme suffering.

What is meant by the norm which demands that autonomy should be respected is far from evident. On the one hand, there is the problem of the *defining properties of autonomy*. On the other hand, there is the question of what *respect for autonomy* involves. With regard to the defining properties of autonomy there are different theories (ten Have et al. 1998). Many theories, however, seem to agree that three conditions are essential to autonomy. First, some kind of independence from controlling influences. Second, the capacity for intentional action. Finally, true information and understanding.

Different opinions also exist on what autonomy involves (see Chapter 8). Immanuel Kant (1724–1804) and John Stuart Mill (1806–73) have been the most influential thinkers in this regard. According to Kant, respect for autonomy requires that autonomous persons should never be treated merely as means. Since autonomous persons are ends in themselves each having the capacity to determine their own destiny, it is morally forbidden to regard them exclusively as a function of the goals of other persons (Kant 1985).

According to Mill (1977), on the other hand, respect for autonomy implies a ban on interfering with the choices and actions of autonomous persons, provided that the latter, in their turn, do not conflict with the freedom of other autonomous persons. Sometimes, however, when other persons act on erroneous beliefs, interference by way of persuasion is morally allowed.

Hence, according to Mill's theory respect for autonomy involves two different duties. First, there is the negative duty of not interfering with the decisions and actions based on the considerations, beliefs and values of an autonomous person. The liberty and freedom to act and think of autonomous persons ought not to be restricted arbitrarily. Second, respect for autonomy implies the positive obligation to interfere in order to enhance or restore the autonomy of persons that have a reduced level of autonomy (Mill 1977).

Returning to euthanasia it is doubtful whether patients' requests for euthanasia in situations in which the only alternative is extreme suffering can be regarded as optimally autonomous (Zylicz 2000). It could be argued that in a situation in which extreme suffering compels patients to ask for euthanasia, their autonomy is limited because there seems to be no independence from controlling influences. The extreme suffering can be regarded as an influence that controls and takes over the will of the patient, thereby effectively reducing the autonomy of the will. For example, on admission to the hospice Mrs D stated that, if her pain could be controlled, she would like to live longer.

But even if we suppose that a patient's request for euthanasia is substantially or even fully autonomous, respect for autonomy would still not demand that euthanasia be conducted. As we have shown, respect for autonomy implies two different duties: a negative duty of not interfering with the freedom of autonomous persons and a positive obligation to interfere in order to enhance or restore the autonomy of persons. Hence, respect for autonomy clearly does not involve an obligation to do anything an autonomous person asks you to do. In the case of a request for euthanasia a patient asks you to interfere with their life. However, a positive obligation to interfere is given only if through this interference enhancement or restoration of the autonomy of a person is possible. Killing a patient would not enhance or restore their autonomy. What is more, it would bring about the annihilation of their autonomy. After all, by taking away the life of the patient, the physician would at the same time destroy the necessary condition for the patient's autonomy. Therefore, a moral obligation for physicians to kill a patient cannot be founded on respect for autonomy, even if the patient's desire to be killed is fully autonomous. If we accept this, the attitude of the physician of Mrs D does not imply any offence against respect for autonomy.

Intentions and unnecessary killing of innocent lives

The ban on killing *innocent* human life is one of the most widely accepted ethical norms of humanity. Hence, in most socially or legally accepted forms of killing the killed victims are not innocent, for example, in self-defence, war or capital punishment. Provoked abortion, which the legislation of many modern countries allows, seems to be the only exception. However, the strategy of advocates of this practice of provoked abortion consists of arguing that fetal life does not entail the same moral status as fully developed human life. Hence, they would not regard provoked abortion as an offence against the norm that innocent human life should never be killed. The same norm of not killing innocent human life forbids euthanasia. Even if someone asks another person to do so, innocent life should not be killed.

What about medically induced death in mainstream palliative care? After all, it is widely accepted that good palliative care can involve using particular means for the relief of suffering that as a secondary effect could significantly shorten the life of the patient. For example, it is acceptable to increase the dose of drugs with the intention of relieving distressing symptoms, even if through this the patient's consciousness may be heavily compromised and dehydration and death follow. The death of the patient is then regarded as a foreseen but undesirable and unintended side-effect.

In general, the principle that often guides us whenever the problem of undesirable and unintended side-effects arises is known as the 'principle of double effect'. Likewise, in palliative care foreseen but undesirable and unintended side-effects of symptom treatment are normally justified using this principle (Janssens 2001). It states that it is licit to posit a cause which is either good or indifferent and from which there follows a twofold effect, one good, the other evil, if a proportionately grave reason is present, and if the end of the agent is honourable, that is, if the agent does not intend the evil effect (Boyle 1980). The principle contains four conditions, all of which together are required for the type of act in question to be licit:

- the agent's end must be morally acceptable
- the cause must be good or at least indifferent
- the good effect must be immediate
- there must be a grave reason for positing the cause.

(Boyle 1980: 528)

In the case of indirect euthanasia in palliative care the first condition is fulfilled: the relief of pain and other agonizing symptoms is certainly a morally acceptable end. Also, there is compliance with the second and the third condition. The cause as such, increase of the dose of drugs, seems to be morally indifferent. Furthermore, the good effect, relief of the symptoms, is immediate. The fourth condition, however, can cause problems. A proportionately grave reason must be present. Here, the following question arises: what kind of suffering justifies a shortening of life and to what extent? It seems clear that extreme suffering justifies an insignificant shortening of the life of the patient as an undesirable and unintended side-effect of its treatment, if there is no alternative to bring about a similar relief of the agony. In contrast, a strong acceleration of the dying process as an undesirable and unintended side-effect of the management of fairly insignificant symptoms would obviously not be proportionate. The reason would not be grave enough for positing the cause and, what is more, there are obviously alternative ways of treating the symptoms. Between these two extremes of the spectrum of possible acts of indirect euthanasia there is obviously a grey zone that has to be discussed within palliative care. It will be difficult to develop any clear-cut guidelines stipulating what kind of suffering is proportionally grave enough to justify a certain acceleration of the dying process. First, suffering being a subjective phenomenon defies straightforward description in objective terms. Second, the extent to which certain measures accelerate the dying process cannot be precisely predicted. Hence, assessment of the distress through good communication with the patient is pivotal (Husebø and Klaschik 1998). Moreover, more research and clarification is needed as to the life-shortening effects of certain forms of pain and symptom treatment.

Slippery slope argument

The slippery slope argument states that in a society in which physicians start to terminate the lives of their patients on request, in the longer term situations could arise that are clearly morally unwelcome (Wilkinson 1990; Prouse 2000). In such a society, palliative care would probably not be developed to the full. In the end, killing would perhaps be the only solution medicine would have to offer in situations of extreme suffering. Thereby, the freedom of terminal patients to choose between different ways of dying would most likely be considerably restricted. Also, increasing cost pressures, as well as greed, laziness, insensitivity and other factors affecting physicians and their institutions might lead to situations in which suffering patients would be more easily killed non-voluntarily or even against their will. This could then involve a suppression of personal choices and individual rights, for example the right to die in a natural way. Hence, the patients' trust in physicians could be undermined.

All these predictions are clearly undesirable. However, they are all fairly speculative and lack a sound basis of empirical research to substantiate them. On the other hand, since societal processes are too complex and too indeterminate to be predicted with certainty, predictions that a practice of terminating patients' lives at their request will not lead to morally undesirable consequences are necessarily speculative as well.

In the Netherlands, there were an estimated 1000 cases of termination of life in 1990. This number was somewhat lower (900 cases) in 1995 (van der Maas et al. 1991; van der Wal and van der Maas 1996). In contrast, the number of cases of voluntary euthanasia went up from 2300 to 3200 during the same period (van der Maas et al. 1991; van der Wal and van der Maas 1996). At first sight, this suggests that the physicians' willingness to perform voluntary euthanasia and their readiness to carry out non-voluntary euthanasia do not grow proportionally. However, in voluntary euthanasia, the patient will have to convince the physician that their suffering is such that euthanasia cannot be seen as a disproportionate measure. If, from the perspective of the physician, the suffering of the patient is not unbearable, they will often abstain from performing euthanasia (van der Wal and van der Maas 1996). Conversely, if an unbearably suffering patient is not able to express a wish to be killed, physicians who are convinced of the excruciating nature of the distress sometimes tend to presuppose a wish to be killed. During the 1990–95 period, the percentage of cases of non-voluntary euthanasia in which a wish to be killed was presupposed by the physician rose from 17 per cent to 30 per cent (van der Wal and van der Maas 1996). Hence, it can be asked whether – in the long run – it is possible to delineate other cases where suffering is more salient, as soon as the traditional defence of voluntary euthanasia based on the wish of the suffering patient is accepted.

Euthanasia and palliative care

Nobody would doubt that relief of suffering is a genuine goal of palliative care. After all, quality of life is one of its most important moral notions (Janssens 2001). Suffering can have very different causes. Pain, other physical symptoms as well as clinical depression can cause extreme forms of suffering. Hence, they can lead to requests for euthanasia (van der Maas et al. 1991; Chochinov et al. 1995; van der Wal and van der Maas 1996). To the extent that these factors do indeed play a role as motives for requesting euthanasia, adequately addressing them with the provision of palliative care can probably take away most of these requests (Gordijn and Janssens 2000).

However, with regard to other forms of suffering such as fear of loss of control and fear of dependency, it can be doubted whether these are readily amenable to a programme of palliative care (Seale and Addington-Hall 1995). Even the best palliative care does not seem to be able to fully prevent the dependency and loss of control that are inherently connected with dying from chronic disease (Zylicz and Janssens 1998; Gordijn and Janssens 2000). These very same factors, however, can also play an important role in developing a wish for euthanasia (Seale and Addington-Hall 1995; Back et al. 1996).

This brings up the question of whether euthanasia should be an option in palliative care. If alternative ways of addressing the suffering of a patient have not been successful, should euthanasia then be considered? One way of approaching this question is the historical argument. It states that medicine inherently has certain goals that physicians should try to achieve. However, killing has never been such a goal. Killing was already prohibited in the Hippocratic oath (ten Have et al. 1998). The physician was bound to save life, not take it. Therefore, physicians should not kill in principle. Hence, euthanasia cannot be an option within palliative care.

However, this argument against euthanasia is flawed in that it jumps from facts to norms. The sheer fact that killing has never been an end of medicine in the past does not imply that it could not be a morally justifiable goal in the future. An empirical thesis cannot substantiate the normative thesis that physicians should under all circumstances abstain from euthanasia.

A more fruitful approach consists in reflecting on the ethos of palliative care. The ideal of a choreographed death on command which is an effect of being-in-control and enjoying-independence has become one of the culturally idealized icons of our time. By abstaining from euthanasia, palliative care takes a critical stance towards these disputable societal developments. After all, the ethos of palliative care admits that life and death are phenomena that are ultimately beyond our control. Hence, if palliative care workers were to start performing euthanasia in situations in which fear of loss of control and fear of dependency play a pivotal role in developing a wish for euthanasia, this would be against the ethos of palliative care. Palliative care would thereby disavow its original ideals. Perhaps instead it should help contribute to a critical reassessment of the idea that life is worth living only as an independent individual fully in control and not in need of any help from others.

Conclusion

Two of the most important arguments that have been brought forward in favour of euthanasia are the arguments of beneficence (compassion, relief of suffering) and respect for autonomy. However, a closer analysis of these arguments has demonstrated that they have serious flaws. In addition, the analysis of the use of the principle of double effect has revealed that the question of what kind of suffering is proportionally grave enough to justify a certain degree of acceleration of the dying process is problematic. Hence, it should be further discussed within palliative care. The reflection on the slippery slope argument against euthanasia, although speculative in principle, demonstrates that as soon as the traditional defense of voluntary euthanasia based on the wish of the suffering patient is accepted, it can be difficult to delineate other cases where suffering is more salient. Finally, it has been argued that palliative care has a role in critically reassessing the culturally idealized icons of being-in-control and enjoying independence.

References

Aulbert, E., Klaschik, E. and Pichlmaier, H. (eds) (1998) *Palliativmedizin – Die Alternative zur aktiven Sterbehilfe. Zur Euthanasie-Diskussion in Deutschland.* Stuttgart: Schattauer.

Back, A.L., Wallace, J.I., Starks, H.E. and Pearlman, R.A. (1996) Physician-assisted suicide and euthanasia in Washington State: patient request and physician responses, *Journal of the American Medical Association*, 275(12): 919–25.

Beauchamp, T.L. and Childress, J.F. (1994) *Principles of Biomedical Ethics*, 4th edn. New York: Oxford University Press.

Bill on certification of life termination on request and PAS (1999) De toetsing van levensbeëindiging op verzoek en hulp bij zelfdoding en tot wijziging van het Wetboek van Strafrecht en van de Wet op de lijkbezorging (TK 26691, vergaderjaar 1998–99).

Birnbacher, D. (2000) Eine ethische Bewertung der Unterschiede in der Praxis der Sterbehilfe in den Niederlanden und in Deutschland, in B. Gordijn and H.A.M.J. ten Have (eds) *Medizinethik und Kultur: Grenzen medizinischen Handelns in Deutschland und den Niederlanden*. Stuttgart-Bad Cannstadt: frommann-holzboog.

Boisvert, M. (1988) All things considered . . . then what?, *Journal of Palliative Care*, 4(1): 115–18.

Boyle, J.M. (1980) Toward understanding the principle of double effect, *Ethics*, 90: 527–38.

Chochinov, H.M., Wilson, K.G., Enns, M. et al. (1995) Desire for death in the terminally ill, *American Journal of Psychiatry*, 152: 1185–91.

Frankena, W.K. (1973) *Ethics*, 2nd edn. Englewood Cliffs, NJ: Prentice-Hall.

Gordijn, B. (1997) Euthanasie in den Niederlanden – eine kritische Betrachtung (Euthanasia in the Netherlands – a critical review), in U. Körner (ed.) *Berliner Medizinethische Schriften. Beiträge zu Ethik und Recht in der Medizin*, Vol. 19. Berlin: Humanitas Verlag.

Gordijn, B. (1998) Euthanasie: strafbar und doch zugestanden? Die niederländische Duldungspolitik in Sachen Euthanasie (Euthanasia: criminal and yet permitted? The Dutch policy of tolerance concerning euthanasia), *Ethik in der Medizin*, 10: 12–25.

Gordijn, B. and Janssens, R. (2000) The prevention of euthanasia through palliative care: new developments in the Netherlands, *Patient Education and Counseling*, 41(1): 35–46.

Gordijn, B. and Visser, A. (2000) Issues in Dutch palliative care: readjusting a distorted image, *Patient Education and Counseling*, 41(1): 1–5.

Husebø, S. and Klaschik, E. (1998) *Palliativmedizin: Praktische Einführung in Schmerztherapie, Ethik und Kommunikation*. Heidelberg and Berlin: Springer.

Janssens, R. (2001) *Palliative Care: Concepts and Ethics*. Nijmegen: University Press Nijmegen.

Janssens, R., ten Have, H.A.M.J. and Zylicz, Z. (1999) Hospice and euthanasia in the Netherlands: an ethical point of view, *Journal of Medical Ethics*, 25(5): 408–12.

Kant, I. (1985) Kritik der praktischen Vernunft, in K. Vorländer (ed.) *Philosophische Bibliothek*, 9th edn, Vol. 38. Hamburg: Felix Meiner Verlag.

Leenen, H.J.J. (1984) The definition of euthanasia, *Medicine and Law*, 3(4): 333–78.

Mill, J.S. (1977) On Liberty, in J.M. Robson (ed.) *Collected Works of John Stuart Mill*, Vol. 18. Toronto: University of Toronto Press.

Overberg, K.R. (ed.) (1993) *Mercy or Murder? Euthanasia, Morality and Public Policy*. Kansas City, MO: Sheed and Ward.

Prouse, M. (2000) Euthanasia: slippery slope or mercy killing?, in P. Webb (ed.) *Ethical Issues in Palliative Care: Reflections and Considerations*. Manchester: Hochland and Hochland.

Roscam Abbing, H.D.C. (1988) Dying with dignity, and euthanasia: a view from the Netherlands, *Journal of Palliative Care*, 4(4): 70–4.

Seale, C. and Addington-Hall, J. (1995) Euthanasia: the role of good care, *Social Science and Medicine*, 40: 581–7.

Ten Have, H.A.M.J. and Janssens, R. (eds) (2001) *Palliative Care in Europe: Concepts and Policies*. Amsterdam: IOS Press.

Ten Have, H.A.M.J., ter Meulen, R. and van Leeuwen, E. (1998) *Medische ethiek*. Houten/Diegem: Bohn Stafleu Van Loghum.

Uhlmann, M. (ed.) (1998) *Last Rights: Assisted Suicide and Euthanasia Debated*. Grand Rapids, MI: Wm B. Eerdmans.

Van den Berg, J.H. (1969) *Medische macht en medische ethiek*. Nijkerk: G.F. Callenbach.

Van der Maas, P.J., Pijnenborg, L. and Delden, J.J.M. (1991) *Medische beslissingen rond het levenseinde: Commissie onderzoek medische praktijk inzake euthanasie* (Medical decisions concerning the end of life: research committee concerning medical practice of euthanasia). The Hague: Sdu Uitgever.

Van der Wal, G. and van der Maas, P.J. (1996) *Euthanasie en andere medische beslissingen rond het levenseinde: De praktijk en de meldingsprocedure* (Euthanasia and other medical decisions concerning the end of life: practice and notification procedure). The Hague: Sdu Uitgever.

Van Dongen, R.T.M., Crul, B.J.P. and de Bock, M. (1993) Long-term intrathecal infusion of morphine and morphine/bupivacaine mixtures in the treatment of cancer pain: a retrospective analysis of 51 cases, *Pain*, 55: 119–23.

Van Dongen, R.T.M., van Ee, R. and Crul, B.J.P. (1997) Neurological impairment during long-term intrathecal infusion of bupivacaine in cancer patients: a sign of spinal cord compression, *Pain*, 69: 206–9.

Wilkinson, J. (1990) The ethics of euthanasia, *Palliative Medicine*, 4(2): 81–6.

Zylicz, Z. (2000) Ethical considerations in the treatment of pain in a hospice environment, *Patient Education and Counseling*, 41(1): 47–53.

Zylicz, Z. and van Dijk, L. (1995) Palliatieve zorgverlening en de vraag naar euthanasie, *Pro Vita Humana*, 6: 161–8.

Zylicz, Z. and Finlay, I.G. (1999) Euthanasia and palliative care: reflections from the Netherlands and the UK, *Journal of the Royal Society of Medicine*, 92(7): 370–3.

Zylicz, Z. and Janssens, M.J.P.A. (1998) Options in palliative care: dealing with those who want to die, in M. Zenz (ed.) *Cancer Pain: Bailliere Clinics of Anaesthesiology*, 12: 121–31.

11 Research ethics in palliative care

FRANZ-JOSEF ILLHARDT AND HENK TEN HAVE

This chapter is concerned with the ethical issues that govern the conduct of research in palliative care. In particular we need to ask what kinds of research questions and research designs might be acceptable and useful, and also under what circumstances do caregivers have the duty to conduct research or to support it for the sake of palliative care?

The status quo

The Cochrane library databases contain information on some 350,000 trials in western biomedicine. Of these a tiny proportion relate to the field of palliative care, as revealed in a keyword search, the results of which can be seen in Table 11.1.

The data summarized in the table are based on searches for 'palliative medicine', 'palliative nursing', 'palliative care', 'terminal care' and 'terminal patients'. The limited number of projects in the field of palliative care compared with the multitude of studies which are listed in the Cochrane library in total is notable. Why do we have such a low number of research projects in the field of palliative care, at least as listed in the Cochrane databases? One reason may be a biomedical prejudice which sees palliative care as a non-biomedical activity. A second reason may refer to moral considerations: conducting clinical trials that are often burdensome for the subjects is ethically problematic, particularly if non-therapeutic studies are performed and if vulnerable persons are included, like children, demented elderly people, and especially persons who cannot be cured or are dying. Accordingly, the

Table 11.1   Search results from Cochrane Library (January 2001)

Search terms	Components of Cochrane database	Date=published between 1995 and 2000			
		No field restriction	Field= abstract	Field= keywords	Field= title
GENERAL SEARCH TERMS					
PALLIATIVE MEDICINE	CDSR[1]	33	1	-	-
	DARE[2]	8	7	1	-
	CCTR[3]	91	4	5	1
	CMR[4]	5	-	-	-
	NHS EED[5]	15	6	2	2
PALLIATIVE NURSING	CDSR	15	-	-	-
	DARE	4	4	-	-
	CCTR	19	-	4	-
	CMR	-	-	-	-
	NHS EED	8	4	2	-
PALLIATIVE CARE	CDSR	51	3	4	-
	DARE	18	11	12	3
	CCTR	414	61	320	20
	CMR	2	2	-	2
	NHS EED	66	31	38	7
TERMINAL CARE	CDSR	42	-	-	-
	DARE	11	10	6	-
	CCTR	75	29	34	6
	CMR	-	-	-	-
	NHS EED	44	24	22	1
TERMINAL PATIENTS	CDSR	58	-	-	-
	DARE	11	10	-	-
	CCTR	371	338	-	17
	CMR	1	1	-	-
	NHS EED	31	26	-	3
	DARE	20	18	-	-
	CCTR	73	41	7	1
	CMR	4	3	-	-
	NHS EED	18	11	6	-
	DARE	2	1	-	-
	CCTR	1	-	-	-
	CMR	-	-	-	-
	NHS EED	-	-	-	-

Notes

1 CDSR = *Cochrane Database of Systematic Reviews*; total entries by the end of May 2001: 1947 (in the table *Complete reviews* and *Protocols* are listed together)

2 DARE = *Database of Abstracts of Reviews of Effectiveness*; total entries by the end of May 2001: 2793 (in the table solely *Abstracts of quality assessed systematic reviews* are listed)

3 CCTR = *Cochrane Controlled Trials Register*; total entries by the end of May 2001: 307,872 (in the table solely *Complete reviews* are listed)

4 CMR = *Cochrane Methodology Register*; total entries by the end of May 2001: 3407

5 NHS EED = *NHS Economic Evaluation Database*; total entries by the end of May 2001: 6822

research output in palliative care may be affected by the view that terminally ill patients should not be harmed or burdened as research subjects. Thus, even if a trial is therapeutic, these patients may be considered unsuitable for entry, on ethical grounds.

The first reason cannot be overcome by rational arguments. At stake here is the debate on concepts and definitions of palliative care which will lead to a more clear and less ambiguous demarcation of the expertise involved in palliative care (ten Have and Janssens 2001; see also Chapter 3). However, it is not really comprehensible why conceptual uncertainties should hinder the development of research projects. In fact, in order to further knowledge in the field and to enable palliative care professionals to improve their expertise, it could be argued that more research needs to be carried out. The second reason, therefore, may be more significant and the analysis of this requires an examination of research ethics.

Research ethics

When a research study is planned within the biomedical paradigm, the process will follow particular stages. An elaboration of the basic idea and the initial hypothesis is followed by the design of the methodological procedure and the production of a protocol for the study. When the proposed study has been assessed and approved by an ethics review committee, it may then be carried out in a healthcare setting. Subsequently, the results will be evaluated and on the basis of the findings new medical interventions and treatments may be justified and implemented in daily clinical practice. Research in healthcare is distinguished from research in other scientific areas because it has a particular objective and because it usually involves human subjects. The first characteristic is the specificity of the objective. Medical research highlights that in medicine everything is focused on finding new methods of treatment and improving existing treatment modalities. There is a continuous effort to generate new data that can be applied to the medical care of patients who are suffering because medical knowledge is deficient and treatment opportunities limited. Although medicine has a long record of scientific studies, new studies are constantly initiated to improve the current standards of treatment (Figure 11.1).

Because of the predominance of treatment issues and the need for practical application in diagnosis, prognostication, therapy and prevention, research should entail the promise of benefiting patients, in the short, or at least long run. Without such a relationship with at least the possibility of tangible health benefits, then studies are hardly justifiable. This of course raises the question of whether a 'study' that merely intends to optimize known methods of treatment can be regarded as a true piece of research.

Figure 11.1 The aim of medical research: improving treatment

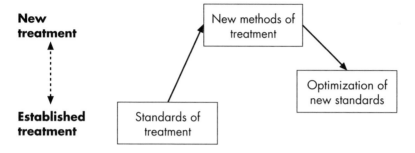

The second characteristic of medical research is the involvement of human subjects. Before clinical research can start, animal experiments have to be done and the results of these have to be documented and approved. Sometimes human subjects have been involved, but the study is not focused on the subjects involved but on specimens of their tissue (blood, material of a biopsy, other body materials) which are to be scrutinized in vitro. The ethical problem, for example for ethics review committees, is the fact that the data can reveal some characteristics of their human donors, and the identity of these donors must be protected.

In reviewing research protocols, committees apply in general two moral rules: informed consent and the risk–benefit ratio. The requirement of informed consent, originating from the moral principle of respect for autonomy (see Chapter 9), implies that extensive information is provided (orally as well as in written form) before consent is asked for participation in a particular study. On the basis of the information, the potential research subject should then be completely free to consent to enrolment in the study. The second rule concerns the analysis of the risks involved and the benefits expected from the projected study. All studies will bring some potential harms and risks to the participating subjects. At the same time, they are conducted in the expectation that they will help to resolve or mitigate specific medical problems, complaints and burdens, for the benefit of patients and of future categories of patients. The balancing of the potential risks versus the expected benefits is not only a task for the research subjects themselves (on the basis of the information provided to them), but also for the ethics committee reviewing the protocol. Even though subjects may consent to participation, the ethics committee can judge that the risks outweigh the potential benefits, and thus not assent to the protocol.

Informed consent, risk–benefit ratio and ethics committee review can therefore be considered the cornerstones of present-day research ethics. However, moral problems may arise with all three, especially when research is planned and carried out in the area of palliative care.

Problems of informed consent

The difficult road to research ethics

The development of present-day research ethics has been difficult and un-easy, in part because of the established status of medicine as a profession. For a long time, it was generally assumed that physicians and healthcare professionals simply know best, and it was they who should decide what is good or bad for patients. Physicians in particular were used to arguing, deciding and intervening on the basis of the 'best-interest' standard. Providing healthcare was regarded as an ethically structured act, the professional always aiming to promote the best interests of the patient and being therefore *per definitionem* acceptable to the person receiving help. Against this background research ethics slowly developed.

One event played a crucial role in formulating one of the basic moral rules, that of informed consent (Faden and Beauchamp 1986). The Nuremberg trials following the defeat of the Nazi regime underlined the unacceptability of a tradition which gave higher value to some other goal than the patient's interests. The doctrine of informed consent was therefore the first answer to a system in which human beings were subordinated to purposes of society, race or war. The widespread practice of using or abusing human beings for extrinsic ends was condemned and it was emphasized that human beings should be regarded as ends in themselves. Even after the Second World War it has been shown that some medical experiments in the United States were conducted without the informed consent of the patients (Beecher [1963] 1977). These experiences led therefore to the incorporation of the principle of informed consent into the Declaration of Helsinki. Subsequently, the World Medical Association was the first to propose the role of ethics review committees for evaluating and controlling medical research (van den Daele and Müller-Salomon 1990). In 1975 the Declaration of Helsinki was in turn revised, urging the medical world to look to ethics review committees for guidance, comment and orientation prior to the commencement of research projects. Such ideas were also stressed in declarations of national societies like the Swiss Academy of Medical Sciences and the American Medical Association, as well as international associations like the World Health Organization.

The freedom of the dying person

The weaker and more ill a patient is, the more they need the help of the caregiver. Following this approach, the ethos of healthcare professionals tends to create a paternalistic attitude. For example in geriatric care it is very difficult to establish a treatment strategy which activates the remaining resources of elderly patients. Irreversibly ill patients experience similar problems. Treatment usually implies compensation for lost functions on the one hand, and mobilization of remaining powers, on the other. It means that paternalistic interventions are apparently necessary to compensate for lost capacities, but that patients still possess freedom to choose and act, although the range of autonomous decision-making may be more and more restricted due to debilitating disease and growing disability. It is also clear that dying patients can become less capable of free choices and acts. The territory of personal autonomy shrinks gradually. Yet freedom is rarely lost completely. The freedom of the dying person is situated between paternalistic care and the autonomy of finite existence.

Freedom has various dimensions that are significant in the case of terminally ill patients. Medical research should acknowledge and be compatible with the ideas of freedom, otherwise it ought not to be done. The terminally ill patient can be free in many dimensions of the notion of 'freedom' and medical research involving these patients has to find adequate ways of safeguarding this multifaceted freedom.

Problems of risk–benefit analysis

The distinction between 'therapeutic' and 'non-therapeutic' research

One proposal for a further revision of the Declaration of Helsinki supported by many scholars is to abandon the traditional differentiation between 'therapeutic' and 'non-therapeutic' medical research (King 1995; Kopelman 1995a; Levine 1999; Vollmann 2000). The point of the distinction was to differentiate the scope, the involved persons and the context in each of the two categories of research. In the case of therapeutic research the goal is to treat an ill person, where those involved are patients who want to recover, and the context is the equipment of a hospital, the experience of the research team and its institutional network. Non-therapeutic research on the other hand aims to obtain basic scientific data, involves healthy subjects (often for financial compensation), and takes place in a research facility, such as a laboratory.

By neglecting the difference between therapeutic and non-therapeutic research with respect to the irreversibly ill patient, the principle of beneficence seems to be in danger. Persons who cannot be cured and have come to a point of no return belong to an especially vulnerable group (Kopelman 1995b; Council for International Organizations of Medical Sciences (CIOMS) 1993). A vulnerable person is somebody who has less access to healthcare facilities or depends on the willingness of others to take into account their interests or even give priority to them. It is not the purpose here to argue for or against the difference between therapeutic and non-therapeutic treatment in general. The point is to consider whether the patients in palliative care can be involved in non-therapeutic settings.

The theory of equipoise

The term 'equipoise' consists of the Latin element *aequus* (just) and a Greek element *poiesis* (work, result of doing). It refers to the equilibrium between the goals of the study (the results) and the conviction of the investigator/physician to help the involved human subject without any bias of personal preference. Many clinical studies seek to compare the efficacy of different combinations of medication. The goal of the study may be the proof that the drug combination A is better than combination B. The conviction that there is a benefit for the patient can be personally, individually, collectively or professionally grounded as right and good. According to this characterization the terms 'personal', 'individual', 'collective' or 'professional equipoise' have been coined (Freedman 1987; Johnson et al. 1991; Illhardt 1996).

We will here outline these four concepts. 'Personal' equipoise refers to the notion that it is fundamental to require that a physician cooperates only in those studies where they can be sure that the established treatment is not as effective as the new and experimental one. This principle depends on the personal moral integrity of the researcher, but it can cause confusion between moral feelings and professional interests (wanting to help someone versus relying on an evidence-based regimen). It therefore prevents the old medical principle of 'wait and see' before doing something and puts under wraps one's real moral feelings. The consequence of this is that the way of orientating the treatment decision according to a principle of equipoise cannot be assessed from outside, it must be based on a personal moral judgment of the investigator who is obliged to weigh the reasons for or against participation in the study. A major disadvantage of this theory of personal equipoise is that a doctor can change treatment plans only by assuming that all decisions made so far were inappropriate. Remember the earlier statement that there can be a moral reason for leaving a well-established treatment regimen only when there are doubts concerning the success of the established treatment. But is it epistemologically possible to arrive at clinical certainty? Only if there is an extremely deep gap between personal and impersonal forms of equipoise, may this theory (and also the next one) seem to have value.

The theory of 'individual equipoise' is also not very strong. The challenge of equipoise can be personal, but not in a strict sense 'individual', because it does not take into account that the doctor's actions are not only the result of individual considerations, but also arise in a mutual climate of science, society, patient, their families, resources and equipment.

The theory of 'collective equipoise' is also not precisely formulated. 'Collective' as an empirical term cannot be proved. What percentage of a population makes a collective? Does 'collective' mean 'all rational people'? There is a hint here of transcendental philosophy, rather than research ethics. Certainly such an idea is not precise enough to result in any recommendations or guidance for the design and conduct of research.

The theory of 'professional equipoise' assumes that whatever the individual doctor believes, she or he must refer to a treatment setting which is based on therapeutic evidence. Yet better treatment has a chance only if the professional community is of the opinion that the optimization of the treatment makes sense and is possible. That means 'professional' equipoise. It is a similar notion to Kuhn's term 'scientific community' (Johnson et al. 1991).

Quality of life assessment

Specific quality of life indices like the Spitzer-Index, EORTC-Index and Kanofsky-Index are nowadays frequently applied in medical research. Sometimes, quality of life is a criterion in comparing the efficacy of two anti-cancer drugs in respect of the well being of the patient. However, it is problematic to use 'quality of life' as an objective standard or criterion. Quality of life essentially has a subjective level; the best person to assess quality of life is the subject involved. By this argument all indices fail because they are not constructed to assess the patient's judgement on their quality of life by the patient themself. One solution has been proposed according to which the indices should be assigned and filled out by doctors and patients simultaneously (Raspe 1990). But do doctors get useful data from patient-oriented indices? The problem here is the role of subjectivity in medicine. The German physician Viktor von Weizsäcker, who founded the movement of psychosomatic medicine in Germany, wrote in 1925 a famous article on the introduction of the subject into medicine (von Weizsäcker 1940). He highlighted two points. First, physicians (and all other caregivers) are subjects themselves. That means that all data are subjectively gained. When they, as professionals, measure the quality of life of the patient, they get subjective judgements as well, although they assume they are getting objective data. The second point of von Weizsäcker is that medicine must be based on the fact that a patient is not only a physiological object, but also a subject. Thus, we have a second reason, why medicine as well as the research it involves, is a subject-based science. The question then is how to characterize medicine: is it an objective science or a subjective mode of treatment? Von Weizsäcker suggested the redefinition of medicine, not as 'psychosomatic' but as 'anthropological' (Eich 1996). Through this renaming he challenged medicine and medical research, both of which appear in danger of losing close contact with the patient.

On this basis we must require of medical research the following:

- Research must be done in the context of the optimal treatment, including that of incurably ill patients.
- Each study must evaluate the status of the patient's quality of life.

- Quality of life assessment not only should cover the activities of daily living but also should include other existential dimensions, like the effectiveness of coping processes, supporting persons and ideas.
- Research without this assessment ought not to be done.

Problems of controlling medical research

Controlling research by a committee

Since the revision to the Declaration of Helsinki in Tokyo in 1974, the World Medical Association requires specially appointed groups to control medical research. Nevertheless, as we have recently seen, the declaration has not prevented studies that are harmful to patients, or frauds in evaluating results (Freedman 1995; Lock 1996; Eser 1999). We must therefore ask whether controlling research by a committee can be effective?

At a first glance it cannot. Three arguments for this can be advanced. First, the researcher controls themself, but this is a pseudo-control, which cannot guarantee that all studies are carried out according to the rules of good clinical practice. Second, the approach is inconsistent because those who do not in general worry about bioethical principles are called upon to apply them in the field of research. Third, the researcher outlines the face of medicine without being entitled to overlook its consequences. What then might be helpful properties of an Institutional Review Board in the process of controlling research?

First, the independence of an ethics committee is a common requirement, found in and endorsed by many statements and declarations. Second, the multidisciplinary composition of the review committee is a further common feature, calling for the development of rules in an interdisciplinary and discursive way. Thus, a continually revised European Community proposal (current version of May 2001) defines an ethics review committee as a working group which consists of persons working in healthcare and other fields (European Parliament and Council Regulation 2001/20/EC, article 2 k). An example may illustrate how committee review works in healthcare practice (Tettenborn 1998) The Ethics Review Committee of the Freiburg University Hospital in Germany is examining 250–350 research projects per year (in 1996 260 proposals came into evaluation). Two-thirds of these projects are drug trials, while one-third concern research for medical products (for example advice for implants), medical procedures (for example surgical methods), genetic treatment (for example adenoviral vector treatment). The committee approves the protocol without further conditions in 34.5 per cent of the cases, 64 per cent are accepted after some amendments or changes have been made, and 1.5 per cent are rejected. In most cases a substantially revised version of the protocol can be submitted again. If the committee demands a change to the protocol, the requirements usually concern the information given to the patient (including their consent form), the methods of evaluating the data, and the weighing of risks and benefits from the side of the investigator.

The preference for a clinical rationale

In the field of medicine research has often been done without a clear clinical justification. However, in order to find out whether a project is justifiable or not one must know whether its results are practically useful. Of course, basic scientific data might be useful, but then those proposing the project must know whether this project is based on a good hypothesis which can and should be applied in the treatment. It is in the interest of medicine itself to prevent any research, which although deemed good for the interests of medical sciences, society, the company, the economic situation of the medical department, is not considered for the good of the patient or for clinical medicine.

The background to many scandals in modern medicine (fraud, manipulation of results, research without licence) is a financial one. The less money the medical departments have for their own goals (and medical research is an important goal) the more comes from industries, first of all from pharmaceutical companies. The medical departments depend on the financial budget, thus they must do some research to raise funds, even if it does not serve the medical task. Further, the university setting generally favours those physicians who are doing a lot of research for whatever reasons, but not those who give priority to 'simple' patient care and treatment.

Room for palliative research?

In the context of this chapter the question is whether patients suffering from an irreversible disease, which is likely to turn out to be fatal, can be involved in medical research. The answer seems affirmative, since the principles of research ethics can protect them sufficiently.

How can terminal patients be protected?

According to a common pharmaceutical practice but not an official guideline, seriously ill patients are enrolled into trials if they meet the following criteria. They must have

- a life expectancy of more than three months
- consented to the trial
- no other concomitant life-threatening diseases.

Regularly, these criteria have been applied to studies in the second-line treatment of cancer. The question is whether they are sufficient to protect especially vulnerable persons like incurably ill patients. There appears to be a consensus 'that the greater the vulnerability and the risk to competent adults, the more specific protections should be adopted' (Kopelman 1995b: 2291).

As regards the first criterion, problems may arise. Patients who come close to the border of three months of life expectancy are to be protected against any kind of exploitation, whether in research or not. Caregivers have the moral (and legal) duty to safeguard the patients' interests. In the final stage of life, terminally ill patients need the devotion and social support of relatives as well as professionals in coping with their fate. Do they also need the progress of science however, from which they may never receive benefits?

As regards the second criterion of 'free consent', many physicians report that irreversibly ill patients consent to be involved in research projects from which they receive no benefits, simply out of a sense of altruism. This altruistic attitude does not necessarily have to be moral at every turn. Most of us have learned that an altruistic ethos is an enhanced ethos. It can be a sign of moral pressure when patients in the last phases of their lives choose for this moral mechanism. They may say: if my life is only a burden for myself and for my loved ones and, thus seems to be without value, I will enhance its value by being altruistic. That is not a sign of moral freedom. It is the caregiver's duty therefore to differentiate between a free altruistic attitude and the fear of being not free disguised as altruism.

The third criterion of 'absence of concomitant life-threatening diseases' is also often problematic. Having only the disease which is the prerequisite of the research helps the researcher to get control over the project. But incurably ill patients usually have many diseases and diseased organs. Thus research with patients in palliative care facilities can easily create situations in which the endpoints of research put risks upon the patient's process of treatment or bring about more inconveniences to him or her than the caregivers can ethically accept.

Refraining from applying the adequate therapy due to the study?

Sometimes, especially in drug trials, a study will produce invalid results, when other drugs have been applied and the amount of drop-outs is too high. In multi-centre and multinational studies, the physicians-researchers are supported by a so-called Data Safety Monitoring Board (DSMB). They take advice from the members of the DSMB to differentiate between serious and non-serious unexpected or adverse events. The DSMB must therefore help to protect the moral commitments of the physician/researcher towards the patients involved. No physician is justified in refusing needed and effective therapy to a patient. It is an essential component of the helping ethos not to do any harm to a patient and not to hinder recovery or cure.

This is consistent with the principles of beneficence and non-maleficence: neither actively nor passively can any harm be done to the patient. This moral reasoning produces a dilemma: no physician can justifiably refuse a patient a treatment which is not proven to be a valid treatment. Or positively formulated: a physician is obliged to provide only such treatment which has shown evidence. It remains unclear which types of evidence (from controlled studies or clinical observation) must be followed. Thus, the physician and the other caregivers have the moral duty to support research, but in each case also to do that on the basis of a concrete risk-benefit-analysis. The greater the risks, the greater the concrete benefits for the involved patient must be. Studies that are likely to provide only small benefits to the patient can be justified only if they also bear very low risks.

A special setting of palliative research

In palliative care it could be argued that controlled studies are impossible, because they do not give direct benefits to the involved person. In order to regard uncontrolled research as valid research however, we must allow exceptions from the medical doctrine that only controlled studies can be valid studies (Pocock and Elbourne 2000). In the recent theory of research, we notice first some arguments for observational studies contra controlled studies. These suggest that observations of clinical application are to some extent as valid as controlled studies (Marquis 1999; Concato et al. 2000). The actual doctrine requires a controlled and prospective design that make a study produce valid data. A 'controlled' design means that a study must have at least two arms, one covering the group with the new medical intervention, the other(s) covering group(s) without that intervention. In cases of severe diseases it is hard to follow this design, as the patients need the treatment. Therefore it can be argued that an observational study is as valid as the controlled and prospective study when it observes the process of treatment and compares the results with 'historical' results, which are gained from charts or clinical reports. If this is right, research involving incurably ill patients becomes possible, as it gives these patients a chance to receive the benefits of the experimental treatment while they are being involved in a study.

The argument against palliative research is therefore related to the current dominance of evidence-based medicine. In palliative care we need a benefit-based medical research, which is designed to

- make clinical observations
- optimize the quality-of-life-situation of the incurably ill patients
- optimize the social support by relatives and caregivers
- strengthen the remaining possibilities for incurably ill patients to control autonomously some procedures in their own bodies as well as in their surroundings.

Conclusion

Research in palliative care is both possible and necessary. Yet we have seen that controlled studies in palliative care have only a limited place in medicine. It is therefore important that we regard irreversibly ill patients as autonomous and capable of consenting in freedom to participate in studies. Consent and autonomy are based on a risk–benefit analysis. Its ratio must be balanced for patients who belong to an especially vulnerable group. Medical research needs therefore the control of a peer review system which can guarantee that research involving irreversibly ill persons respects their interests and rights.

Acknowledgement

Frank-Josef Illhardt would like to thank Tobias Fischer, Barbara Frisch and Petra Schweier for their assistance in solving some special problems.

References

Beecher, H.K. ([1963] 1977) Ethics and clinical research, in S.J. Reiser, A.J. Dyck and W.J. Curran (eds) *Ethics in Medicine: Historical Perspectives and Contemporary Concerns*. Cambridge, MA: MIT Press.

Concato, J., Shah, N. and Horwitz, R.I. (2000) Randomized, controlled trials, observational studies, and the hierarchy of research designs, *New England Journal of Medicine*, 342(25): 1887–900.

Council for International Organizations of Medical Sciences (CIOMS) (1993) International Ethical Guidelines for Biomedical Research Involving Human Subjects (in collaboration with the World Health Organization), in W.T. Reich (ed.) *Encyclopedia of Bioethics*, Vol. 5. New York: Macmillan, Simon and Schuster.

Eich, W. (1996) Psychosomatische Medizin als anthropologische Medizin: Die Heidelberger Tradition, in H. Schott (ed.) *Meilensteine der Medizin*. Dortmund: Harenberg.

Eser, A. (1999) Die Sicherung von 'Good Scientific Practice' und die Sanctionierung von Fehlverhalten (Anhang 'Selbstkontrolle in der Wissenschaft'), in H-D. Lippert and W. Eisenmenger (eds) *Forschung am Menschen: Der Schutz des Menschen – die Freiheit des Forschers*. Berlin: Springer.

European Parliament and Council (2001) Directive 2001/20/EC of 4 April 2001 on the approximation of the laws, regulations and administrative provisions of the Member States relating to the implementation of good clinical practice in the conduct of clinical trials on medicinal products for human use, *Official Journal of the European Communities* L 121/34.

Faden, R.R. and Beauchamp, T.L. (1986) *A History and Theory of Informed Consent*. Oxford and New York: Oxford University Press.

Freedman, B. (1987) Equipoise and the ethics of clinical research, *New England Journal of Medicine*, 317: 141–5.

Freedman, B. (1995) Unethical research, in W.T. Reich (ed.) *Encyclopedia of Bioethics*, Vol. 4. New York: Macmillan, Simon and Schuster.

Illhardt, F.J. (1996) Bewertung und Motiv der Randomisierung: Ethische Eckdaten im Medizinischen Experiment, *Onkologie*, 19: 184–90.

Johnson, N., Lilford, R.J. and Brazier W. (1991) At what level of collective equipoise does a clinical trial become ethical?, *Journal of Medical Ethics*, 17: 30–4.

King, N.M.P. (1995) Experimental treatment: oxymoron or aspiration?, *Hastings Center Report*, 25(4): 6–15.

Kopelman, L.M. (1995a) Controlled clinical trials, in W.T. Reich (ed.) *Encyclopedia of Bioethics*, Vol. 4. New York: Macmillan, Simon and Schuster.

Kopelman, L.M. (1995b) Risk and vulnerable groups, in W.T. Reich (ed.) *Encyclopedia of Bioethics*, Vol. 4. New York: Macmillan, Simon and Schuster.

Levine, R.L. (1999) The need to revise the Declaration of Helsinki, *New England Journal of Medicine*, 341(7): 531–4.

Lock, S. (1996) Research misconduct: a résumé of recent events, in S. Lock and F. Wells (eds) *Fraud and Misconduct in Medical Research*, 2nd edn. London: BMJ.

Marquis, D. (1999) How to resolve an ethical dilemma concerning randomized clinical trials, *New England Journal of Medicine*, 341(9): 691–3.

Pocock, S.J. and Elbourne, D.R. (2000) Randomized trials or observational tribulations?, *New England Journal of Medicine*, 342(25): 1907–9.

Raspe, H.H. (1990) Zur Theorie und Messung der 'Lebensqualität' in der Medizin, in P. Schölmerich and G. Thews (eds) *'Lebensqualität' als Bewertungskriterium in der Medizin*. Symposium der Akademie der Wissenschaften und der Literatur, Mainz. Stuttgart: G. Fischer.

Ten Have, H.A.M.J. and Janssens, R. (eds) (2001) *Palliative Care in Europe: Concepts and Policies*. Amsterdam: IOS Press.

Tettenborn, S. (1998) *Profil und Effizienz einer Ethik-Kommission*. Med. Diss Freiburg. Freiburg: Hochschulverlag.

Van den Daele, W. and Müller-Salomon, H. (1990) *Die Kontrolle der Forschung am Menschen durch Ethikkommissionen*. Stuttgart: Enke.

Vollmann, J. (2000) 'Therapeutische' versus 'nicht-therapeutische' Forschung – eine medizinethisch plausible Differenzierung?, *Ethik in der Medizin*, 12: 65–74.

Von Weizsäcker, V. (1940) *Der Gestaltkreis: Theorie der Einheit von Wahrnehmen und Bewegen*. Leipzig: Thieme.

12 Futility, limits and palliative care

HENK TEN HAVE AND RIEN JANSSENS

Since its emergence as an effective science and powerful healthcare practice, modern medicine has also attracted a multifaceted complex of criticisms, manifested in various guises and with different theoretical emphases. Some examples are contained in 'holistic' care, alternative medicine, anthropological medicine and psychosomatic medicine. It can be argued that present-day bioethics as well as the modern hospice movement and palliative care have also originated within this same critical realm. Bioethics developed from the 1960s as a theoretical effort to transform medicine into a humane activity through critique and revision of its underlying moral framework (ten Have and Gordijn 2001). In the same period, the hospice movement evolved as a practical response to cure-orientated aggressive hospital-based medical treatment, dependent upon technology and scientific knowledge, and aimed at prolonging patients' lives (Maruyama 1999; see also Chapter 1).

The bioethical literature has elaborated two strategies to resist the growing power of medicine, and to safeguard medicine as a human enterprise. The first strategy is the emphasis on the moral principle of autonomy (see Chapter 8). The second strategy focused on the need for limiting medical interventions. The notion of 'futility' has a crucial role in these debates and policies. Just as interventions can have 'utility', that is work for the benefit of the patient, so they can also be characterized as 'futile' in particular circumstances. In this chapter we discuss the notion of 'futility' in relation to palliative care. At first sight it seems that palliative care begins as soon as medical treatment has become futile. Palliative care itself therefore can never be futile. However, in the context of palliative care many activities are initiated which may become futile at a particular point in time. The interesting question then becomes: are there any limits to palliative care itself?

The notion of 'futility'

Although the notion of 'futility' was first introduced into the bioethical debate in the late 1980s, the underlying view is as old as medicine itself. One of the duties of the physician has always been to recognize when treatment is useful or not. The adage summarizing this duty 'to refuse to treat those who are overmastered by their diseases, realizing that in such cases medicine is powerless' has been attributed to Hippocrates. Literally, 'futile' means 'useless', 'ineffective', 'vain', 'serving no useful purpose'.

The notion of futility encompasses two different cases. The first case concerns treatment that is unlikely to work. The purpose intended can simply not be achieved with the methods employed. The treatment will not work because it has no effect. The problem is that very few interventions have no effect at all. The example of resuscitation of a brain-dead patient illustrates such 'physiological futility' (Youngner 1988). More common are situations where there is some potential effect but of low probability. On the basis of existing scientific knowledge and accepted professional standards it is unlikely that the treatment will produce the desired effect in a given patient. The concept of 'quantitative futility' is introduced here:

> when physicians conclude (either through personal experience, experiences shared with colleagues, or consideration of reported empiric data) that in the last 100 cases, a medical treatment has been useless, they should regard that treatment as futile.
>
> (Schneiderman et al. 1990: 951)

In such cases, medical professionals have no ethical obligation to provide the treatment. They also have no obligation to disclose the possibility of such treatment. If the treatment is widely accepted to be ineffective, then it is the physician's obligation to discontinue it. If a treatment is highly unlikely to work, it is even immoral to prescribe it to patients. For example, laetrile treatment should be denied to cancer patients.

The second case involves treatment that is effective, but controversial regarding the end supported. Here the notion of 'qualitative futility' has been introduced. Based on the distinction between an effect and a benefit, it is argued that a treatment that has an effect on the patient, is not necessarily to the benefit of that patient. The idea is that although the treatment may be successful in achieving an effect, that effect is not worth achieving. For example, Schneiderman and colleagues propose

> that any treatment that merely preserves permanent unconsciousness or that fails to end total dependence on intensive medical care should be regarded as nonbeneficial and, therefore, futile.
>
> (Schneiderman et al. 1990: 952)

This notion of 'qualitative futility' is controversial since it involves a judgment about the quality of life of the patients. Here the question is: What sort of life is worth preserving? It is not at all clear that the physician is the person best qualified to make such a determination, and thus be allowed to withhold or withdraw the treatment (Harper 1998).

Although during the 1990s several hundreds of articles on futility were published in the medical literature, the notion of 'futility' has remained ambiguous. No consensus has been achieved on the concept, and the underlying problem of making decisions about treatments that are of minimal benefit has continued to exist (Helft et al. 2000). The first reason for the persistence of the problem is that advances in medical technology continue to stimulate efforts to prolong life and life-supporting technologies continue to provide patients with the 'illusion of control' over life and death (Youngner 1994). Some interventions, however, only prolong the dying process. The second reason is the problem of resource allocation, obliging physicians to control costs and to discontinue treatments that are expensive and of marginal benefit to patients. The same reasons still exist today. The conclusion after a decade of debate, regardless of the conceptual controversies, therefore is:

> Doctors all recognize clinical situations in which intervention will be futile and should tell patients and families when they believe further treatment is futile.
>
> (Helft et al. 2000: 296)

Futility and autonomy

One of the leading motivations in the futility debate is the desire to redress the balance between the autonomy of the patient and the autonomy of the medical professional. The notion of 'futility' can support an effective response to demands from patients and families for treatment, while physicians consider this treatment to be inappropriate. Futility is a professional judgment that takes precedence over patient autonomy. Because continuation or initiation of treatment is regarded as inappropriate, patient approval to decide to forgo treatment is unnecessary. Physicians do not have an obligation to provide healthcare that they believe has no benefit. Medicine is a moral activity focused on the benefit of patients, not a morally neutral service enterprise where providers respond to patients' wishes. The concept of 'futility' is useful therefore in demarcating the area of professional autonomy.

This view is highly contested. Except for treatment that has no effect, it is unclear why physicians should have the ability and the power to decide what is beneficial to patients. No one is better able to make such judgments than patients themselves (Lantos et al. 1989). If futility implies the weighing of benefits and burdens of the proposed intervention, the subjective views of the patient concerning what constitutes benefits and burdens are important, but so too is the determination of the various goals that the interventions aims to achieve. Even physiologically futile treatments may offer some psychological benefits to patients and families. For example, a patient in the advanced stages of a terminal illness, hospitalized far from home, wants his former wife by his side before he dies. His treatment goal is to gain some time so that his wife can reach the bedside before death occurs. Blood transfusions are continued for a limited time although the transfusions do not alter the course of disease. Such compassionate use of futile therapy is justifiable as long as the treatment goals of the patient have priority.

Because of the potential antagonism between patient's autonomy and the medical prerogative of determining what is futile, many efforts have focused on developing procedures and policies to resolve disputes and conflicts over futility (Council on Ethical and Judicial Affairs 1999). The ethical debate has thus shifted from conceptual clarification to pragmatic mediation. Instead of articulating the decision-making power of physicians against the autonomous wishes of patients, it is argued that futility is the starting point for discussions regarding the benefits of (further) treatment:

> The judgment that further treatment would be futile is not a conclusion – a signal that care should cease; instead, it should initiate the difficult task of discussing the situation with the patient.
>
> (Helft et al. 2000: 296)

What is primarily needed is shared decision-making. The concept of futility locates the power of decision-making unilaterally in the medical professional. Controversies arise because of discrepant values or goals of care. Now it is recognized that the physician's feeling that treatment is futile should lead to extensive communication about these values and goals.

Palliative care and futility

It is interesting to observe that the notion of 'futility' is frequently used in the context of end of life care, but rarely in the context of palliative care. As we saw argued in Chapter 1, during the 1970s the impact of intensive treatments was growing rapidly. Newly discovered life-supporting technologies, such as respirators, dialysis machines, cardio-pulmonary resuscitation, cardiac surgery and transplantation gave physicians a real chance to postpone death in a significant way. The duty to preserve life, emphasized in medical ethics at the beginning of the modern period, became the driving force of technological interventions primarily aimed at the prolongation of life. However, many efforts to preserve life failed, or did so at the price of suffering and degradation. Preservation of life was possible but often with horrible side-effects. Gradually, many people came to question whether these interventions were justified, and eventually rejected the notion that it is morally necessary to preserve life in all cases and by all means. In this context of intensive treatment with its focus on cure and preservation of life, the hospice movement and palliative care have emerged, in fact as an analogue of intensive care (see Chapter 1). In the same context, however, the notion of 'futility' has been introduced, as a counterforce against efforts to postpone death by prolonging the suffering of the patient or against efforts aimed at prolonging life that is no longer meaningful for the patient. This specific context may explain why 'futility' is not useful as far as palliative care is concerned, since medical interventions to prolong life are no longer relevant in palliative care. In this argument, the judgment that medical interventions are futile demarcates the moment when palliative care should begin. In other words, the recognition that medical treatment is futile, provides at the same time the motivation to initiate palliative care. Comfort care should follow when treatment is futile (Schneiderman et al. 1994).

Practice, however, is more complicated. Although studies and relevant literature are scarce, the notion of 'futility' has been applied in the context of palliative care. For example, it has been reported that family members of deceased patients indicated futilities in 28 per cent of the cases. Most common was unnecessary medication (21 per cent), followed by unnecessary diagnostic examinations (19 per cent), treatments (18 per cent) and caring processes (17 per cent). These unnecessary interventions caused suffering to the dying patients, most frequently in hospitals (50 per cent) and less often at home (8 per cent) (Miettinen and Tilvis 1999). Of course, these findings can be considered as an indication that the quality of palliative care has been poor. However, what is disturbing here is that even caring processes are regarded as futile, although it is unclear what is meant here; no examples are provided. Reports of futility in this study are also associated with a lack of adequate information and communication. The notion of 'futility' is also used in guidelines and statements of palliative care organizations, for example when it is stated that there is no ethical obligation to discuss cardiopulmonary resuscitation with palliative care patients for whom such treatment is judged to be futile; this apparently is the case for the majority of these patients (National Council for Hospice and Specialist Palliative Care Services and Association for Palliative Medicine 1997).

Within the palliative care literature, 'futility' has been discussed extensively by Dunphy (2000), who criticizes the use of the notion, blaming advocates for promoting 'futilitarianism': the opinion that 'futility is a sufficient ethical ground for the unilateral withholding/withdrawing of treatment from patients' (Dunphy 2000: 314). 'Unilateral' means that the doctor takes the decision, does not discuss the treatment with the patient and does not provide it. Without denying the notion of 'quantitative futility', Dunphy explicitly focuses on 'qualitative futility'; he deconstructs this notion and proposes a more sophisticated model of futility scenarios, based on three values: the chance of benefit of an intervention, the chance of harm, and its costs. If the benefit of an intervention is low and the harm high, then, regardless of the costs, there is no duty to disclose the treatment option. The same is true when benefit and harm are low, but the costs are high. In cases of low benefit with the chance of harm and with high costs, there is, however, a duty to disclose the option. In all scenarios with high benefit, a similar duty to disclose exists.

Although the model is more differentiated, therefore, the conclusion is more or less the same as with the earlier criticized futilitarianism: there are specific cases in which the physician may withdraw treatment unilaterally. However, the justification of such a decision is based on an assessment of benefits, harms and costs, rather than on qualities of survival (such as being dependent or unconscious). The underlying assumptions of Dunphy's approach are problematic. Obviously it is assumed that physicians in palliative care can make an assessment of benefits for patients, and decide when these benefits are marginal. What precisely counts as benefit is unclear; only once does Dunphy briefly refer to 'benefits and harms being specified with respect to the goals of the patient' (2000: 318). It is assumed furthermore that palliative care decision-making should be orientated towards costs. If providing a treatment will reduce the availability to others, it should not be provided.

What is evident from these writings is that the notion of 'futility' is indeed used in the context of palliative care. Whatever definition is employed, it seems that even here professional efforts can be marginal, non-beneficial, useless or harmful to patients. For a further analysis of this finding it is helpful to make a distinction between care and treatment. Futility primarily seems to refer to treatment. In response to a report of the American Medical Association (Council on Ethical and Judicial Affairs 1999), Halevy and Brody warned that the term 'futile care' should be avoided: 'We believe that appropriate care of the patient, especially at the end of life, is never futile. Rather, particular interventions may be futile and medically inappropriate' (Halevy and Brody 1999: 1331).

The use of the term 'futile care' in the report seems to us a mistake since the examples provided refer to 'futile treatment' (life-sustaining intervention for patients in a persistent vegetative state, resuscitation efforts for the terminally ill, haemodialysis for advanced fatal illness). The distinction articulates the point that care itself cannot be futile, and thereby withheld. When life-sustaining interventions are deemed futile, full palliative care is or will remain necessary.

What is not articulated is why this distinction is made. Why can the notion of futility not be applied in care? One reason is that the vocabulary of 'use', 'effect' or 'purpose' is not appropriate when care is concerned. At least, care is not provided to achieve particular effects or to accomplish a purpose. Care is an activity in a different domain of human existence from the domain of production and action where the results of activities can be measured, calculated and quantified in terms of specific output. Even if care has no effect at all, it should be provided simply because it endows a patient with dignity and it acknowledges the patient as a fellow human being. Care is provided because it affirms the relations between human beings, as described in Chapter 7. This characteristic of care explains why the quantitative notion of futility applies to palliative treatments but not to palliative care. Care can have no effect at all and yet still be necessary.

It is more problematic to explain why the notion of 'qualitative futility' is not applicable to care. Is care always beneficial? Can the benefit of palliative care never become marginal or low, so that care itself becomes 'futile' in this sense of the term? Here also there seems to be an opposition between two fundamentally different ethical approaches: consequentialist versus deontological (or in the terminology of Chapter 5 of this volume: *Erfolgsethik* versus *Gesinnungsethik*). Consequentialist ethics assumes that an action is morally right if the consequences are good. Accordingly, morality is a matter of weighing benefits and harms as to the effects of our acts. What is morally relevant are the consequences of what we do. The notion of futility presupposes this consequentialist approach. Deontological ethics on the other hand assumes that certain moral duties hold independently of any probable or actual benefit. Regardless of the consequences of our acts, what counts morally is whether we are morally bound to act or not. According to this approach, caring activities should be explained, not because they have particular consequences, but because they are required in a network of human relationships. Drawing on this moral framework, palliative care has been inspired by conviction ethics. Nowadays, however, as argued in Chapter 5, the ethics of palliative care is changing from conviction ethics to responsibility ethics. But again, the question is whether there are limits to our duty to care or our responsibility to care.

In the following sections of this chapter, we first focus on the issue of forgoing treatment in the context of palliative care. Medical treatments are provided in palliative care; they can be futile and therefore withheld or withdrawn. The problem is that the demarcation of treatment and care is not always clear. We subsequently discuss the question whether care can ever be non-beneficial. In other words, is palliative care always good, or are there certain limitations?

Withholding and withdrawing treatment

Forgoing life-sustaining medical treatment with the subsequent death of the patient is relatively common. Data from a Dutch study of medical decision-making at the end of life show that in 1995 over 20 per cent of the total number of deaths were preceded by a decision to withdraw or withhold medical treatment (van der Maas et al. 1996). As described in Chapter 4, a survey in the *Pallium* project indicated that the majority of palliative care professionals accept that withholding and withdrawing mechanical ventilation can be a component of palliative care. On the other hand it is remarkable that 20 per cent of the respondents agree that forgoing mechanical ventilation, but also dehydration, should not be a part of palliative care. This agreement should probably not be interpreted as an assertion that such treatments should always be applied in the context of palliative care. Precisely because of this context, these treatments are aiming at specific goals, not primarily prolonging life (like outside the context of palliative care), but rather enhancing quality of life, relieving symptoms and providing comfort care. If these latter goals are at stake, then such treatments cannot be withheld or withdrawn. This interpretation points to an important assertion: the utility or futility of a treatment cannot be assessed without relation to the goals of the treatment. In Chapter 3 of this volume it is argued that palliative care is characterized by four specific goals: enhancing quality of life, relief of suffering, promotion of 'good death', and prevention of euthanasia. Although each goal is in need of further clarification, it is significant that the background of the futility discussion in this context is therefore different from similar discussions in other areas of medicine, simply because preservation or prolongation of human life is no longer a goal of medical intervention.

A second point regarding forgoing treatment in the context of palliative care is that withholding and withdrawing treatment will hasten the death of the patient, although the death of the patient is not intended, and not actively brought about. Death follows after forgoing treatment, but the decision to discontinue treatment is not the cause of the death of the patient. This makes forgoing treatment different from euthanasia. Similar reasoning is used to distinguish palliative sedation from euthanasia (see Chapter 9). The problem, of course, is that many practitioners do not make clear distinctions. As discussed in Chapter 4, it is paradoxical that a substantial number of palliative care professionals agree that euthanasia cannot be part of palliative care, and at the same time agree that forgoing treatment with the intention to shorten life can be. This finding is remarkable since other studies showed that healthcare practitioners largely accept (in contradistinction to many bioethicists) that a significant moral difference exists between stopping treatment and euthanasia or assisted suicide, although the consequences of both actions may be the same (Dickenson 2001).

A final observation regarding the survey data in Chapter 4 is that the large majority of respondents do not consider withholding or withdrawing ventilator treatment without the consent or without the knowledge of the competent patient to be a part of palliative care. We know that in the context of palliative care, the role of the patient is extremely important. The utility or futility of a treatment cannot be assessed without the input and participation of the patient, contrary to the claims of Dunphy (2000) discussed above. Whether a treatment is beneficial or not can be determined only in relation to the goals of the treatment, and the goals need to be indicated by the patient themself.

The significance of goals, consequences and the role of the patient is acknowledged in the ethical argumentations justifying withholding or withdrawing medical treatment (Verweij and Kortmann 1999). In order to create clarity in the muddied waters of the futility debate, a distinction can be made between three ethical arguments. The first concerns the autonomous refusal of the patient, the second concerns the (in)effectiveness of the medical treatment, and the third argument concerns the (dis)proportionality of the medical treatment.

The patient refuses medical treatment

The moral principle of respect for autonomy implies that autonomous decisions should be respected, as long as they do not infringe the autonomy of other persons. Individuals have the liberty to choose their own goals and make choices to achieve these goals (see Chapter 8). These choices need to be respected. The consequence of this view is that autonomous persons may not be forced to undergo medical treatment unless exceptional circumstances occur in which for instance refusal of medical treatment is likely to cause serious harm to others. Forcing medical treatment upon someone against their autonomous wishes is considered inhumane as it is a violation of the bodily integrity of the patient and disrespectful to their autonomy. Even if the caregivers are convinced that the proposed treatment is effective and meaningful, it is in the end the patient who has the final say.

In palliative care practice, cases in which a patient persists in their refusal of an effective and, in the opinion of the caregivers, meaningful treatment, are probably scarce. The goals of the treatment, determining whether it will be useful, will most probably in the context of palliative care be discussed in advance. Since the treatment will be focused on, for example, symptom relief or better quality of life, it is unlikely that the patient will refuse it. If adequate information is provided and the purposes, benefits and harms of the treatment are well communicated, most patients will eventually be convinced by the caregivers, even if they have initially been reluctant. However, even in such circumstances, patients may refuse treatments that are clearly beneficial according to the caregivers. The following case occurred during a participant observation study in a hospice setting (Janssens et al. 1999).

Mrs E

A widow of 86 years is admitted to the hospice with a vulva carcinoma as a consequence of radiotherapy on a previous gynaecological tumour. The wound around the perineum is vast, smelly and bleeding. Her wound needs cleaning many times a day, especially after defecation. The patient suffers a lot of pain but refuses to take any pain medication apart from some paracetamol tablets. Probably her refusal comes forth from a wish to die. The patient is convinced that any medication will postpone her death. Adequate medication would be successful in relieving her pain. However, she says that if this is forced upon her, she will run away from the hospice. In the past, at least twice she has run away from the nursing home where she was staying. She argues that she is able to bear the pain. Attempts by the nurses to negotiate and explain the use and meaning of the medication do not make her change her mind. All caregivers are convinced that she has more pain than she is willing to admit. The patient, however, explains that she has had the pain for 20 years now and that it is not useful to treat it. She is angry because the nurses are too persistent.

After some time the situation deteriorates. The patient does not want to go to the shower, possibly because that is too painful, and wants to be washed in her bed. Still she refuses any medication. At night, she often screams because of the pain, keeping her fellow patients awake. The team decides to call for a psychiatrist who will have to decide whether or not she can be regarded as an autonomous person, and whether or not her refusal to take medication should be accepted. During the consultation with the psychiatrist she refuses to talk. However, as she reacts adequately for a person unwilling to communicate, it is decided to treat her as an autonomous person.

Finally, she starts to suffer from dyspnoea. The decision is taken to involve her family in this dilemma. The daughters' opinions are asked and they say she should be treated with adequate pain medication. Following the family's wishes, and in line with the patient's explicit refusal of morphine, she is administered 20 mg ketamine. After increasing the dose to 30 mg the pain decreases. The patient becomes more tired and sleeps most of the day. For the last two days of her life, the patient is sedated in order to be sure she will not be in any pain. She dies quietly in the hospice.

The argument that any patient may refuse medical treatment is morally valid. But, as this case indicates, there can be times in which the refusal of the patient is hard to bear for the caregiving team as well as for fellow patients. Both are confronted time after time with a screaming patient suffering from intense, unnecessary pain. Attempts to inform the patient about the absence of any life-prolonging effects of morphine fail. In the end the patient becomes angry with the team for being so 'pushy'. When the family members insist that pain medication must be given, the situation becomes even more complex from a moral point of view. Based on the moral notion of beneficence, much can be said in favour of administration of medication. Based on the notion of autonomy the patient's refusal seems to carry at least as much weight.

Ineffective medical treatment

Effectiveness of medical treatment is usually proven through research. The effects of the treatment are documented and the chances of success can be expressed in terms of a percentage. Because of this, Schneiderman et al. (1990) proposed that a treatment is ineffective if the probability that it will achieve its goal is less than 1 per cent. Helft et al. (2000) found that in the literature most authors clustered around 5 per cent. In palliative care, the most common goal of medical treatment is the relief of pain and symptoms. It sounds commonplace: if a specific medical treatment is considered ineffective, it should be withheld; if the effectivity of a medical treatment that has been provided so far falls below a certain threshold, the treatment should be withdrawn. In such cases the conversation with the patient on an ineffective medical treatment has merely an informative character. The physician decides. On further consideration, however, the decision to consider a certain medical treatment ineffective gives rise to many questions.

First, it should be noted that in palliative care, as probably in other medical practices, treatments that are effective for one patient, may be ineffective for others, and vice versa. This makes it problematic to base decisions on clear-cut statistical data. Percentages, if they are available at all, deal with groups of patients instead of individual persons. Second, if it is possible to express the chance of success of a medical treatment in a percentage, it is arbitrary to establish a threshold for decisions about effectiveness. Proposed percentages in the literature range from 0 per cent to 60 per cent (Helft et al. 2000). Third, the criterion to measure effectiveness can also be subject to debate. Is chemotherapy effective if life prolongation of not more than one month can be expected? Should such treatments be negotiated with the patient at all? What counts as effect? Do only the physiological effects of the treatment count, or can also a couple of days of rest for the patient and relatives count as effect?

An example of a case in which the (in)effectiveness of medical treatment was heavily debated in the Dutch media occurred in July 1999.

Mr F

An 80-year-old man received palliative surgery as a consequence of a malignant intestinal tumour. Due to unexpected complications the patient

did not wake up. Incapable of expressing himself, one of his daughters
spoke on his behalf. According to her (and contrary to what the other
daughters thought), her father had arranged with the physicians that in
case of complications during the surgery, everything would be done to
sustain his life, including admission to an intensive care unit. The
physicians of the university medical centre, where the patient had surgery,
held the opinion that referral from a medium care ward to an intensive
care unit would be medically futile: doomed to fail and, at the most,
leading to only a very limited life prolongation.

In September, the daughter of the patient, a lawyer herself, went to
court. She demanded that her father be transferred to an intensive care
unit of another hospital. Ventilation and cardio-pulmonary resuscitation
should not be withheld. In October the court ruled that the professional
judgment that medical treatment is futile weighs heavier than the wish to
live on the side of the patient. In the end, according to the court, the
decision about medical futility is guided by medical professional criteria.

The physicians and the court, using the terminology of futility, in fact
are referring to the ineffectiveness of treatment. Here all the difficulties
of ineffectiveness are illustrated. Is intensive care treatment in this case
really without effect? Perhaps a few weeks or maybe just a few days would
have been won by intensive care treatment. From the perspectives of
the physicians this limited effect may not have been worthwhile. But if
the goal of treatment is prolongation of life, however limited, then this
treatment is clearly not ineffective. If the goal of treatment is otherwise, for
example relief of suffering, then intensive treatment will be ineffective, and
palliative care is indicated. But who determines what is the proper goal of
treatment?

Disproportional treatment

Most decisions to forgo medical treatment are based on an assessment of
the benefits and burdens of the treatment. In this case, the patient does not
refuse the treatment but is requesting it. The treatment, if initiated, will not
be without any or minimum effect. However, the point precisely is that
there is a chance of some beneficial result but also the chance that the
treatment will have side-effects and will be burdensome to the patient. In
this case, what is at stake is the burden–benefit proportion. The argument
to discontinue or not to start the treatment is that the magnitude of the
benefit, in whatever way it contributes to the patient's treatment goals, is
disproportionately small in relation to the magnitude of the risks and harms,
thus worsening the patient's condition. This argument requires an analysis
of the benefits versus burdens proportion. The risks, harms, benefits and

probable outcomes of the treatment option need to be reviewed and discussed. In the context of palliative care such analysis and balancing requires communication between physician and patient, where the patient primarily determines which treatment goals are acceptable, and which effects of treatments will be beneficial and non-beneficial. When a patient decides that the benefits of a treatment do not weigh up to the harms, they can ask the physician to withhold or withdraw the treatment. It is argued that this is of course a personal judgement of the patient; the physician may not agree or may think that the judgement is wrong. At the same time, the best person to make a judgement on the meaning or value of a treatment in the context of their own life, is the patient since they are most capable of assessing their quality of life. The implication is that medically effective treatments can be considered disproportionately burdensome by one patient but proportionately beneficial by other patients. Conversations between the physician and patient are dialogues within which in the end it is the patient who decides whether a certain medical treatment is worthwhile for themselves. But again, what seems trivial at first sight can become complicated in daily practice. Patients who are ready to die may receive medical treatment with life-prolonging (side-)effects without their knowledge. For them, life prolongation would be considered a harm. And it is questionable to what extent physicians are willing to inform such patients of the life-prolonging effects of the medication they receive and of the possibility that they may be withdrawn. The conversation on futile medical treatment is a dialogue within which, first and foremost, it is the patient who is dependent on the information received from the physician. Some physicians may, from the perspective of autonomy, inform patients on for instance the life-prolonging effects of medication and the possibility of having these medications withdrawn and replaced by others, once the patient is ready to die. Others may find this kind of information unnecessary or even tendentious. They do not want to give the patient the idea of being better off dead. Consider for example the following case (Janssens et al. 1999).

Ms G

A woman of 58 years was suffering from lung carcinoma. When the patient was informed of her diagnosis, the first thing she said to the oncologist was that, when her suffering became unbearable, she would want to have euthanasia (which under certain conditions is legalized in the Netherlands: see Chapter 11). Sixth months later she contacted a hospice physician, asking for information about hospice care. She was told that euthanasia was not performed in the hospice but that, independent of her decision, the caregivers would never abandon her. Thirteen months after the diagnosis, the woman was admitted to a university hospital with pain in her back. Metastases in the brain and

*spinal column were diagnosed. Radiotherapy and chemotherapy aimed at
life prolongation and the palliation of symptoms were initiated. Sixteen
months after the diagnosis, she decided to discontinue chemotherapy
and, at her request, she was admitted to the hospice. It appeared that the
dose of opioids she was receiving was far too high. After the dose was
decreased, her symptoms alleviated. Corticosteroids were prescribed
to alleviate the headache and nausea. During the first weeks in hospice
she acted in a rather detached manner. But one morning, during a
conversation with the hospice physician, she said frankly that she was
afraid to die and that she felt guilty about her children, whom she had
never been able to take care of. She mentioned that, after her divorce,
one daughter had been living with her ex-husband and one daughter with
her. After this conversation, her relations with the people around her
improved and she started to enjoy the care she received. Nineteen months
after her diagnosis, she re-established contact with her sister, who lived in
India. The patient then felt reassured that she had done all the things she
needed to. Apart from fatigue, she did not suffer from any symptoms. She
had enjoyed her months in the hospice and had accepted her fate. During
one of her last discussions with the hospice physician, she repeated her
request for euthanasia. She wanted to die. She was afraid that the dying
process would be endless and that she would deteriorate slowly. The
hospice physician proposed an alternative, namely to discontinue the
corticosteroids and start sedative medication. She said that she needed a
day to consider this option. She phoned a schoolfriend, a rheumatologist,
who confirmed the rationality of this option. She agreed and felt relieved.
Four days after the withdrawal of the corticosteroids, she died semi-
consciously in the presence of her daughters.*

The decision of this patient to have chemotherapy and radiotherapy withdrawn was rather unproblematic. The harms of the treatment outweighed
the benefit of life prolongation. The decision to have the corticosteroids
withdrawn however may be considered more problematic. This time, life-
sustaining medical treatment had become a harm in the opinion of the
patient. The reason why the corticosteroids were withdrawn and sedatives
were administered was her request to die. If the physician had not proposed
this alternative to euthanasia, she probably would have had euthanasia
in another healthcare facility. The question that can be asked is whether
withdrawal of the corticosteroids in this case should be considered the
withdrawal of a disproportionate treatment, or whether the physician's
proposal is actually a positive response to the patient's request to die?
Crucial here again is the moral difference between the active shortening of
the patient's life and the decision to stop life-sustaining treatment at the
patient's request.

From care to treatment

These ethical arguments all concern examples of medical treatment. It is controversial whether nutrition and hydration can be located within the area of futility, so that they can be withdrawn or withheld if ethical arguments justify so doing. Or are these activities of care, so basic and special that they cannot be discontinued or refused? If nutrition and hydration are basic care, they must be provided to all patients regardless of their wishes and regardless of whether they offer benefits that exceed the benefits of refusal. Over the years in many countries courts have decided that nutrition and hydration should be regarded as treatments, so that they can be refused by competent patients or discontinued if futile. For example, in the United States, the cases of Claire Conroy in 1985 and Nancy Cruzan in 1990 were the first to redefine nutrition and hydration from care into treatment. Similar legal processes have occurred in other countries.

Ineke Stinissen

In 1974, Ineke Stinissen was admitted to a Dutch hospital for a simple surgical operation. Due to unexpected complications, a cardiac arrest occurred. The patient did not wake up and remained comatose. After several weeks, she was transferred from the hospital to a nursing home. In 1985, after 11 years of coma, a public debate started. Her husband advocated withdrawal of artificial hydration and nutrition. The physicians of Ineke Stinissen did not agree. In 1987, the case was brought to court. The lawyer of the patient's husband argued that any further medical treatment, including artificial hydration and nutrition, was futile according to medical standards. The nursing home argued that the patient had the right to all medical care that the nursing team could offer her. The ruling of the court was ambivalent. It refused to make a decisive statement. Following this ruling, the husband appealed to a higher court. In 1989, this court decided that decisions with regard to medical futility should be considered as part of the physician's competence. After this ruling, attempts to have the patient transferred to another hospital or nursing home failed since the nursing home would consider this an act of complicity. After extensive deliberations among the staff, the nursing home changed its opinion in 1990. Artificial hydration and nutrition were withdrawn; 11 days later, 16 years after her surgery, Ineke Stinissen died from dehydration.

In the public debate about this case two opposing ethical arguments were defended. The first emphasized that artificial hydration and nutrition should be considered as medical treatment that can become futile if it no longer contributes to the patient's quality of life. Eating and drinking in the context of healthcare are not different from other professional activities; their primary aim is to serve the interests and well-being of the patient. The other argument stipulated that artificial hydration and nutrition should be considered as elements of basic care. The provision of nutrition and hydration is not aimed to achieve particular effects; these are common ways among human beings to demonstrate love and affection. Withdrawal of such care should therefore be considered inhumane; patients, no matter how seriously ill they are, should never be allowed to die from starvation or dehydration. Moreover, withdrawal of artificial hydration and nutrition was said to be comparable to 'direct euthanasia' (Pranger 1992).

The crucial point in the debate about care versus treatment is the transition from 'natural' to 'artificial'. Nobody argues that normal eating and drinking should be subjected to the criteria of futility. It appears strange to argue that we eat and drink in order to prolong our lives or to assess foods for their life-sustaining qualities. If we assist ill people to eat and drink, then we engage in a basic activity of care, outside the realm of futility judgments. As soon as we try to take over the patient's abilities to eat and drink by tube feeding, we try to remedy the natural deficiencies with artificial substitutes (Gallagher-Allred and Amenta 1993). At that moment, we initiate a medical intervention with a specific purpose. This intervention can then be assessed according to its effectiveness and usefulness. If artificial nutrition and hydration is subsequently evaluated, it turns out to have adverse consequences. Tube feeding in patients with advanced dementia for example has documented adverse effects, challenging the reasons often used to start it (McCann 1999). There is a lack of evidence that tube feeding makes patients live longer, improves quality of life, or makes patients more comfortable (Finucane et al. 1999). In the hospice setting, keeping dying patients well hydrated with intravenous fluids often adds to patient discomfort by worsening respiratory secretions and dyspnoea (Schmitz and O'Brien 1986; Printz 1992). The conclusion then is that artificial nutrition and hydration cannot be assumed to be effective treatment; often they have serious adverse effects. Finucane et al. (1999: 1369) conclude that for a demented patient with eating difficulties 'a comprehensive, motivated, conscientious program of hand feeding is the proper treatment'. Given the recent history of thinking about tube feeding, this is an ironic conclusion. First, it has been argued that artificial feeding is not care but treatment; then it can be evaluated according to its effect, and forgone if it is futile. Subsequently, it cannot be proven to be effective treatment. Finally, the best approach to eating difficulties is simple basic care, with increased personal assistance with meals, and efforts to alter the size and frequency of meals according to the needs and capacities of the patient. In conclusion, the transformation of eating and drinking into artificial activities is questionable.

Limitations of palliative care

The futility debate as well as the framework of ethical arguments discussed here applies to treatments. With these arguments it is possible to justify withholding and withdrawing treatment, thereby limiting medical interventions in healthcare for terminally ill patients. But what about palliative care itself? Is it without any limits? Prima facie, when life-saving treatments have become futile, efforts should be redirected toward strategies for maximizing comfort, relieving symptoms, and easing pain.

Obviously, palliative care has limitations. In principle two types of limits can be distinguished: external and internal limits.

External limits are due to circumstances that restrict the implementation of good palliative care. For example, a lack of resources. In the Netherlands, it is estimated, for example, that the demand for palliative care up to 2015 will increase by 20 per cent because of health determinants such as the growing prevalence and mortality of chronic diseases, and the ageing of the population (Francke and Willems 2000). Since palliative care is already insufficient to cover the demands of the existing population, scarcity will increase and palliative care will experience ever more stringent limitations. Another limitation is the lack of adequately trained and experienced physicians and nurses in palliative care in many countries. Dissemination of expertise in the healthcare system is therefore limited, and palliative care is not provided to patients who might benefit from it. Finally the organizational setting for palliative care services may be insufficient, so that there is not a coherent delivery of services (Chapter 2 illustrates the differences in service development in European countries; see also ten Have and Janssens 2001). The inertia of health policy may then result in an unequal distribution of palliative care services, limiting the delivery of palliative care in specific areas or for particular patient populations. The above limitations are external to palliative care. They are not inherent in the concept or methods of palliative care, but mainly due to inadequate external conditions. In principle, they can be ameliorated and removed. More resources may be allocated, better training facilities and educational programmes may be established, and health policies may initiate more coherent and well-organized palliative care services.

Internal limits are related to the concept and value structure of palliative care itself. These are limits inherent in palliative care. Perhaps palliative care has specific assumptions about what is a good patient and these are intrinsically limited because not all patients will accommodate these assumptions. Joanne Lynn observes for example that 'in the United States, institutions such as hospice, developed for those who are dying assume that dying persons take to their beds, reflect on life's meaning, and proceed to die "on time"' (Lynn 2001: 928). Because of these assumptions a dying person is not expected to do frivolous things, make long-term investments or run a business. These stereotypes of what is a good patient will necessarily imply limitations. Some terminally ill patients will resist being labelled as 'dying' or accepting hospice care. Some patients will not behave 'appropriately' or conform to the assumptions of palliative care.

Other internal limits seem related to the goals of palliative care. In Chapter 3, four goals are distinguished: achieving the best quality of life, relief of suffering, good death, and prevention of euthanasia. None of the goals as such is questionable (though further clarification is needed), but each goal seems to articulate its limits. The main reason of course is that dying ultimately is tragic, although it can be accepted and comforted by good care. There is no way to eliminate this basic tragedy. While the goals of palliative care might be valuable to most terminally ill people, they might be rejected by some. Thus some people would find the fact of impending death so painful, that they simply cannot accept it. They are not willing to forgo the options of high-tech life-prolonging or experimental curative care, even if it is explained to them that these are most probably futile and ineffective (Ackerman 1997). Palliative care apparently assumes particular attitudes towards its goals, taking for granted that these goals are universally appreciated. This assumption is questionable, particularly with regard to different cultures. For example, in present-day Japan, death is regarded as the defeat of medical science. Death is the enemy; no surrender can be allowed. The diagnosis is concealed from terminally ill cancer patients. Interest in palliative care is therefore limited. It is also questionable whether the potential of palliative care can be fully explored in a context where only 49 per cent of patients know their true diagnosis (Maruyama 1999).

A third type of internal limit is related to assumptions about what is a good caregiver. As explained in Chapters 1 and 5, palliative care increasingly demands an ethics of care focusing on responsibility for the patient and family, relatives or close ones. These demands set very idealistic requirements for the professionals who are expected to provide good care. They need to be able to work with various professions. They must communicate with patient and relatives. They must have the best technical expert knowledge available, but at the same time possess excellent humane qualities and virtues such as empathy, compassion and courage. It is clear that in many cases, these idealistic expectations cannot be met. One reason is that the standards are perhaps set too high and we always have to deal with mostly down-to-earth human beings. Physicians for example tend to focus on medical-technical issues, whether or not they are working in a palliative care setting. Even if improving quality of life is one of the goals of palliative care, quality of life issues are not more frequently discussed in outpatient palliative care consultations than in other treatment settings (Detmar et al. 2001). Another reason why the expectations may be unrealistic is because some of the required professional qualities are elusive, not instrumental and intrinsically limited. For example, virtues such as compassion, are not manageable and teachable; they are present in some persons and some situations or not; it cannot be expected that all professionals all the time provide compassionate care. Even if it was possible to make a protocol for compassionate care, and teach professionals how to work according to this protocol, something would be missing. We do not want professionals to be compassionate because the protocol or management requires it, but because they really are compassionate.

Conclusion

It was not until the end of the 1980s that the notion of futility was introduced into bioethical discourse. At the same time, questions regarding the beneficial effects of medical technology have been central in modern bioethics since its origins at the end of the 1960s. Modern bioethics has come forth out of a moral discomfort with the disproportionate use of medical technologies, especially in the context of the care for dying people. Against the power of the physician, bioethics stressed the self-determination of the patient. Thus, the moral principle of autonomy became central and served as a defence mechanism to protect patients from potentially harmful treatment. It is not coincidental that in the same period of time individual cases, such as the Quinlan case in the United States and the Stinissen case in the Netherlands, led to heated public debates about the utility of life-sustaining medical treatment. The view that effective medical treatment (such as use of the ventilator with a patient in persistent vegetative state) is not always beneficial, is on the one hand as old as medicine but on the other hand of a particular urgency in the context of increasing technological possibilities.

It is remarkable that the notion of futility has not been extensively reflected upon within the palliative care movement. The explanation may be that palliative care only starts at the moment when medical treatments have become futile. The recognition that medical treatment has become futile provides the motivation to initiate palliative care. Still, the concept of futility is not absent in palliative care. It relates for instance to treatments with life-prolonging (side-)effects. Sometimes, patients who are ready to die receive such treatments and the question is whether the physician should inform the patient of the option of withdrawing the treatment (as a possible alternative to euthanasia) with the consequence that the patient's life will be substantially shortened. The notion of futility has also been debated with regard to palliative care itself. Can care ever be futile? From a deontological point of view, even if care is ineffective, it can never be futile since it is reflective of human solidarity and compassion. Self-evidently, strict utilitarians will argue that it can be futile if the care given does not result in increased benefit or decreased harm.

Much unclarity still circles around the notion of futility. Sometimes it is used to indicate ineffectiveness of treatment, sometimes it is used to indicate the beneficence and non-maleficence of treatment, sometimes it is considered useless since it depends fully on the autonomous will of the patient. It is imperative that such distinctions are reflected upon, specifically in the area of palliative care. At the same time, argumentation models, such as those set out here, can serve as provisional guidelines. No more no less, for there is a sense in which they will never provide clearcut norms for everyday practice, since practice is always more complex than theory.

References

Ackerman, F. (1997) Goldilocks and Mrs. Ilych: a critical look at the 'Philosophy of Hospice', *Cambridge Quarterly of Healthcare Ethics*, 6: 314–24.

Council on Ethical and Judicial Affairs (American Medical Association) (1999) Medical futility in end-of-life care, *Journal of the American Medical Association*, 281(10): 937–41.

Detmar, S.B., Muller, M.J., Wever, L.D.V., Schornagel, J.H. and Aaronson, N.K. (2001) Patient–physician communication during outpatient palliative treatment visits, *Journal of the American Medical Association*, 285(10): 1351–7.

Dickenson, D. (2001) Practitioner attitudes in the United States and United Kingdom toward decisions at the end of life: are medical ethicists out of touch?, *Western Journal of Medicine*, 174: 103–9.

Dunphy, K. (2000) Futilitarianism: knowing how much is enough in end-of-life healthcare, *Palliative Medicine*, 14: 313–22.

Finucane, T.E., Christmas, C. and Travis, K. (1999) Tube feeding in patients with advanced dementia: a review of the evidence, *Journal of the American Medical Association*, 282(14): 1365–70.

Francke, A.L. and Willems, D.L. (2000) *Palliatieve zorg vandaag en morgen: Feiten, opvattingen en scenario's.* Maarssen: Elsevier.

Gallagher-Allred, C. and Amenta, M.O. (1993) *Nutrition and Hydration in Hospice Care: Needs, Strategies, Ethics.* New York: Haworth.

Halevy, A. and Brody, B.A. (1999) Medical futility and end-of-life care, *Journal of the American Medical Association*, 282(14): 1331.

Harper, W. (1998) Judging who should live: Schneiderman and Jecker on the duty not to treat, *Journal of Medicine and Philosophy*, 23(5): 500–15.

Helft, P.R., Siegler, M. and Lantos, J. (2000) The rise and fall of the futility movement, *New England Journal of Medicine*, 343: 293–6.

Janssens, M.J.P.A., Zylicz, Z. and ten Have, H.A.M.J. (1999) Articulating the concept of palliative care: philosophical and theological perspectives, *Journal of Palliative Care*, 15: 38–44.

Lantos, J.D., Singer, P.A., Walker, R.M. et al. (1989) The illusion of futility in clinical practice, *American Journal of Medicine*, 87: 81–4.

Lynn, J. (2001) Serving patients who may die soon and their families: the role of hospice and other services, *Journal of the American Medical Association*, 285(7): 925–32.

McCann, R. (1999) Lack of evidence about tube feeding – food for thought, *Journal of the American Medical Association*, 282(14): 1380–1.

Maruyama, T.C. (1999) *Hospice Care and Culture: A Comparison of the Hospice Movement in the West and Japan.* Aldershot: Ashgate.

Miettinen, T.T. and Tilvis, R.S. (1999) Medical futility as a cause of suffering of dying patients – the family members' perspective, *Journal of Palliative Care*, 15(2): 26–9.

National Council for Hospice and Specialist Palliative Care Services and Association for Palliative Medicine (Great Britain and Ireland) (1997) Ethical decision-making: CPR for people who are terminally ill, *European Journal of Palliative Care*, 4: 125.

Pranger, D. (1992) *Het beëindigen van kunstmatige voeding bij aanhoudend vegeterende patiënten.* Amsterdam: Thesis Publishers.

Printz, L.A. (1992) Terminal dehydration, a compassionate treatment, *Archives of Internal Medicine*, 152: 697–700.

Schmitz, P. and O'Brien, M. (1986) Observations on nutrition and hydration in dying cancer patients, in J. Lynn (ed.) *By No Extraordinary Means.* Bloomington, IN: Indiana University Press.

Schneiderman, L.J., Jecker, N.S. and Jonsen, A.R. (1990) Medical futility: its meaning and ethical implications, *Annals of Internal Medicine*, 112: 949–54.

Schneiderman, L.J., Faber-Langendoen, K. and Jecker, N.S. (1994) Beyond futility to an ethic of care, *American Journal of Medicine*, 96: 110–14.

Ten Have, H.A.M.J. and Gordijn, B. (eds) (2001) *Bioethics in a European Perspective.* Dordrecht: Kluwer.

Ten Have, H.A.M.J. and Janssens, M. (eds) (2001) *Palliative Care in Europe: Concepts and Policies.* Amsterdam: IOS Press.

Van der Maas, P.J., van der Wal, G., Haverkate, I. et al. (1996) Euthanasia, physician-assisted suicide, and other medical practices involving the end of life in the Netherlands, 1990–1995, *New England Journal of Medicine*, 335: 1699–705.

Verweij, M.F. and Kortmann, F. (1999) Abstineren: Staken of afzien van leven-sverlengend handelen, *Nederlands Tijdschrift voor Geneeskunde*, 143: 145–8.

Youngner, S.J. (1988) Who defines futility?, *Journal of the American Medical Association*, 260: 2094–5.

Youngner, S.J. (1994) Applying futility: saying no is not enough, *Journal of the American Geriatrics Society*, 42: 887–9.

13 Conclusion: ethics and palliative care

HENK TEN HAVE AND DAVID CLARK

As the preceding chapters have shown, there are some interesting connections between palliative care and ethics. On the one hand, palliative care gives rise to specific moral dilemmas and problems, needing clarification, explanation and resolution from the perspectives of ethical theory and methodology. On the other, ethics itself may benefit from the peculiarities of palliative care as a movement and philosophy of care, introducing new moral notions of wider relevance in the healthcare context. These fascinating interactions and possible mutual benefits are now beginning to be discovered and explored by scholars and professionals in palliative care as well as in ethics. The rather late interest is surprising, for palliative care and ethics have at least three features in common. First, it is the case that both have a long-standing tradition within healthcare and have been part and parcel of medicine since its origins. Palliation was indeed the most significant goal of medical care until the recent development of effective therapies and preventive strategies. Ethics has also been an essential component of medical practice since Hippocrates established medicine as a profession separated from religion and philosophy. Second, although ideas relating to what we now call palliative care and also to ethics have always been intrinsic dimensions of medicine, they have enjoyed a resurgence of interest since the 1960s. Modern medicine developed rapidly in the decades after the Second World War. For the first time in its history, effective treatment was available to eradicate many life-threatening diseases; innovative technologies expanded the diagnostic and therapeutic abilities of physicians; and life-saving technologies and advanced surgery were used to counteract the impact of emergencies and also to prevent death from acute illness. This explosion of medical innovations, technologies and therapies instigated the emergence of bioethics in the late 1960s with controversial cases and public scandals in relation to medical research, dialysis treatment and resuscitation policies, first in North America, and somewhat later in Europe. This is a controversial history and we should beware an uncritical acceptance of the notion that up to this point physicians had few ethical standards and that the contribution of bioethics to the debate has somehow been disinterested and objective (Martensen 2001). At the same time, death and dying have been a special focus of critical attention because the expansion of medicine has increasingly transformed not only the location of death (from the home to the hospital) but also the management of death (from care to intervention). Palliative care, and especially the hospice movement, developed as an effort to improve healthcare for dying patients and to redirect the emphasis of a medicine driven by therapy and technology. The new interest in ethics as well as palliative care is therefore not simply a reiteration of long-existing but forgotten dimensions but also an attempt to redefine the core of medicine itself, to influence its development, and to at least remedy a one-sided interest in technological interventions primarily aimed at curing illness and prolonging life. This observation points to a third common feature: bioethics and palliative care seem to share similar objectives: to maintain or if necessary reinstitute a humane medicine, primarily focused on the human person in need. Instead of being driven by technology and the possibilities and promises of science, medicine from this perspective is committed first and foremost to the patient and their particular interests. Accordingly, medicine should acknowledge that technology and science can easily distort the proper view of what is really appropriate in certain circumstances, for example when frail and vulnerable patients are admitted to the intensive unit, when patients with advanced cancer are included in another clinical trial, or when medical interventions for the demented elderly are continued without critical assessment.

New connections

Notwithstanding these features held in common, there has also been a notable disjunction between ethics and palliative care, at least until recently. Bioethics developed as a separate discipline, certainly interested in issues of death and dying, and particularly in controversies about euthanasia and the forgoing of medical treatment, but not specifically focused on the area of palliative care. At the same time, palliative care emerged as a new approach to and philosophy of care, creating structures and arrangements of care, and developing into a discipline with textbooks, chairs, academic and clinical departments, educational programmes and special services. In palliative care journals, moral dilemmas and issues have featured strongly and have been widely discussed by clinicians, but paradoxically professional bioethicists have been rather slow to make their contribution to these debates (Hermsen and ten Have 2001). While the professional literature tends to show that palliative care practitioners frequently experience moral issues and dilemmas, we can see from the chapters in this volume that many of these moral queries also arise in other healthcare areas, though some are undoubtedly specific to the palliative care setting. Bioethics can contribute to the analysis and clarification of these problems, as well as to the development of practical approaches and methods which can support palliative care practitioners in coping and dealing with them. In this regard, palliative care presents itself, albeit rather late, as a new area of bioethical research and consultation. As medical knowledge grows and medical practice evolves, new areas and topics require ethical analysis. Usually, we tend to refer to technology and to science as key generators of new moral queries, for instance stem cell research, genetic screening technologies or xenotransplantation. Palliative care is important because it shows that transformation and innovation within healthcare practice can also introduce new moral issues. Practice changes are driven by new perceptions of patient needs resulting from demographic changes, the increasing burden of chronic disease, or the need to improve the quality of care, rather than the necessities of science and technology.

Even more important than the opening up of new areas for bioethical research, is the prospect that palliative care may offer a reconsideration of some of the basic notions and approaches of bioethics itself. Many chapters in this book have shown that the moral values incorporated in palliative care practice are not easily compatible with the dominant conception of bioethics. While palliative care may benefit from the contributions of bioethicists, therefore, it is our contention that bioethics can in turn also learn from the experiences of palliative care practitioners.

Ethics *in* and *of* palliative care

Pellegrino (1976) introduced a distinction that can clarify the various connections between ethics and palliative care. Explaining how philosophy can engage with medicine, Pellegrino distinguished two models of engagement: philosophy *in* medicine, and philosophy *of* medicine. The first mode refers to the application of the traditional tools of philosophy, such as critical reflection, dialectical reasoning, the uncovering of value and purpose, or asking first-order questions, to some medically defined problems (Pellegrino 1976: 20). In this vein we can refer to ethics *in* palliative care as the application of the tools of ethics to the problems of palliative care. The bioethicist is thereby called upon to serve a useful function in the context of palliative care practice. Such an approach seeks to illuminate and examine critically what palliative care practitioners do in their day-to-day work. Likewise it can make contributions in teaching, research and consultation that can enhance the further development of palliative care. From this perspective bioethics is deployed in the service of palliative care to resolve those problems which palliative care has defined and identified as in need of attention.

From Pellegrino (1976) however the philosophy *of* medicine, on the other hand, examines the conceptual foundations, the ideologies and the ethos which pervades the medical realm. Medicine thereby generates philosophical issues in regard to its meaning, its nature, concepts, purposes and value to society. From this critical perspective the practical context of medicine is no longer taken for granted, but is rather considered to be an object of further philosophical inquiry, transcending the narrower medical context itself and producing questions that are of wider significance to philosophy as a discipline. Analogously, we suggest, the ethics *of* palliative care can be regarded as the critical examination of the meaning of palliative care, its nature, concepts, purposes and value to society. This analysis assumes that palliative care as a practical human activity has a trans-medical meaning which has important implications for bioethics itself. Reflection on experiences in palliative care may thereby produce insights that influence and change current notions and approaches to bioethics.

In principle both kinds of ethical reasoning are worthwhile and possible; it is important however that bioethicists are clear at any one time about in which mode they are operating. Exactly the same point holds true in the cognate field of medical sociology, where scholarly endeavour may be either applied to the problems which medicine defines, or alternatively may seek to problematize medicine itself as an object of enquiry.

Conceptions of bioethics

The evolution of bioethics into an autonomous discipline has been presented as an unprecedented story of success, though histories produced from within are inclined to overstate the extent of this (Jonsen 1998, 2000). Not only have the moral problems of medicine and health burgeoned during the 1970s, 1980s and 1990s, but also the preferred methods and concepts for a 'scientific' approach to these problems have been moulded into a separate discipline (Rothman 1991). Two developments are usually regarded as crucial to the rise of bioethics. First, enormous advances in biotechnology, molecular biochemistry and pharmacology have led to drastic changes in medical knowledge and practice, yet many people are quite unaware of how relatively novel some of the benefits of present-day medicine actually are. Before 1960 the major medical journals were silent on such topics as fibreglass endoscopy, coronary contrast radiology, artificial lens implantation, cardio-resuscitation techniques and oral contraceptives. New and more or less effective diagnostic and therapeutic interventions have increasingly called into question the goals of medicine. The second development that has transformed the traditional notion of medical ethics is the changing sociocultural context of medical practice. Not only has a plurality of values emerged, but also a non-religious, secular-grounded normative view of human life has become more influential, which emphasizes personal autonomy and each patient's right to make their own healthcare decisions.

Whatever the precise determinants, traditional medical ethics has evolved rapidly into bioethics. 'Medical ethics' used to refer to the deontology of the medical profession. In this manner, it formed a system of moral rules, codes of etiquette and structures governing professional conduct. This system is immediately intelligible to the medical practitioner, since it emerges from the internal morality of medicine, those values, norms and rules intrinsic to the actual practice of healthcare. It is a system which is endorsed through the entry of new practitioners into the medical profession, so that being a physician implies the acceptance of particular moral views. From this viewpoint medicine is not considered as merely a technical enterprise that can be morally evaluated from some external standpoint. Rather, the professional practice of medicine always presumes and implies a moral perspective or point of view; good clinical practice is determined by the shared rules and standards of the profession.

The emergence of modern bioethics and the concomitant atrophy of medical ethics in the traditional sense, is visible in at least two ways. First, it has produced a new expert, the 'bioethicist' or the healthcare ethicist. Bioethicists make claims to a specific body of knowledge and particular cognitive skills which are in turn disseminated in specialized journals and newly formed societies, and are taught in special centres, institutes and departments. Second, it has produced a growing public interest in medico-moral matters; so that whenever issues of reproduction, education, relationships, sexuality, suffering or disability lead to public concerns, ethicists become spokespersons to analyse, explain and resolve these matters. 'Bioethics' has therefore come to be regarded as a major public platform from which to address, explicate and give meaning to a range of problems generated by science and technology.

It is important to note that the evolution of bioethics has been associated with a specific conception of ethics (ten Have 2001). Ethics in healthcare is regarded as *applied ethics*. The standard textbook of Beauchamp and Childress therefore defines biomedical ethics as 'the application of general ethical theories, principles and rules to problems of therapeutic practice, healthcare delivery, and medical and biological research' (Beauchamp and Childress 1983: ix–x). The relevant concepts in this definition of ethics are 'application' and 'principles'. Instead of the theoretical abstractions of traditional moral philosophy, applied ethics can contribute to the analysis of dilemmas, to the resolution of complex cases and to the clarification of

practical problems arising in the healthcare setting. This practical 'usefulness' of applied ethics not only manifests itself in biomedicine, but also has
a wider scope. Applied ethics can extend to almost any area of life where
ethical issues arise. 'Application' here has a double connotation: it indicates
that ethics is available for what we usually do, it applies to our daily problems; but it is also helpful and practical, in the sense that ethics has something to do, it works to resolve our problems. The second characteristic
of the dominant conception of medical ethics is the focus on *principles*.
If ethics is conceived as applied ethics, then subsequent reflection is needed
on what is being applied. The emerging consensus that principles should
provide the answer to this question is consistent with the moralities of
obligation that have dominated modern ethical discourse, especially since
the Enlightenment philosopher Immanuel Kant. Behaviour in accord with
moral obligations is considered morally right. The morality of behaviour is
a morality of duty. Morality is thereby understood as a system of precepts
or rules that people are obliged to follow. Particularly in the early days
of bioethics, when medical power was strongly criticized, the rights of
patients were vehemently emphasized as requiring respect, the moralities of
obligation presented themselves as a common set of normative principles
and rules that should be followed in practice. As Gracia (2001) points out,
the Belmont Report in the United States in 1978 was influential because it
was the first official body to identify three basic ethical principles: autonomy, beneficence and justice. A basic principle was defined as a general
judgement serving as a justification for particular prescriptions and evaluations of human actions. From these principles, ethic guidelines were
derived that could be applied to the biomedical area. About the same time,
Beauchamp and Childress, in the first edition of their book, introduced the
four-principles approach, adding 'non-maleficence' to the list. In their view,
principles are normative generalizations that guide actions. However, as
general guides they leave considerable room for judgement in specific cases
and various types of rules are needed in order to specify the principles as
precise guides to action.

Although Beauchamp and Childress have considerably nuanced their theoretical framework in later editions, their work has contributed to a conception of medical ethics that is currently dominating the practical context, in
ethics committees, clinical case-discussions, ethics courses, and compendia
and syllabi. This conception is sometimes called 'principlism': the focus is
on the use of moral principles to address ethical issues and to resolve conflicts at the bedside (DuBose et al. 1994). So for example British physician-
ethicist, Raanan Gillon, can argue that the advantage of the four principles
is not only that they are defensible from a variety of theoretical moral
perspectives, but also that 'they can help us bring more order, consistency,
and understanding to our medico-moral judgements' (Gillon 1986: viii).
Principlism apparently is a universal tool; it provides a method to resolve

all moral issues in all areas of daily life, whatever the personal philosophies, politics, religions or moral theories of the persons involved.

Since the early 1990s, this dominant conception of applied ethics has come under critical scrutiny. As experiences in palliative care have shown, it is a conception which is inattentive to the particularities of the practical setting. Moral theories and principles are necessarily abstract and are not therefore immediately relevant to the particular circumstances of actual cases, the concrete reality of clinical work, and the specific responsibilities of healthcare professionals. By appealing to principles, norms or rules, applied ethics may fail to realize the importance of the concrete lived experience of healthcare professionals and of their patients. The moral agent is taken to have an abstract existence. This point is elaborated critically by several contemporary philosophers. According to Bernard Williams (1988), ethics does not respect the concrete moral subject with their personal integrity. It requires that the subject gives up their personal point of view and exchanges it for a universal and impartial point of view. This, Williams argues, is an absurd requirement, because the moral subject is requested to give up what is constitutive for their personal identity and integrity. The same point is made by Randall and Downie (1996) when they characterize the art of palliative care. The idea that knowledge of normative theories and principles can be applied to medical practice simply ignores the fact that moral concerns tend to emerge from experiences in medical settings themselves. A similar issue is raised by Charles Taylor (1989) in his *Sources of the Self*, in which morality and identity are considered two sides of the same coin. To know who we are is to know to which moral sources we should appear and the community, the particular social group to which we belong, is usually at the centre of our moral experience.

As several authors in this volume argue, the hitherto dominant conception of bioethics is revealed as inadequate when faced with the dilemmas of palliative care practice. Instead, the actual experiences of patients and healthcare practitioners, as well as the context in which physicians, nurses, patients and others experience their moral lives – for example the roles they play, the relationships in which they participate, the expectations they have, and the values they cherish – these should all be taken into consideration when addressing moral problems (Zaner 1988). The physician–patient relationship is neither ahistorical nor acultural. It is not an abstract rational notion: persons are always persons-in-relation; they are always members of communities; they are immersed in traditions and participants in culture. Experiences in palliative care also create interest in alternative conceptions of ethics in order better to explain the moral experiences of patients and professionals. We can list several of these, for example: narrative ethics which emphasize the stories of individual patients (Newton 1995), care ethics which attend to the context of support and care (Tronto 1993), responsibility ethics as described by Gracia (Chapter 5 in this volume), virtue ethics which look to qualities of character, such as compassion, in both individuals and communities (Pellegrino and Thomasma 1993) and the new casuistry drawing from the classical casuistic mode of moral reasoning (Jonsen and Toulmin 1988). These conceptions attempt to provide a more comprehensive understanding of the nature, scope, method and application of ethics in the contemporary healthcare context. We can see from this that palliative care aptly illustrates the contemporary criticism of the principlist approach in bioethics. It demonstrates that a proper understanding of the moral problems and dilemmas of healthcare practice requires first and foremost a conception of *interpretative* ethics. The role of interpretation is generally underlined in 'hermeneutics'. Originally, hermeneutics refers to the art of interpreting and the science of interpretation. As such, it was used in theology, law and philosophy, in each case with a concern for interpreting the meaning of texts. It also came into prominence in the nineteenth century as a methodology characterizing the humanities and social sciences. Philosophers such as Schleiermacher and Dilthey showed that not only texts but also all human products need interpretation, and that hermeneutics involves both the interpretandum (what is interpreted) and also the interpreter (who is interpreting). Then in the twentieth century, through the works of Heidegger, Gadamer and Ricoeur, hermeneutics evolved into a philosophy for understanding and explaining human existence. Some have argued that medicine must appropriately be considered as a hermeneutical enterprise, presuming that medicine is not or is not merely a natural science (Daniel 1986; Leder 1988; Svenaeus 1999). The modern emphasis on information and empirical data has contributed to new understanding of diagnosis and treatment as the physician's *interpretation* of what concerns the patient and what can be done to help the patient. Metaphorically, the patient is then conceived as a 'text' that may be considered on different interpretative levels. It is important to reflect upon the typical preconditions of interpretation in medicine. The patient is usually understood through an anatomico-physiological model. The patient's body is made 'readable' by the use of technology. The biomedical language of diagnosis and treatment reduces the overwhelming amount of information presented by the patient so that the standard medical case report reflects not the story of the patient's life but of the physician's relationship with the patient's illness (Poirier and Brauner 1988). It is also important to look at the effects of medical interpretation upon the interpreter. Interpretation seems to bring understanding and empathy. Interpreting symptoms involves understanding what is actually wrong with a patient and appreciating what they are going through. Interpreting the patient's illness arouses therefore an 'affiliative feeling' in the physician-interpreter (Zaner 1988). Finally, it is argued that ethics is best considered to be a hermeneutical discipline (Leder 1994). Ethics can therefore be defined as the hermeneutics of moral experience. Complex bioethics problems must be understood within the broader framework of an interpretative philosophical theory. Such theory, one of us has argued, should concentrate upon four characteristic parameters (ten Have 1994): experience, attitudes and emotions, community, and ambiguity.

Experience

The starting point of medical activity is the moral experience of the patient. Through illness and the possible prospect of death, the patient is confronted with ruptures in the fabric of daily life and thereby presents to the physician as both puzzling and meaningful. The patient's symptoms are deeply textured by the biographical situation, beliefs, values, habits and lifestyle. To ascertain what is wrong requires an interpretation, the more so since there is an initial distance between patient and physician.

Attitudes and emotions

Randall and Downie emphasize that we have to recognize not only the cognitive dimension, but the affective as well: 'the morally good person is not just principled, but also compassionate' (1996: 13). An argument can be made that for ethics the fundamental question is not so much 'What to do?' but rather 'How to live?' It is *praxis* not *poiesis* that is important (van Tongeren 1988). The moral relevancy of our actions should not be reduced to their effects; it is also determined by an evaluation of what we do in executing our actions. For example, the problem of conducting research with terminally ill patients should not be settled by reference to future results, but should also raise the question: 'Why are we interested in scientific research?' The problem of euthanasia should not be reduced to the question of whether it will eliminate suffering or respect the autonomy of the patient. It should also focus attention on how we deal with suffering, and what the meaning is of a medicine which saves the lives of patients and at the same time terminates human life; is it ever possible for medicine not to act? This change of focus implies a reorientation from activity to passivity, from acts to attitudes and emotions, from speaking to silence. Moral experience involves feelings of indignation, confusion or contentment; secondarily, these emotional responses can be made the object of moral thinking (Callahan 1988). A sharing of moral experiences of patients and physicians, and of the emotions and attitudes involved, is therefore required in order to elucidate the relevant ethical issues of the case or situation. Understanding and defining the morally relevant facts of a case does not involve the identification of relevant general principles and the deduction of a set of rules from which the correct response to the problem can be derived. The role of medical ethics is not so much to explicate and apply ethical theories and principles but to interpret and evoke what is implied in moral experience. The notion of 'applied ethics' suggests wrongly that we already know which moral principles and rules to apply. Conversely, rules and principles might be seen as answers to what is evoked or appealed to in a particular case. First, we need to understand what the moral experience of vulnerability and the appeal to assistance really means in this case. We need to discover why particular principles will motivate us; why is there a particular ideal, rule or obligation? Close scrutiny is required therefore of the medical situation in all its complexity.

Community

The interpretative reading of a patient's situation is not an individual doctor's affair. The medical prior understandings that orientate the interpretation are the sediments of cultural assumptions concerning the nature of the world, the body, life and death, and the results of a specific historical evolution of medical knowledge. This is especially true for palliative care, with its emphasis on particular goals such as the 'good death'. Interpretation presupposes a universe of understanding. This is a consequence of the so-called hermeneutic circle: in order to interpret the meaning of a text, the interpreter must be familiar with the vocabulary and grammar of the text and have some idea of what the text might mean (Daniel 1986). As social beings, our understanding is always a community phenomenon, a matter of understanding in communication with others. The continuous effort to reach consensus through a dialogue with patients, colleagues and other health professionals, induces us to discover the particularities of our own prior understanding, and through that, to attain a more general level of understanding.

Ambiguity

Ethics primarily aims at interpreting and understanding moral experience. But moral experience is complex and versatile. It implies that every interpretation is tentative; it opens up a possible perspective. Definitive and comprehensive interpretation is non-existent. An interpretative approach always has an ambiguous status in which more than one meaning is admitted. As Zaner points out: 'Every life is linguistically inexhaustible, there is always a richer tale to be told that can never be wholly captured in words, no matter how evocative they might be' (Zaner 1988: 272). We can see from this that moral judgments and decisions framed on the basis of understanding the thematic moral ordering of a person's life are fundamentally uncertain.

Using these four notions, we suggest that an interpretative conception of bioethics can be further developed and experiences in palliative care can help, not only to underline the need for such a new conception, but also to clarify and expand its characteristic parameters.

Autonomy and community

In the dominant conception of bioethics, individual autonomy has a peculiar role. As we have seen, respect for autonomy is one among, usually four, moral principles but at the same time it is often considered as overriding the other ones. This emphasis on individual autonomy is understandable since it seems to be such an effective counterbalance to medical power. Moral issues arise in the context of an almost exclusively technological orientation to the world and a predominant scientific conceptualization of human life. At the same time human beings resist the tendencies of medicine to focus primarily on their bodies and biological existence. They protest against the overwhelming power of health professionals and healthcare institutions, which reduce patients to cases, numbers or objects. They object to the lack of individual involvement in decision-making processes, as well as to an inattention to the authenticity and subjectivity of individual patients. Bioethics, it claims, has emerged as a movement to reintroduce the subject of individual patients into the healthcare setting, emphasizing patients' rights, respect for individual autonomy, and the need to set limits to medical power. In this sense, as Frank (2000) puts it, bioethics has become the new way of being moral.

However, the emphasis on individual autonomy has two consequences which are often criticized in the context of palliative care. First, it is associated with a mechanistic view of the human body, whereas palliative care makes claims to the rhetoric of 'whole person care'. Second, it focuses on the individual person, whereas palliative care also seeks to include the family members, associates and companions of the patient.

The role of the human body in bioethical discourse is paradoxical. Bioethics as a critical movement has originated from the argument that medicine separates the individual person into subject and object, and that the human subject must somehow be reintroduced into medical discourse. The best way to focus attention on the patient as a 'whole person' and as an agent 'in control' of their own life, is to stress the autonomy of the individual subject and to demand moral respect for this autonomy. However, the emphasis on individual autonomy tends to neglect the significance of the human body. In most ethical discourse, there is little recognition of the special experiences of embodiment; rather a picture of a disembodied human subject emerges in which complete priority is given to mental processes and actions. The body becomes merely the instrument through which the subject is interacting with the world. The subject is in full control of its body. It is imperative therefore that the integrity of the body should be respected, as it is the prime vehicle of the autonomous person. The moral principle of respect for autonomy in healthcare ethics therefore seems to be associated with a popular image of the body as property (ten Have and Welie 1998). When the individual person is regarded as an autonomous subject, then the body becomes private property. And the person is the sovereign authority with property rights over their body.

At the same time, the concept of body ownership is morally problematic. For as the sociologist Brian Turner (1996) points out, we both 'have' and 'are' bodies. The distinction between person and body is therefore contrary to our existential identification with our bodies and to our experience of ourselves as embodied selves. In drawing on the notion of the autonomous subject as the owner of a body, and of the body as private property, bioethics seems therefore to be proceeding from the same dualism which it criticized in its early days. Moreover, it is apparently using a dualistic distinction between person and body, subject and object, which has led to the emergence of bioethics itself. Paradoxically, whereas medicine tends to neglect the subject, bioethics tends to neglect the body (ten Have 1998; Zwart 1998). This dualism was also rejected by the early founders of the hospice movement. Dualism proposes a view that medical interventions should focus on the human body since this is the vehicle for prolonging life; as long as the body is functioning, medical interference and activities will be justified. Separating object and subject and differentiating between an objective, real world which is independent from an isolated, individual subject, leads to an almost exclusive preference for the methods of the natural sciences in the context of healthcare. These methods are focused on intervention, control and manipulation, introducing the technical point of view of the engineer into the domain of disease, suffering and death. A dualistic view leads to a one-sided approach to suffering which is regarded as merely a bodily phenomenon. Cicely Saunders' (1967) concept of 'total pain' sought to go beyond this in a view which encompassed physical, emotional, social and spiritual components (Clark 1999) and saw all of these as interrelated phenomena. In this context, in which a dualistic view is unwarranted, the primacy of the medical approach, primarily targeted on the human body, should disappear to be replaced by a multi-professional approach to the dying patient and family.

The focus on individual autonomy is of course also central in palliative care. Autonomy, however, tends to isolate the person as sovereign decision-maker. It neglects dimensions of human vulnerability, dependency and fragility which are characteristic of human existence and which are experienced particularly when confronting serious illness, suffering and debilitating conditions. In an ethics of care, however, these dimensions are recognized. It is suggested therefore that the notion of *authenticity* better conforms to moral experiences in palliative care than does the notion of autonomy (Janssens et al. 1999). Authenticity underlines the notion that the individual's decisions need to be interpreted within the perspective of personality and biography. It also acknowledged that individual existence is fragile and dependent (Welie 1998). Yet authenticity needs to be fostered and sustained. Patients should be aware that they can be themselves despite their suffering because vulnerability and dependency are shared with professional and non-professional caregivers as conditions common to all human beings. This awareness links authenticity with community. Individuals are social beings; they have the potential to be autonomous decision-makers only in so far as the community provides the proper conditions and adequate circumstances. Palliative care aims to create such conditions and circumstances in order to enable patients to experience their humanity as members of a community, particularly at the moment of death. The patient is not an 'unencumbered self' as postulated in the liberal tradition emphasizing individual autonomy (Sandel 1996). On the contrary, the cloak of palliative care demonstrates that the dying person is essentially related to others and is situated in a set of social and communal relations.

Different images of human beings

Our critique of the moral principle of autonomy shows a further area where palliative care can make a contribution to bioethics. Not only does palliative care serve to demonstrate the inadequacy of the current conception of bioethics and the need for alternative approaches, as well as the one-sidedness of the principle of respect for autonomy, but also it indicates that in healthcare an image of human beings is necessary that is more comprehensive than the images which predominate in everyday life.

The postmodern person has been characterized through the image of tourist:

> the life of the men and women of our [postmodern] times is . . . like that of the tourists-through-time: they cannot and would not decide in advance what places they would visit and what the sequence of stations would be; what they knew for sure is that they will keep on the move, never sure whether the place they reach is their final destination.
>
> (Bauman 1994: 20)

In postmodern existence there is no final state, no state of perfection which may be realized in search of improvement; life has only local and transitory achievements. The defining feature of postmodern existence is the fear of being fixed. Persons avoid fixation, commitment and stable relationships. They like to keep their options open. Contingency, episodicity and fragmentation are the marks of human life. Human 'being' is construed as an image which is perpetually changing. The postmodern person is also, in the words of Bauman, 'a conscious and systematic seeker of experience, of a new and different experience, of the experience of difference and novelty' (Bauman 1995: 96). For the person as tourist it is, in the end, not clear where home is; having a home becomes a mere postulate. The tourist belongs nowhere, but paradoxically dreams of belonging.

We do not need necessarily to agree with this diagnosis of postmodernity in order to recognize the consequences. The postmodern person is an interest-seeking subject for whom objects in the world are not relevant as entities in their own right. What matters is whether they are pleasing or not pleasing, satisfactory or unsatisfactory. The tourist does not want to change the world, but rather to lead an enjoyable life. Reality poses no challenge and does not provoke rectification, improvement, transformation. Postmodern life strategies are instead focused on rendering human relations fragmentary and discontinuous. Doing so, they promote a distance between the individual and the other in which the other is considered primarily as the object of aesthetic, not moral evaluation. The effect of these postmodern strategies of disengagement and commitment-avoidance is the suppression of the moral impulse. However, what transforms experiences into moral experiences has much to do with responsibility for the other, engagement in the fate of the other, and commitment to the other person's welfare.

Palliative care seems to operate with another image of the human being, emphasizing notions like authenticity and community, as well as responsibility and engagement. Palliative care builds on a concept of human beings as dynamic, adapting to the world, reconstructing and redefining their identity in order to make it solid and stable, considering life as a project, an individual task to accomplish the goals that have been set, and to give meaning to the various stages and experiences. This is the image of human life as pilgrimage (Bauman 1994, 1995). For the pilgrim, the true place is always some time, some distance away. What makes life worthwhile is a proximity between the true world and this world; destined to be elsewhere, the pilgrim's life is worthwhile to the extent that the journeying continues, and the closer the goal becomes, the more worthwhile becomes the life. In postmodern times, if life has been transformed into a pilgrimage, it receives meaning. It is the destination that makes a whole out of the fragmentation, that lends continuity to the episodic. Human life therefore becomes a continuous story, and although it is an individual project, it is carried out in an orderly, determined, predictable world.

Healthcare aims at providing care and shelter for persons who journey through life. The hospice movement in particular has developed a discourse focusing on aspects of journeying, pilgrimage and the meaning of suffering (Clark and Seymour 1999). Even if this image of the human being as pilgrim is open to challenge, it appears useful as an antidote to the fragmentary existence portrayed in some postmodern philosophy. It is an image that delineates specific characteristics central to human life: such as goal-directedness, the deliberate choosing of successive steps in life, and a changing world requiring adaptation, unity and continuity within the life project. It may be more difficult for postmodern human beings to realize these characteristics, but this observation does not diminish their relevancy. Perhaps it is a function of healthcare, specifically in the context of chronic, incurable and terminal illness, to provide a niche within the hectic, disengaged social environment of today in order to allow 'wandering' and vulnerable people to find peace and tranquillity, and finally to be 'home' (Dekkers 2001; see also Rumbold 1998).

Another powerful image of human beings nowadays is that of the consumer. This image is connected with the notion of individual autonomy. Barber (1995), for example, argues that postmodern individuals are members of a worldwide community, so-called McWorld, the global theme park of MTV, Macintosh and McDonald's, a world tied together by communication, information, entertainment and commerce. In this world everyone is a consumer, defined by needs and wants. McWorlds' therefore is not really a community: the significant relations are exchange relationships among individual consumers and individual producers: society is privatized and commercialized. In the context of palliative care, this image of consumer is brought into question, at least in part. If the hospice is a 'place of rest and nurture for those wearied at the end of life's journey' (Hockley 1997: 84), considering the suffering patient as a consumer until death seems obscene. The discourse of choice and consumption appears inappropriate in such circumstances. Of course, palliative care itself may increasingly be affected by economic values, and thus the discourse of consumption, particularly with its growing integration into mainstream health services. Nonetheless, it remains important to underline, as Street (1998: 79) argues, 'the non-economic values of acceptability, appropriateness of service, community participation and community development as being essential elements of the palliative care approach'. The central notion here, again, is community. Palliative care services, and hospice services, particularly in the United Kingdom and the United States have initially emphasized community-based inpatient programmes or home care, in each case with considerable involvement on the part of volunteers. The concern was to spread hospice principles into the wider community, offering a 'good death' as compared with the options for dying provided in mainstream health services. The image advocated here therefore is that of a human being related to other human beings. This interrelatedness of human existence, as argued by Schotsmans (Chapter 7), is also the basis of morality. It is the face of the other that makes us moral beings, whether we choose to act accordingly or not. At first reading, the postmodern conception that human beings are tourists, consumers, free and independent selves, seems plausible. But in a second-order reading, the very condition of making such a conception possible and understandable, reveals the social embeddedness of individual life. It shows that our selves are constituted through the practices of community. Cultural context and community are therefore constitutive of the values and goals of individuals. Communal relatedness falsifies the idea of the unencumbered self, the idea of self-ownership assuming that the individual as an entity exists prior to the ends which are affirmed by it. According to this second-order reflection, the idea that the self designs its life-project from some asocial or presocial position, and subsequently participates in the community, is self-defeating. Without societal culture our potential for self-determination, choice and consumption will remain empty. Therefore, the individual self is fundamentally dependent on community.

But at this point problems arise. When palliative care assumes the communal basis of human existence, in what way is this assumption culturally determined, and therefore different in varying social, cultural and historical contexts? It is precisely at this point that the philosophical struggle is located in recent works in social and political philosophy: if the postmodern human being is not an unencumbered individual or an autonomous consumer, but part of an encompassing community, how as a reflective moral being is it possible to escape the universal dominance of the community? Sandel (1996), for example, argues against the moral claims of 'cosmopolitan citizenship' with its emphasis on the community of all human beings; in this view, universal identities take precedence over particular ones; ideally, the distinction between friends and strangers should be overcome in a truly ethical point of view. Sandel points out that most of the time we live our lives by smaller solidarities; we learn to love humanity not in general but through its particular expressions. What is morally relevant, therefore, is not the community of all human beings but the particular communities that locate us in the world. What is typical, furthermore, is that we live in a range of different communities, some overlapping, others contending. Moral reflection then becomes necessary to decide which of one's identities is properly engaged. Postmodern individuals are not unencumbered by moral ties they have not chosen; but they are also not encumbered in a universal community with obvious encompassing loyalties. They are, however, citizens who can think and act as 'multiply-situated selves'. Ethical reflection is primarily needed to cope with the ambiguity associated with multiply-encumbered selves; it should give us 'the capacity to negotiate our way among the sometimes overlapping, sometimes conflicting obligations that claim us, and to live with the tension to which multiple loyalties give rise' (Sandel 1996: 350). A similar argument is developed by Barber (1995). Interposed between the state and the market is where community exists, where we are more than clients or consumers, where we are public beings having regard for the general good, where we as citizens relate in the co-operative, non-coercive pursuit of public goods. Barber defines a citizen as 'an individual who has acquired a public voice and understands himself to belong to a wider community, who sees herself as sharing goods with others' (Barber 1995: 286). But also Barber agrees that humankind depends for its liberty on variety and difference; we live in several spheres, in a many-sectored civil society. Whereas market choices are private and speak about individualistic goals and individual preferences, citizens speak about the social consequences of their private choices; they speak the public language of the common good; but at the same time, this public language is multiple and heterogeneous; civil society has many narratives about the common good. It appears therefore that the *universal* human condition of existence as a communal-cultural being can be realized only in *particular* ways; the communal self is constituted by particular cultural characteristics. A richer medical ethics can therefore result from taking seriously the basic idea of moral community and concomitantly, the various narratives about the particularities of people as communal beings. As it is currently developing in many countries and cultures, palliative care, in advocating the image of human beings as citizens rather than consumers, can offer important lessons to the task of ethical reflection.

Conclusion

In this concluding chapter, we have pointed out that palliative care and ethics are nowadays entering into a new and fascinating phase of interaction and cooperation. On the one hand, many moral issues and dilemmas arise in the practice of palliative care. Ethics can help to analyse and elucidate these particular problems. Ethics can also provide models and methods to address systematically and discuss practical cases in order to facilitate clinical decision-making. We have argued that this level of interaction is ethics *in* palliative care. On the other hand, bioethics may be enriched by experiences in palliative care practice and through reflection upon palliative care as a historical and social movement. This second level of interaction we have called the ethics *of* palliative care. Here the approaches, concepts and values in palliative care may be relevant to a critical reflection of bioethics itself, and may provide new ideas and richer views. So both ethical orientations *vis-à-vis* palliative care appear worthwhile. We have argued that in three areas palliative care may give significant inspiration to enrich bioethics. First, palliative care practice demonstrates the inadequacy of the current dominant conception of bioethics as applied ethics. It shows the need for an interpretative ethics which is a better accommodation to healthcare practice. Second, palliative care illustrates the one-sidedness of the major moral principle of today: that of respect for autonomy. From the perspective of care, although individual autonomy is important, it is necessary not to disconnect the autonomous subject from the objective human body with its ailments, deficiencies and suffering. It is also necessary to regard the individual patient as a member of some form of community that can support him or her. Third, palliative care also points attention to certain images of human beings that tend to be neglected in postmodern society, in particular the image of the human person as pilgrim rather than tourist, and as a citizen rather than consumer. In short, palliative care is more than another healthcare context in which moral issues emerge. It is an incentive for philosophers, theologians and ethicists generally to evaluate the notions and models of present-day bioethics itself.

References

Barber, B.R. (1995) *Jihad vs McWorld*. New York: Ballantine.

Bauman, Z. (1994) *Alone Again: Ethics after Certainty*. London: Demos.

Bauman, Z. (1995) *Life in Fragments: Essays in Postmodern Morality*. Oxford: Blackwell.

Beauchamp, T.L. and Childress, J.F. (1983) *Principles of Biomedical Ethics*, 2nd edn. New York: Oxford University Press.

Callahan, S. (1988) The role of emotion in ethical decision-making, *Hastings Center Report*, 18: 9–14.

Clark, D. (1999) 'Total pain', disciplinary power and the body in the work of Cicely Saunders, 1958–67, *Social Science and Medicine*, 49(6): 727–36.

Clark, D. and Seymour, J. (1999) *Reflections on Palliative Care*. Buckingham: Open University Press.

Daniel, S.L. (1986) The patient as text: a model of clinical hermeneutics, *Theoretical Medicine*, 7: 195–210.

Dekkers, W. (2001) Coming home: on the goals of palliative care, in H.A.M.J. ten Have and M.J.P.A. Janssens (eds) *Palliative Care in Europe: Concepts and Policies*. Amsterdam: IOS Press.

DuBose, E.R., Hamel, R. and O'Connell, L.J. (eds) (1994) *A Matter of Principles? Ferment in U.S. Bioethics*. Valley Forge, PA: Trinity Press International.

Frank, A. (2000) Social bioethics and the critique of autonomy, *Health*, 4(3): 378–94.

Gillon, R. (1986) *Philosophical Medical Ethics*. Chichester: John Wiley.

Gracia, D. (2001) History of medical ethics, in H.A.M.J. ten Have and B. Gordijn (eds) *Bioethics in a European Perspective*. Dordrecht: Kluwer.

Hermsen, M.A. and ten Have, H.A.M.J. (2001) Moral problems in palliative care journals, *Palliative Medicine*, 15(5): 425–31.

Hockley, J. (1997) The evolution of the hospice approach, in D. Clark, J. Hockley and S. Ahmedzai (eds) *New Themes in Palliative Care*. Buckingham: Open University Press.

Janssens, M.J.P.A., Zylicz, Z. and ten Have, H.A.M.J. (1999) Articulating the concept of palliative care: philosophical and theological perspectives, *Journal of Palliative Care*, 15(2): 38–44.

Jonsen, A.R. (1998) *The Birth of Bioethics*. New York: Oxford University Press.

Jonsen, A.R. (2000) *A Short History of Medical Ethics*. New York: Oxford University Press.

Jonsen, A.R. and Toulmin, S. (1988) *The Abuse of Casuistry*. Berkeley, CA: University of California Press.

Leder, D. (1988) The hermeneutic role of the consultation-liaison psychiatrist, *Journal of Medicine and Philosophy*, 13: 367–78.

Leder, D. (1994) Toward a hermeneutical bioethics, in E.R. DuBose, R. Hamel and L.J. O'Connell (eds) *A Matter of Principles? Ferment in U.S. Bioethics*. Valley Forge, PA: Trinity Press International.

Martensen, R. (2001) The history of bioethics: an essay review, *Journal of the History of Medicine and Allied Sciences*, 56(2): 168–75.

Newton, A.Z. (1995) *Narrative Ethics*. Cambridge, MA: Harvard University Press.

Pellegrino, E.D. (1976) Philosophy of medicine: problematic and potential, *Journal of Medicine and Philosophy*, 1(1): 5–31.

Pellegrino, E.D. and Thomasma, D.C. (1993) *The Virtues in Medical Practice*. New York: Oxford University Press.

Poirier, S. and Brauner, D. (1988) Ethics and the daily language of medical discourse, *Hastings Center Report*, 18: 5–9.

Randall, F. and Downie, R.S. (1996) *Palliative Care Ethics: A Good Companion*. Oxford: Oxford University Press.

Rothman, D.J. (1991) *Strangers at the Bedside: A History of How Law and Bioethics Transformed Medical Decision Making*. New York: Basic Books.

Rumbold, B.D. (1998) Implications of mainstreaming hospice into palliative care services, in J.M. Parker and S. Aranda (eds) *Palliative Care: Explorations and Challenges*. Sydney: MacLennan and Petty.

Sandel, M.J. (1996) *Democracy's discontent: America in Search of a Public Philosophy*. Cambridge, MA: Belknap Press of Harvard University Press.

Saunders, C. (1967) *The Management of Terminal Illness*. London: Hospital Medicine Publications.

Street, A. (1998) Competing discourses with/in palliative care, in J.M. Parker and S. Aranda (eds) *Palliative Care: Explorations and Challenges*. Sydney: MacLennan and Petty.

Svenaeus, F. (1999) *The Hermeneutics of Medicine and the Phenomenology of Health: Steps towards a Philosophy of Medical Practice*. Linköping, Sweden: Linköping University.

Taylor, C. (1989) *Sources of the Self: The Making of Modern Identity*. Cambridge: Cambridge University Press.

Ten Have, H.A.M.J. (1994) The hyperreality of clinical ethics: a unitary theory and hermeneutics, *Theoretical Medicine*, 15(2): 113–31.

Ten Have, H.A.M.J. (1998) Health care and the human body, *Medicine, Health Care and Philosophy*, 1(2): 103–5.

Ten Have, H.A.M.J. (2001) Theoretical models and approaches to ethics, in H.A.M.J. ten Have and B. Gordijn (eds) *Bioethics in a European Perspective*. Dordrecht: Kluwer.

Ten Have, H.A.M.J. and Welie, J.V.M. (eds) (1998) *Ownership of the Human Body: Philosophical Considerations on the Use of the Human Body and its Parts in Healthcare*. Dordrecht: Kluwer.

Tronto, J.C. (1993) *Moral Boundaries: A Political Argument for an Ethic of Care*. New York: Routledge.

Turner, B. (1996) *The Body and Society*, 2nd edn. London: Sage.

Van Tongeren, P. (1988) Ethiek en praktijk, *Filosofie en Praktijk*, 9: 113–27.

Welie, J.V.M. (1998) *In the Face of Suffering: The Philosophical-Anthropological Foundations of Clinical Ethics*. Omaha, NB: Creighton University Press.

Williams, B. (1988) Consequentialism and integrity, in S. Scheffler (ed.) *Consequentialism and its Critics*. Oxford: Clarendon.

Zaner, R.M. (1988) *Ethics and the Clinical Encounter*. Englewood Cliffs, NJ: Prentice-Hall.

Zwart, H. (1998) Medicine, symbolization and the 'real' body – Lacan's understanding of medical science, *Medicine, Health Care and Philosophy*, 1(2): 107–17.

Index

Complementary studies available include:

Parental Perspectives in Cases of Suspected Child Abuse
Hedy Cleaver and Pam Freeman (The Dartington Team)
HMSO 1995. ISBN 0 11 321786 2

Child Protection Practice: Private Risks and Public Remedies
Elaine Farmer and Morag Owen (The University of Bristol Team)
HMSO 1995. ISBN 0 11 321787 0

The Prevalence of Child Sexual Abuse in Britain
Deborah Ghate and Liz Spencer (Social and Community Planning Research)
HMSO 1995. ISBN 0 11 321783 8

Development After Physical Abuse in Early Childhood: A Follow-Up Study of Children on Protection Registers
Jane Gibbons, Bernard Gallagher, Caroline Bell and David Gordon (University of East Anglia)
HMSO 1995. ISBN 0 11 321790 0

Operating the Child Protection System
Caroline Bell, Sue Conroy and Jane Gibbons (University of East Anglia)
HMSO 1995. ISBN 0 11 321785 4

Working Together in Child Protection
Elizabeth Birchall (The University of Stirling)
HMSO 1995. ISBN 0 11 321830 3

Paternalism or Partnership? Family Involvement in the Child Protection Process
June Thoburn, Ann Lewis and David Shemmings (University of East Anglia)
HMSO 1995. ISBN 0 11 321788 9

Message From Research
HMSO 1995. ISBN 0 11 321781 1

M. *Managing Human Services*. Washington DC: International City Management Association.

Wistow, G. (1982) Collaboration between health and local authorities: why is it necessary? *Journal of Social Policy and Administration*, 16, 1, 44–62.

Wistow, G. (1989) untitled contribution in (ed) Mocroft, I. *Collaboration in planning and working: the voluntary sector, local authorities and health authorities*. Association of Researchers in Voluntary Action and Community Involvement (ARVAC) Occasional Paper No 10.

Wistow, G. and Fuller, S. (1986) *Collaboration since restructuring: the 1984 survey of joint planning and finance*, Centre for Research in Social Policy and the National Association of Health Authorities in England and Wales.

Yin, R. (1989) *Case Study Research*. London: Sage.

Zeifert, T. and Faller, K. (1981) Interdisciplinary team and the community in Faller, K. (ed) *Social work with abused and neglected children*. New York: Free Press.

Printed in the United Kingdom for HMSO
Dd301478 10/95 C10 G3397 10170